The Expanding Continuum of GENDER-BASED VIOLENCE

Trauma-Informed Care

Presentation, Assessment, & Intervention

Volume 1

STM **Learning,** Inc.

Leading Publisher of Scientific, Technical, and Medical Educational Resources
Saint Louis
www.stmlearning.com

The Expanding Continuum of

GENDER-BASED VIOLENCE

Trauma-Informed Care

Presentation, Assessment, & Intervention

Volume 1

Paul Thomas Clements, PhD, RN, AFN-C™, ANEF, DF-IAFN, DF-AFN
Clinical Professor
Center for Excellence in Forensic Nursing
Texas A&M University
College Station, Texas

David Solomon, PhD, HSP-P
Associate Professor
Department of Psychology
Director
Health Services Psychology PsyD Program
Western Carolina University
Cullowhee, North Carolina

Kaleigh Mancha, MS, LMFT, Certified Full Spectrum Doula
Co-Founder
Heart and Sol Collective
Founder, Licensed Marriage and Family Therapist
Kay and Me
Las Vegas, Nevada

Mitzy D. Flores, PhDc, MSN, RN, AHN-BC, CHSE, COI, Caritas Coach®, Introspective Hypnosis Practitioner
Academic and Clinical Nurse Educator
Visiting Professor
School of Nursing
University of South Florida
Tampa, Florida

Christopher A. Mallett, PhD, Esq, LISW-S
Professor
School of Social Work
Cleveland State University
Cleveland, Ohio

STM **Learning,** Inc.

Leading Publisher of Scientific, Technical, and Medical Educational Resources
Saint Louis
www.stmlearning.com

Publishers: Glenn E. Whaley and Marianne V. Whaley
Managing Editor: Samantha Brown
Graphic Design Director: Glenn E. Whaley
Graphic Designer: Connie H. C. Wang
Curriculum Developer: Samantha Brown
Associate Editors: Katie Slaten, Miya Russell, Tammy Arnow, Gracie York, Megan Farmer
Copy Editors: Miya Russell, Katie Slaten, Megan Farmer, Tammy Arnow, Gracie York

Printed in the United States of America.

Publisher: STM Learning, Inc.
Saint Louis, Missouri 63033
Phone: (314) 434-2424
http://www.stmlearning.com orders@stmlearning.com

Print ISBN: 978-1-953119-23-0
eBook ISBN: 978-1-953119-30-8

Library of Congress Cataloging-in-Publication Data

Names: Clements, Paul T. (Paul Thomas), 1962- author. | Solomon, David T., author. | Mancha, Kaleigh, author. | Flores, Mitzy D., author. | Mallett, Christopher A., author.
Title: The expanding continuum of gender-based violence : trauma-informed care / Paul Thomas Clements, David Solomon, Mitzy D. Flores, Kaleigh Mancha, Christopher A. Mallett.
Description: Saint Louis : STM Learning, Inc., [2024] | Includes bibliographical references. | Contents: v. 1. Presentation, assessment, & intervention -- v. 2. Applying responsive practices. | Summary: "The first volume of The Expanding Continuum of Gender-Based Violence: Trauma-Informed Care is a thorough examination of current knowledge on the way gender impacts both group and individual risk of violence. In this volume, interdisciplinary professionals focus on the presentation and assessment of trauma with a special focus on trauma-informed approaches. Special emphasis is placed on inclusive language recommendations in order to guide clinicians and care providers in current best practices. Together, with Volume 2, this text intends to do the following: Define the problem Identify causes and risk factors Design interventions Disseminate information Educate students and future professionals"-- Provided by publisher.
Identifiers: LCCN 2024039425 (print) | LCCN 2024039426 (ebook) | ISBN 9781953119230 (v. 1 ; paperback) | ISBN 9781953119247 (v. 2 ; paperback) | ISBN 9781953119308 (v. 1 ; ebook) | ISBN 9781953119315 (v. 2 ; ebook)
Subjects: MESH: Gender-Based Violence--prevention & control | Psychological Trauma--therapy | Sex Offenses--prevention & control | Culturally Competent Care
Classification: LCC RC569.5.V55 (print) | LCC RC569.5.V55 (ebook) | NLM WM 172.5 | DDC 616.85/820081--dc23/eng/20241010
LC record available at https://lccn.loc.gov/2024039425
LC ebook record available at https://lccn.loc.gov/2024039426

Contributors

Gerica Alvarado, MD, FAAFP
Physician
Optum, Department of Family Medicine
Valley Health System Family Medicine Residency
Las Vegas, Nevada

Kelsey Arias, MSW, Peer Support Specialist
Confidential Advocacy Program Director
Department of Student Affairs
Oregon Health and Science University
Portland, Oregon

Erin M. Aschman, BSN, RN, SANE-A, GFN-C
Associate Nurse Manager
Forensic Nurse Examiner Program
University of Colorado Health
Aurora, Colorado

Patrick C. Barton, PsyD
Detective
Brevard Police Department
Department of Psychology
Western Carolina University
Hendersonville, North Carolina

Kathy Bell, MS, RN, AFN-C, SANE-A, SANE-P, IVSE-C, DF-AFN
Adjunct Professor
Center for Health Sciences
Oklahoma State University
Tulsa, Oklahoma

Paul Thomas Clements, PhD, RN, AFN-C™, ANEF, DF-IAFN, DF-AFN
Clinical Professor
Center for Excellence in Forensic Nursing
Texas A&M University
College Station, Texas

Theresa Fay-Hillier, DrPH, MSN, PMHCNS-BC
Associate Clinical Professor
College of Nursing and Health Professions
Drexel University
Philadelphia, Pennsylvania

Mitzy D. Flores, PhDc, MSN, RN, AHN-BC, CHSE, COI, Caritas Coach©, Introspective Hypnosis Practitioner
Academic and Clinical Nurse Educator
Visiting Professor
School of Nursing
University of South Florida
Tampa, Florida

Christine Foote-Lucero, MSN, RN, CEN, SANE-A, SANE-P, AFN-C, DF-AFN
Forensic Program Manager
Emergency Department
University of Colorado
Aurora, Colorado

Kimberly Fuller, PhD, LISW-S, CST
Associate Professor
BSW Director
School of Social Work
Cleveland State University
Cleveland, Ohio

Nilesh Neil Gokal, MD, FAAFP
Senior Medical Director
Department of Population Health and Education
Optum
Associate Program Director
Valley Health Systems Family Medicine Residency Program
Las Vegas, Nevada

Christina Hall, MSW
Director
Jean Nidetch Care Center
University of Nevada, Las Vegas
Las Vegas, Nevada

Bibiana Lopez, BA
Case Management Coordinator
Department of Student Wellness
Jean Nidetch Care Center
University of Nevada, Las Vegas
Las Vegas, Nevada

Christopher A. Mallett, PhD, Esq, LISW-S
Professor
School of Social Work
Cleveland State University
Cleveland, Ohio

Kaleigh Mancha, MS, LMFT, Certified Full Spectrum Doula
Co-Founder
Heart and Sol Collective
Founder
Licensed Marriage and Family Therapist
Kay and Me
Las Vegas, Nevada

Ash Moomaw, MA
Department of Counseling Psychology
Ball State University
Muncie, Indiana

Jae A. Puckett, PhD
Assistant Professor
Department of Psychology
Michigan State University
East Lansing, Michigan

Holly Ramella, MA
Prevention and Education Manager
Department of Student Affairs
OHSU Confidential Advocacy Program
Portland, Oregon

Oak Reed, PhD
Licensed Clinical Psychologist
Regional Director of Eastern Virginia
Active & Connected Family Therapy
Palmyra, Virginia

David Solomon, PhD, HSP-P
Associate Professor
Department of Psychology
Director
Health Services Psychology PsyD Program
Western Carolina University
Cullowhee, North Carolina

Natasha T. Stewart, MPA
Nonprofit Programs Management
Stewart Counseling, LLC
Chesapeake, Virginia

Deborah St. Germain, DNP, RN, AFN-C, SANE-A, SANE-P
Lecturer
Graduate Forensic Nursing
College of Nursing
Texas A&M University
College Station, Texas
Sexual Assault Nurse Examiner
Sexual Assault Services
Jefferson Parish Coroner's Office
Harvey, Louisiana

Justine Suba-Cohen, DO, MS, DABOM, FAAFP
Physician
Associate Program Director
Department of Family Medicine
Southwest Medical Associates
Las Vegas, Nevada

Kasey E. Vigil, MA
Department of Educational, School, and Counseling Psychology
University of Kentucky
Lexington, Kentucky

Gaurav Zirath, MD, MBA, DABOM, FAAFP
Associate Program Director
Optum
Las Vegas, Nevada

Our Mission

To become the world leader in publishing and information services on child abuse, maltreatment, diseases, and domestic violence. We seek to heighten awareness of these issues and provide relevant information to professionals and consumers.

Foreword

Gender-based violence, formerly known as violence against women, is an expansive topic that now encompasses all peoples, regardless of their nationality, culture, or sexual diversity.[1] The aftermath of violence, whether from childhood, adolescence, adulthood, or in older persons, has the potential to change a person's physiology,[2] influence behavioral choices to relieve stress, and consequently enhance physical and psychological disease development[3] and potential for diminished health and early mortality.[4] Health care providers without the understanding of trauma and trauma's aftermath as it relates to health contribute to the dearth of healthy solutions available to all people. As such, this book brings together the next generation of expert authors who cite current publications to inform future providers about the importance of trauma-informed principles[5] that are culturally humble, without extrinsic bias, and in keeping with the current understanding of the providers' role in creating a safe environment that is transparent and inclusive, enticing the person toward empowerment, exercising the person's voice in mutuality that respects the person's choices, even if the person's choice is to decline the choices offered from the published research.[6] Nursing ethics inform providers about common values that reject stereotypes or judgements and look beyond, accepting all human conditions, including a person's choices to manage their complex situations with their resources, including their unique reactions and behavioral adaptations to traumatic situations.[7] By accepting the science of a person's adaptations to trauma, the provider forms analytical rationales for treatment options with which to guide the person in a mutually beneficial journey toward health after trauma. The inclusive collection of topics reveals the evidence for trauma reactions to situations, whether child maltreatment, domestic or intimate partner abuses, coercion, or neglect and exploitation in older persons. Across the lifespan there is 1 common thread—as humans, we overcome or we die.[8,9] The purpose of the book, *The Expanding Continuum of Gender-Based Violence: Trauma-Informed Care,* is to utilize gathered evidence to enhance understanding about application of trauma-informed principles in the care of all persons in the aftermath of violent and traumatic events in a person's lived-experience. Whether a victim of wars or bullying in the schoolyard, recovery is possible, and this book provides an opportunity to integrate trauma-informed strategies that prevent, mitigate, and manage the care of persons across the lifespan who have or are currently experiencing violence.

> *"You did what you knew how to do, and when you knew better, you did better."* (M. Angelou, 1995 per O. Winfrey).

Let's do better.

Respectfully,

Patricia M. Speck, DNSc, CRNP, FNP-BC, AFN-C, IVSE-C

Distinguished Fellow, International Association of Forensic Nurses (DF-IAFN)
Fellow, American Academy of Forensic Sciences (FAAFS)
Distinguished Fellow, Academy of Forensic Nurses (DF-AFN)
Fellow, American Academy of Nurse Practitioners (FAANP)
Fellow, American Academy of Nursing (FAAN)

1. A new era of conflict and violence. United Nations. Accessed July 16, 2022. https://www.un.org/en/un75/new-era-conflict-and-violence
2. Scattolin MAA, Resegue RM, Rosário MCD. The impact of the environment on neurodevelopmental disorders in early childhood. *J Pediatr (Rio J)*. 2022;98(Suppl 1):S66-S72. doi:10.1016/j.jped.2021.11.002
3. D'Amico D, Amestoy ME, Fiocco AJ. The mediating role of allostatic load in the relationship between early life adversity and cognitive function across the adult lifespan. *Psychoneuroendocrinology*. 2022;141:105761. doi:10.1016/j.psyneuen.2022.105761
4. Anda RF, Dong M, Brown DW, et al. The relationship of adverse childhood experiences to a history of premature death of family members. *BMC Public Health*. 2009;9(106). doi:10.1186/1471-2458-9-106
5. Substance Abuse and Mental Health Services Administration. *Trauma-Informed Care in Behavioral Health Services: Part 3: A Review of the Literature, Treatment Improvment Protocol: Tip 57*. US Department of Health and Human Services; 2014. https://store.samhsa.gov/system/files/sma14-4816_litreview.pdf
6. Dowdell EB, Speck PM. CE: trauma-informed care in nursing practice. *Am J Nurs*. 2022;122(4):30-38. doi:10.1097/01.NAJ.0000827328
7. Speck PM, Robinson LS, Johnson K, Mays L. Care for women with past trauma using trauma-informed care. *Advances in Family Practice Nursing*. 2023; 5(1):119-135. doi:10.1016/j.yfpn.2022.11.002
8. McEwen BS. Sex, stress and the hippocampus: allostasis, allostatic load and the aging process. *Neurobiol Aging*. 2002;23(5):921-939. doi:10.1016/s0197-4580(02)00027-1
9. McEwen BS. Neurobiological and systemic effects of chronic stress. *Chronic Stress*. 2017;1:247054701769232. doi:10.1177/2470547017692328

Preface

The concept of *gender* has become a proverbial hotbed of controversy and conflict in contemporary society. In its many forms—noun, adjective, or even verb—it remains partly arbitrary, based on distinguishable characteristics (such as body shape, social rank, manner of existence, or presumed sex) and often assumes a predetermined agreement with established social constructs on the behavioral, cultural, or psychological traits typically associated with 1 biological birth sex. The words *sex* and *gender* have had a long and intertwined history—including attempts at parsing out a clear delineation between the 2 terms.[1] "In the past, sex was the preferred term for biological forms while gender generally involved behavioral, cultural, and psychological traits. Within this overarching dichotomy, the terms male and female related only to biological forms (sex), while the terms masculine/masculinity, feminine/femininity, woman/girl, and man/boy related only to psychological and sociocultural traits (gender)."[2] Often, when comparisons explicitly between male and female people were made, the term gender was employed, with that term dominating in such collocations as gender differences, gender gap, gender equality, gender bias, and gender relations. It is likely that gender was applied in such contexts because of its psychological and sociocultural meanings.

In the present era, despite a societal interest in exploring what many now see as the continuum of gender, rather than the presumed dichotomy, many of these sociological underpinnings remain intact and are still applied. In such cases, when "gender" is employed against the prescribed use, there may subsequently be a "bristled" response. This indicates that the ultimate definitions, translations, usages, and applications of the terms sex and gender are by no means universally agreed upon. There is much evidence of resistance to using gender-neutral pronouns.[3,4] According to Pew Research Center, almost 1/2 of all Americans say they feel "somewhat or very uncomfortable" using they/them pronouns. The level of discomfort has a lot to do with age and where the respondents fall on the political spectrum.[3] Another common explanation for those resisting the use of "they/them" to describe individual people is that doing so is "poor grammar." This is not technically correct, as people use they/them to describe singular individuals frequently, often without realizing. As in, "Who parked their car here? They did a terrible job."[4] Furthermore, many professional organizations, such as the American Psychological Association[5] and the Modern Language Association,[6] have endorsed the use of the singular pronoun "they" when referring to either a person of unknown or irrelevant gender or a person who specifically identifies with "they/them" pronouns, as has Merriam-Webster's Dictionary.[7] Additionally, we do currently have well-ingrained, socially constructed conventions of which pronouns to use for a person based on their perceived gender expression that may be difficult for some individuals to initially overcome. However, this does not mean that we cannot or should not work to change those conventions and resist the habit of assuming a person's gender identity and pronouns based on their gender expression. Discomfort or difficulty with grammatical use is one thing, but when the issue of pronouns turns into stereotypes, threats, and gender-based violence, it becomes an issue in need of addressing on a larger scale.

Gender-based violence is unique and specific in its categorization, as it involves harassment directed against a person because of their gender or threats and violence that disproportionately affect persons of a particular gender.[8] Notably, women and girls statistically remain the main victims of gender-based violence[9] that continues to contribute to the significant levels of severe harm to families and communities.[10-12] To truly understand and eliminate gender-based violence, it is vital to recognize and address the intersecting forms of discrimination, marginalization, and oppression that too many individuals and communities still face. Acts of gender-based violence are rooted in social identity, status, and power. At its core, gender-based violence is an abuse of power and is a reflection and manifestation of power imbalances across different groups of people, especially related to sexual orientation, gender identity or expression, and sex characteristics; race and ethnicity; age; socioeconomic status; nationality; disability; religion; and citizenship or refugee status.[13]

In direct response, this book explores and examines these unique issues from both a broad theoretical and evidence-based approach, as well as a translational hands-on interdisciplinary and clinically focused practitioner perspective. The topics reviewed range from microaggression and systematic trauma in trans and nonbinary health care, to the intersectionality of gender-based violence impact, to the myriad of groups and subgroups affected across the fluid gender expression spectrum. In doing so, multiple treatment approaches, both preventative and post-trauma, are interwoven throughout the text to guide both the student and the practitioner toward enhanced awareness, sensitive assessment, and targeted intervention. There are also many specific groups, some easily identifiable and others less visible, discussed in the text, including those with HIV, victims of hate crimes, older adult victims, sex trafficking victims, and those involved in sex work.

As a collective, the lead authors of this book embraced the foundational pillars of trauma-informed care (TIC) to be interwoven throughout all the chapters. The first tenet is that all assessment and treatment approaches be held to the highest standard of *do no harm* when working with those who have experienced gender-based violence. The related tenets of the TIC approach utilized are set forth by the Substance Abuse and Mental Health Services Administration (SAMHSA)[14] which include:

— Understanding that traditional service-delivery models of care may trigger, silence, or disempower those who have experienced trauma, which can exacerbate poor outcomes and lead to disengagement from care;

— Employing strategies that avoid traumatization or retraumatization;

— An awareness that retraumatization is often unintentional—and that there are some "obvious" practices that could be retraumatizing, such as physical exams; however, less obvious practices or situations that involve specific smells, sounds, or types of interactions may cause individuals to feel retraumatized;

— Much harm can be avoided through awareness; appropriate preparation and ethical standards; and a critical reflective stance.

Finally, this is a book for the professional in need of a thorough, evidence-based resource check, and a source for the student who is just learning about the scope of gender-based violence and related traumas. It is not limited to a particular discipline or a particular part of the globe. Specifically, in direct response to the overarching and overwhelming needs of at-risk populations, *The Expanding Continuum of Gender-Based Violence: Trauma-Informed Care* intends to do the following:

— **Define** the problem of gender-based violence conceptually and numerically, using statistics that describe the state of violence and the characteristics of those most affected by it.

— **Identify** causes and risk factors that appear to affect susceptibility to gender-based violence, such as factors that increase a person's risk of violence or obstacles to delivering effective services.

— **Design** interventions that are trauma-informed, sensitive, and developmentally targeted.

— **Disseminate** information about the evidence and effectiveness of these interventions to increase the profile for their usage in clinical practice.

— **Educate** students and future professionals in psychology, medicine, nursing, social work, creative arts therapies, and others to mitigate the effects of gender-based violence for future generations.

Some may continue to ask about the importance to respect which pronouns people want to use. Ultimately, what it comes down to can be summed up in 2 words that are not pronouns: safety and respect. Pronouns signal to the world our gender identity. Part of respecting each other's humanity is honoring how we all identify. We hope that the words contained within this book will empower you, the reader, to empower your patient, not *regardless* of their pronouns, but because they have entrusted you *with* their pronouns.

Paul Thomas Clements, PhD, RN, AFN-C™, ANEF, DF-IAFN, DF-AFN

David Solomon, PhD, HSP-P

Kaleigh Mancha, MS, LMFT, Certified Full Spectrum Doula

Mitzy D. Flores, PhDc, MSN, RN, AHN-BC, CHSE, COI, Caritas Coach®, Introspective Hypnosis Practitioner

Christopher A. Mallett, PhD, Esq, LISW-S

References

1. Vaidakis N. Conceptual controversies regarding the terms gender and sex. *Psychiatriki.* 2020;31(3):271-274. doi:10.22365/jpsych.2020.313.271

2. Introduction and background. In: Becker T, Chin M, Bates N, eds. *Measuring Sex, Gender Identity, and Sexual Orientation.* National Academies Press (US); 2022. https://www.ncbi.nlm.nih.gov/books/NBK581050/

3. Geiger AW, Graf N. About one-in-five US adults know someone who goes by a gender-neutral pronoun. Pew Research Center. September 5, 2019. https://www.pewresearch.org/short-reads/2019/09/05/gender-neutral-pronouns/

4. Luu C. They're here, they're genderqueer, get used to gender neutral pronouns. JSTOR Daily. May 12, 2015. https://daily.jstor.org/theyre-here-theyre-gender queer-get-used-to-gender-neutral-pronouns/

5. Singular "they". American Psychological Association. July 2022. Accessed October 6, 2023. https://apastyle.apa.org/style-grammar-guidelines/grammar /singular-they

6. How do I use the singular they? Modern Language Association. March 4, 2020. Accessed October 6, 2023. https://style.mla.org/using-singular-they/

7. They pronoun. Miriam Webster Dictionary. Accessed October 6, 2024. https://www.merriam-webster.com/dictionary/they

8. *US National Plan to End Gender-Based Violence: Strategies for Action.* The White House. May 2023. https://www.whitehouse.gov/wp-content/uploads/2023/05/National-Plan-to-End-GBV.pdf

9. Violence against women. World Health Organization. 2023. https://www.who.int/health-topics/violence-against-women#tab=tab_1

10. Gender-based violence in emergencies. UNICEF. Updated November 11, 2022. https://www.unicef.org/protection/gender-based-violence-in-emergencies

11. What is gender-based violence? European Commission. 2023. https://commission.europa.eu/strategy-and-policy/policies/justice-and-fundamental-rights/gender-equality/gender-based-violence/what-gender-based-violence

12. Release of the national plan to end gender-based violence: strategies for action. The White House. May 25, 2023. https://www.whitehouse.gov/gpc/briefing-room/2023/05/25/release-of-the-national-plan-to-end-gender-based-violence-strategies-for-action/

13. United States strategy to prevent and respond to gender-based violence globally 2022. Office of Global Women's Issues, US Department of State. 2022. https://www.state.gov/reports/united-states-strategy-to-prevent-and-respond-to-gender-based-violence-globally-2022/

14. Trauma-informed care in behavioral health services: a treatment improvement protocol. Substance Abuse and Mental Health Services Administration, US Department of Health and Human Services. 2014. https://store.samhsa.gov/sites/default/files/sma14-4816.pdf

Reviews

Gender-Based Violence *is a 2-volume set that will provide a thorough examination of current knowledge on the way gender impacts both group and individual risk of violence. Applying the principles of trauma-informed care reaches far beyond professional and student practice and is a skill that can be utilized by all.*

Examples of interdisciplinary professionals that focus on the presentation and assessment of trauma with a special focus on trauma-informed approaches are included.

These books will also examine the impact of violence on contemporary populations which may previously have been overlooked. A special focus is given to the intersectionality of vulnerable groups and the impact of marginalization on assessment and treatment. These books promise to educate students and future professionals in gender-based violence. It is a must-have for your library.

Diana Faugno, MSN, RN, CPN, AFN-C, IVSE-C, FAAFS, SANE-A, SANE-P, DF-IAFN, DF-AFN

Gender-Based Violence *is an invaluable resource for understanding this pervasive issue. This well-researched guide is especially beneficial for professionals in various disciplines, particularly in health care. Nurses, uniquely positioned to prevent, identify, and respond to gender-based violence, will find this text particularly useful. Practical insights and evidence-based solutions will empower the reader to respond to gender-based violence.*

Justin Schneider, DNP, RN, AGPCNP-BC, CNEcl, CNE
Assistant Professor, Nursing
California State University
San Bernardino

The Gender-Based Violence *series is a comprehensive exploration of the complex dynamics surrounding violence that affects individuals based on gender. One of the strongest features of this series is its in-depth examination of intersectionality, emphasizing how gender-based violence intersects with race, class, sexual orientation, age, and other social identities. The authors intentionally underscore how these overlapping identities contribute to different experiences of violence and access to support systems. This nuanced approach encourages deep reflection and engagement by any professional invested in addressing systemic violence.*

Hannah Hyun Whiter, PhD
REEDS Postdoctoral Research Fellow
College of Education
University of Arizona

Gender-Based Violence *stands out for its dedicated focus on trauma-informed care. The series offers a thoughtful and empathetic approach, highlighting the importance of recognizing trauma's impact on survivors' lives. Practical frameworks and case studies make the material highly accessible, offering valuable insights into developing policies and practices. This series is a vital tool for health care professionals, social workers, and educators committed to fostering healing and resilience in their work with survivors.*

Samuel J. Hickson, PhD, LCSW, NPT-C
Psychotherapist
Serenity Counseling and Support Services

Contents in Brief

Contents in Detail

The Expanding Continuum of
GENDER-BASED VIOLENCE
Trauma-Informed Care

Presentation, Assessment, & Intervention

Volume 1

STM **Learning,** Inc.

Leading Publisher of Scientific, Technical, and Medical Educational Resources
Saint Louis
www.stmlearning.com

Section I

Biological/Presentation

Chapter 1

Contemporary Views of Gender and Implications for Affirming Practice with Transgender and Gender Diverse Communities

Jae A. Puckett, PhD

Key Points

1. *Because conceptualizations of gender have evolved significantly in recent decades, professionals need to be informed on contemporary gender terminology to provide affirming care.*
2. *The impact of gender-based violence on mental health and wellbeing in transgender and gender diverse (TGD) communities is compounded by higher prevalence rates, limited access to resources, and additional minority stress.*
3. *To aid in providing more affirming care to survivors of gender-based violence, practitioners and service providers must critically evaluate the level of inclusion of their services and take steps to reduce cisnormativity.*

Background and Significance

TGD communities have many strengths and resilience, although they also experience substantial hardship. Despite high rates of gender-based sexual and physical violence experienced by TGD individuals,[1,2] practitioners are often ill-equipped to work with this population due to lack of training.[3-5] This lack of training may lead to practitioner microaggressions (ie, subtle, often unintentional forms of discrimination)[6] or even more overt harm. This discrimination may prevent TGD people from seeking help following experiences of gender-based violence or may cause further harm to those who do seek help.[7] Additionally, TGD people's experiences may be minimized, as a recent randomized experiment found that when a sexual assault survivor was described as being a transgender man, the crime was rated as being less severe than when the survivor was described as a cisgender woman.[8] Given that TGD people may understandably be fearful of seeking services in the aftermath of violence due to previous negative stigmatizing experiences from both society more widely and helping professionals specifically, it is critical that practitioners and service providers take steps to improve levels of inclusivity in their treatment spaces and reduce cisnormativity (ie, assuming that cisgender identities are "the norm" and that individuals they encounter in their practice will all be cisgender).[9] Cisnormativity may be evident in service providers' actions, forms, and physical spaces. This chapter includes suggestions for how to improve services in general to be more inclusive of TGD people, as well as guidance on frameworks that may aid practitioners and service providers in understanding the contextual factors that influence exposure to gender-based violence and mental health for TGD people.

Terminology

Many TGD people report challenges in health care and other contexts due to providers' assumptions of their gender or misgendering when providers equate their sex assigned at birth to their gender.[10] Because sex assigned at birth and gender identity are often conflated, disentangling these concepts allows for a fuller understanding of TGD people's experiences and creates a space where TGD people can be more likely to be affirmed.[11] Sex assigned at birth generally refers to whether a person was assigned as male or female at birth and is typically based on physical sex characteristics, but it can also include internal reproductive organs and chromosomes. In addition to these binary designations of being assigned male or female at birth, other individuals may be intersex or have a difference of sex development. There are many ways that a person may be intersex, such as variations in internal and external reproductive organs or chromosomal differences. Due to birth record processes in the United States, individuals born intersex are still given a binary sex designation, although they may update their identification in some states to indicate being intersex.

Gender identity refers to a person's self-understanding of their gender experience as a woman or man, transgender or cisgender person, or many other identities that exist beyond binary understandings of gender (eg, genderqueer, nonbinary, agender, genderfluid).[12] A person who is TGD has a gender identity that differs from the gender typically associated with their sex assigned at birth, whereas for cisgender people, their gender identity aligns with that which is typically associated with their sex assigned at birth. Transgender or the term TGD are commonly used in the literature as umbrella terms to recognize the vast range of identities within these communities, as there is not a single term that best reflects the nuances in identity that can exist across individuals. Even so, it is important to note that TGD communities may use other language, such as transgender, nonbinary, or other iterations, instead of TGD, which is more common in academic communities.

Table 1-1 offers brief definitions of gender terminology, such as transgender (or trans) woman and other labels. Even though these are common definitions, it is important to recognize that gender experiences vary across individuals even if a shared label may be used. For instance, even though some TGD people may identify with a single label such as trans woman, the depth of their experience may be better described with multiple terms, such as a nonbinary trans femme person. However, TGD people often must choose single labels to describe their experience on forms or record-keeping systems that prioritize simplicity rather than allowing for more richness in their gender descriptors. Given this, it is important for clinicians to have a broad understanding of gender terminology and to recognize that a single label may not describe the complexity of a client's experience. Providers should also refrain from making assumptions about a TGD person's desire for or history of medical gender affirmation based on gender identity. For example, an individual who is a transgender man may or may not wish to use hormone therapy or any surgical treatments to affirm their gender.

Gender also differs from sexual orientation. Sexual orientation is complex and can include sexual attraction, sexual behaviors, and sexual identity. Cisgender and TGD people can have any sexual orientation. Despite common misconceptions, some TGD people will identify as heterosexual, whereas others may identify as lesbian, gay, bisexual, queer, or other identity labels. Again, it is crucial not to make assumptions about a person's sexual orientation or what a particular identity label means about who they may have had sex with or who they are attracted to. For instance, someone who identifies as a lesbian may report having sex with people of various genders, not just women. Ultimately, providers do not know information about sexual attraction and behaviors unless they ask rather than relying on assumptions based on identity labels.

Table 1-1. Gender-Related Terminology

Term	Definition
Cisgender	A person whose gender aligns with the gender that is typically associated with their sex assigned at birth (eg, a person who was assigned female at birth and identifies as a woman).
Transgender and Gender diverse	Umbrella terms to recognize any individual whose gender is different than the gender typically associated with their sex assigned at birth (eg, someone who was assigned female at birth and identifies as agender).
Transgender woman/trans woman	A person who was not assigned female at birth and identifies as a woman or transgender woman.*
Transgender man/trans man	A person who was not assigned male at birth and identifies as a man or transgender man.*
Genderqueer or Nonbinary	A person whose gender identity does not fall into binary categories of being a man or a woman. Genderqueer or nonbinary individuals may identify with multiple genders, no gender, as somewhere on a spectrum of gender experiences, or as having fluctuation in their gender experiences. There are also other specific terms that people may use to describe their experiences such as agender, bigender, genderfluid, and others that may fall under these umbrella terms.

*Note: This table represents a selection of gender identity terms and is not exhaustive. *Not all TGD people will identify with the prefix of "trans" and may instead simply identify with the gender term best aligned with their experiences (eg, identifying as a woman instead of as a transgender woman).*

Basics of Affirming Practice

In practice, providers (meant to broadly refer to any service provider, including health care staff, doctors, nurses, therapists, and advocates) may learn about clients' gender, sex assigned at birth, sexual orientation, and other demographics via their paperwork. However, TGD people's information is often inaccurate. Paperwork may assume, for instance, that a person's legal name is the name they go by, which can result in marginalization for TGD people who go by an affirmed name that they have not been able to legally change from their given name. This may result in deadnaming, which occurs when a TGD person is referred to by a previous name they no longer use. Office questionnaires may also only inquire about a person's "sex" without making clear whether the information being sought is about a person's sex assigned at birth, current legal designation, or their gender identity. Paperwork may also lack a space for a client's pronouns, which can result in providers making assumptions about what the client's pronouns are (note that language such as "preferred pronouns" is outdated and can be marginalizing). These issues can all be addressed through thoughtful reflection and adapting paperwork and processes to take into consideration the needs of TGD people. When providers do not work to make these changes, they are contributing to an atmosphere that further marginalizes TGD people, inhibits their engagement in care, and potentially hinders their ability to seek services to address gender-based violence. Furthermore, these experiences of marginalization disempower TGD people and replicate systems of oppression that manifest at the broader sociopolitical level.

Although paperwork is a starting place, there is much more that a provider can do to demonstrate affirming care. **Table 1-2** includes a few examples of ways to shift health care settings to be more TGD-inclusive and affirming. In addition, Queering

Table 1-2. Examples of Broad Opportunities to Improve TGD Client Care

Area or Situation	Do	Do Not
Demographic forms	Do ask about gender in inclusive ways – see the resource from Queering Medicine for recommendations. This may include asking gender via an open-ended question instead of force-choice options.	Do not assume that asking about sex or sex assigned at birth equates with gender.
General consent forms	Do use gender-neutral pronouns of they/them throughout.	Do not assume that all services are for people whose pronouns are she/her or he/him.
Restroom access	Do provide clearly labeled access to a gender-neutral restroom, and ensure this restroom is ADA accessible.	Do not only provide gendered restrooms for "women" and "men," or provide a gender-neutral restroom only in a hard-to-access, concealed, or wheelchair prohibitive location.
Record-keeping system	Do include a dedicated field to record a client's pronouns and their affirmed name.	Do not record pronouns based on the person's appearance or gender identity or assume that a legal name is the name that a person goes by.
Privacy and confidentiality	Do ask clients what name to use on mail or when calling or leaving voicemails to avoid unintentionally outing TGD people to others in their home environments.	Do not assume client preferences around name or permission to disclose this information.
Body diagrams	Do provide options for body diagrams, including a gender-neutral option.	Do not assume what body diagram a person would like.
Reports	Do ask clients what name and pronouns they would like used in any forensic reports or documentation.	Do not assume what name or pronouns to use for the individual in documentation or reports.
Referrals	Do properly vet referrals based on their competence and training in working with TGD people.	Do not assume that all referrals are safe and affirming for TGD people.
Websites and promotional materials	Do directly state the types of training and education that staff have obtained related to TGD people's experiences and inclusivity.	Do not make blanket statements regarding your competence to communicate skill level in working with TGD people. Knowing that you work with TGD people generally or that you are an ally can be less helpful than knowing the specifics of your training and background actually working with TGD people.

Note: Many other steps can be taken to create an inclusive health care space. For brevity, the topics in this table represent just a few areas; service providers should take initiative to seek out additional readings and trainings about creating TGD-inclusive and affirming services.

Medicine, a Lansing, Michigan-based coalition focused on LGBTQIA+ health, provides in-depth guidance about how to construct inclusive intake forms (see **Additional Resources**).

Mistakes

Some of the health care marginalization experienced by TGD people is intentional, and other times it may be as a result of a mistake, assumption, or misunderstanding.[10] Service providers should be prepared to acknowledge and address mistakes when they are made, without getting defensive or trying to justify their actions when TGD clients bring up issues or point out provider mistakes. This type of behavior further harms TGD people and can be seen as an assertion of provider power in professional relationships. Instead, efforts to empower TGD clients to provide feedback, validate concerns, and address mistakes by correcting that behavior or misstep can increase the trust, rapport, and quality in the provider-client relationship.[11]

Ultimately, service providers need to expect to make mistakes and be able to name when they have made a mistake. Glossing over these experiences is often invalidating to TGD people and demonstrates a lack of awareness about how deeply these mistakes, even when inadvertent, can impact TGD clients. At the same time, it is vital that service providers not focus on their own discomfort or make dramatic displays of overcorrection that attempt to portray them as competent and affirming. For example, providers who have made mistakes will sometimes take up a significant amount of time explaining how hard they are trying, how difficult it is for them, or all the ways they believe they are a great ally. These statements often represent attempts to quell the provider's anxiety, centering their experience rather than that of the client. To address mistakes, it is often helpful to keep apologies direct and to the point and to make intentional, concerted efforts not to repeat the act of marginalization again in the future. To prepare for these discussions, **Table 1-3**

Table 1-3. Reflection Questions to Prepare for Repairing Relationships after Mistakes

- **Have you ever made a mistake while interacting with a TGD person in the past, such as using the wrong name or pronouns (either when working with clients or more generally in your life)?**

If so:

  - What was your initial emotional response (eg, guilt, shame, anger, sadness)?
  - What happened in that situation? How did you respond? How did your response influence the other person's experience?
  - If you could redo this experience, is there anything you would change or do differently?

- **Imagine that you just used the wrong pronouns for a person seeking services. What is your immediate emotional response? What behaviors or interactions do you think this emotional response will prompt from you (eg, excessive apologizing, avoidance of discussing the issue)?**
- **Has a TGD person ever pointed out to you a mistake you made related to your interactions with them or other TGD people?**

If so:

  - What was your initial emotional response (eg, guilt, shame, anger, sadness, gratitude)?
  - What happened in that situation? How did you respond? How did your response influence the other person's experience?
  - If you could redo this experience, is there anything you would change or do differently?

continued

Table 1-3. Reflection Questions to Prepare for Repairing Relationships after Mistakes *(continued)*

If not:

- — Why do you think this is? Do you think that you create a safe and open space for others to bring mistakes to your attention?
- — Are there any things that you could change about your interactions with others that would communicate greater receptivity to these types of discussions?

Note: If you found it difficult to answer the questions above because you have not interacted with any TGD people in your life, it may be helpful for you to reflect about how that affects your knowledge and awareness of TGD people's life experiences. In addition, you can take steps to become more involved with the TGD community via volunteering with your local LGBTQIA+ community center, reading books and memoirs by TGD people, and so forth.

includes a few questions that service providers can use for their personal reflection. Taking the time to write and reflect on answers to these questions can help service providers to identify areas they may need to work on in the future.

Research Evidence on Gender-Based Violence in TGD Communities

The previous sections provided general information that could apply to most TGD individuals, but it is important for practitioners to note TGD communities are uniquely impacted by gender-based violence. One could assume that much of the violence and other types of victimization experienced by TGD individuals is based on their gender. As such, this section is meant to provide a broad overview of research related to TGD people's experiences of gender-based violence. Specific rates of violence also vary by the type of violence being measured and the specific definitions used by authors, but overall, rates of victimization are high for TGD people. For instance, Barr and colleagues found that 78.9% of their sample reported at least 1 experience of victimization (eg, experiences of sexual assault and threats or actual experiences of physical assault) related to their gender.[13] Furthermore, they found that 93.1% of their participants had experienced a potentially traumatic event related to being transgender.[13] Other research specifically exploring experiences of Black and Latinx transgender women has found similarly high rates of exposure to victimization; 91.4% of participants reported at least 1 form of violence (identified as threats or actual experiences of physical or sexual violence) and 86.8% reported multiple types of victimization.[14] Other studies have likewise found high rates of experiences of violence in TGD communities.[15,16]

Considering intimate partner violence (IPV), a high proportion (41.4%) of TGD people also report a history of physical violence within current relationships or from prior partners.[17] In addition, rates of stalking vary substantially across studies with 1 systematic review finding that anywhere between 7% and 53% of sexual and gender minority participants reported being stalked; the authors of this systematic review noted that the rates varied in part based on the definition of stalking, including if they considered cyberstalking or if emotional distress of the victim was required.[18] Furthermore, in a recent meta-analysis, TGD people were shown to be 1.7 times more likely to experience any form of IPV, 2.2 times more likely to experience physical IPV, and 2.5 times more likely to experience sexual IPV compared to cisgender people.[19] These experiences of violence accumulate over the lifetime of TGD people, particularly transgender women.[20] In addition, TGD people of color may be more likely to experience violence, stalking, and other forms of assault compared to White TGD people.[21]

Some research also has suggested that experiences of physical violence have increased for TGD people. For instance, Arayasirikul and colleagues conducted repeated cross-sectional studies with trans women in 2010, 2013, and 2016.[22] Experiences of verbal abuse and physical violence were overall high, with more than 83% and more than 56.7% of participants reporting each type of targeting across each time point respectively. After accounting for the effects of demographics, the study found that the odds of experiencing physical violence were significantly higher in 2016 than in 2010.

TGD people also experience significant barriers to accessing services in the aftermath of violence.[20] In addition to experiencing disproportionate rates of violence, TGD people may also be less likely to report this violence to the police due to valid concerns about being targeted or mistreated by police officers.[16] TGD people may also be discriminated against in spaces for people of a specific gender (eg, "women's shelters").[20] Overall, TGD people may be reluctant to utilize services that could aid in recovery due to fears of being further victimized or targeted.[23]

The high rates of violence and mistreatment TGD people experience are also associated with mental health issues in this marginalized community. For instance, Barr and colleagues found that close to 1/2 of their sample had clinically significant levels of post-traumatic stress disorder (PTSD) symptoms.[13] In addition, 44.2% of the sample likely met criteria for a possible diagnosis of PTSD.[13] TGD people's exposure to multiple types of victimization has also been associated with depression symptoms and PTSD.[14] Gender-based victimization has also been shown to drive suicidality in TGD children and adolescents[24] and TGD adults.[25] Likewise, experiencing sexual violence has been associated with suicidal ideation and history of suicide attempts for TGD people.[17] In addition, gender-related violence and stigmatization can also lead to delays in gender affirmation or coming out to others.[26] The impacts of gender-based violence on TGD people's mental health and wellbeing are substantial.

Models to Further Understand TGD People's Experiences

It may benefit service providers to be familiar with models of minority stress, as these factors can perpetuate gender-based violence and may simultaneously impact TGD people in care settings. The minority stress model was originally developed with the experiences of lesbian women and gay men in mind, but broadly refers to the unique stressors that minority groups experience, above and beyond general stressors that nonminorities endure.[27-29] This model proposes that various stressors help explain mental health disparities that sexual and gender minorities may experience. These stressors are broadly characterized as distal stressors and proximal stressors. Distal stressors include external actions such as rejection, victimization, and discrimination. Proximal stressors include experiences that are often reactions to distal stressors, such as internalized stigma, expectations of rejection, and identity concealment.

Although TGD people experience the stressors outlined in the minority stress model, there are nuances to TGD people's experiences that are not reflected in the original version due to differences across populations. For example, TGD people experience misgendering (also referred to as gender nonaffirmation; ie, deliberately or accidentally referencing TGD people with pronouns, names, or gendered terms that do not align with their gender identity).[30] Recent research has also identified other variables that can be integrated into this model. Some examples are binary normativity (ie, the belief and enforcement of there being only 2 genders),[31] burdening (ie, expectations of mental and emotional labor to educate cisgender people or comfort them after their perpetration of stigma),[31] gender dysphoria,[32] and hypervigilance (ie, being on guard for mistreatment by others).[33] These concepts can potentially play out in the interactions of TGD people with practitioners. For example, many TGD clients experience hypervigilance in early interactions with practitioners as they are bracing themselves for cisnormativity. Furthermore, if a practitioner expresses confusion over the gender identity of a nonbinary client, the client has experienced binary normativity and burdening when they then may feel the need to explain the concepts to the clinician.

Other research has also integrated advancements in understanding minority stressors with other frameworks, such as socioecological models[34] and frameworks of stigma.[35] These additional studies have identified minority stressors of gender binarism (ie, the cultural norms and enforced beliefs in there only being binary genders),[35] bodily vigilance (ie, being on alert for how others are reading or interpreting one's gender),[34,35] and others. Collectively, this growing literature has provided a more nuanced understanding of minority stressors TGD people may experience.

Experiences of gender-based violence must be considered in concert with these models of minority stress. For instance, there are unique forms of stalking that sexual and gender minority people may experience that particularly focus on their gender or sexual orientation.[18] Within romantic relationships, TGD women may be dehumanized or objectified in the context of gender-based violence.[36] Other TGD-specific forms of violence may include threats to disclose the person's sexuality or gender identity to others against their will, belittling TGD people as unworthy of another partner, or withholding access to gender-affirming medical care (eg, hormones or surgeries to affirm someone's gender). Furthermore, some experiences of minority stress, even those that are not necessarily classified as traumas in diagnostic terms, may be experienced as traumatic and associated with PTSD and other mental health challenges.[37] By having a fuller understanding of the types of minority stressors TGD people experience, service providers will be better able to validate the experiences of clients and understand factors that may be influencing access to resources, mental health, and overall wellbeing.

TGD people develop ways of coping with gender-related stressors, such as avoidance, learning to appropriately externalize these experiences (ie, not taking responsibility for cisnormative and transphobic comments made by others), and utilizing social supports to cope.[38] Research has found other ways that TGD people cope with violence, including self-protecting behaviors (eg, changing gender expression to decrease likelihood of violence) and self-affirming behaviors (eg, validating one's own experiences and gender).[39] When considering the effects of gender-based violence on the lives of TGD people, taking into account unique forms of coping may help to expand clinicians' and service providers' understandings of how they can best help clients.

Case Studies

Case Study 1-1

Ari was a 27-year-old Asian trans man. He was a college student and came to the campus health care services with complaints about abdominal pain. Ari recently got into a physical altercation with his partner, Quinn (a cisgender woman), which resulted in the physical pain he came in to address.

Although Ari identified as a trans man, he had not been able to change his name legally or update his gender marker. The university did not have an inclusive name or gender marker policy, which resulted in Ari's records only having his legal name and gender marker. Ari had been hesitant to seek medical care in the past because he knew he would have to give his birth name to the front desk. His birth name is traditionally associated with femininity, so he has often encountered challenges when front desk staff or others look at him with scrutiny due to discrepancies between his masculine gender expression and the name, ask interrogating questions as if he is lying about his identity, or joke about his birth name either to his face or to other employees. Ari also knew that staff and medical providers would likely misgender him, because he was listed as "female" in the records. These inaccuracies in his file might then lead to other uncomfortable conversations.

The doctor Ari was seeing had made many assumptions in the past about Ari's sexual orientation and the gender of his partners. Ari did not have the emotional bandwidth for this conversation or to engage in the emotional labor of correcting the doctor about Quinn's pronouns when the doctor assumed that Ari's partner was a man due to him being assigned female at birth. Given all of this, Ari instead decided to say that he got into a fight at a bar with a stranger rather than sharing that his partner physically assaulted him. The assault also included verbal slurs about Ari's gender, threats to out him to his family, and throwing away Ari's testosterone. However, none of this was discussed with the provider.

Discussion

As a result of institutional policies that omit the needs of TGD students, Ari's experiences of violence remained unheard, and he returned to a context where he continued to be unsafe and at risk for continued violence. This missed opportunity to address the violence may not have occurred if the setting and providers had been more competent in TGD-inclusive health care practices on a broad level.

Case Study 1-2

Amber was a 27-year-old Black trans woman who had been experiencing homelessness for about 3 months, following a series of adverse events that resulted in her losing her apartment. While working as a delivery driver for a local restaurant, a few customers complained to the owner about Amber delivering their food orders. She was often called slurs by customers or given looks of disgust. She even once had a customer refuse to take the order and demand a refund. Amber experienced many other instances of mistreatment in the past, so this was not new to her. She developed a tough exterior to protect herself from the bias and prejudice of others. Unfortunately, her boss did not support her after these experiences and fired Amber. She spent the next month looking for employment but could not find a job. She either was not selected for an interview, or she did not move further along in the interview process once she was recognized as being a trans woman. Given that Amber had held service work positions, she did not have a lot of savings. In addition, her family was no longer in her life due to their disapproval of her gender identity and so she could not reach out to them for support. These events culminated in Amber being evicted from her apartment due to not paying rent.

Amber found a few areas in the city where she felt safe, but one night a group of strangers began antagonizing her with slurs related to her race and gender. She was physically attacked, and one of the men in the group sexually assaulted her. An acquaintance of Amber's saw her afterwards, and she was taken to an emergency room for care. Amber's identification documents still had her gender marker as male and her given name rather than her affirmed gender and name. Her state had stringent requirements and processes for updating identification documents and it would have cost about $400 to legally change one's name in her state. The logistical and financial barriers prohibited her from legally affirming her gender.

The nurse examining Amber took the time to ask the name and pronouns she used, updated Amber's chart to include this information, and let the other staff know to use the correct name and pronouns for her. All of the staff had been educated during their employment onboarding and on a yearly basis about the importance of these basic steps to ensuring better quality care for TGD people at the hospital, so they were quick to take in this information. Amber was relieved by this experience. The nurse provided Amber with advance notice about how she may need to examine Amber's body and the physical wound on her forehead, which required stitches. Amber did not disclose information about the sexual assault to the nurse or any other medical staff because she was nervous about their potential reactions given mistreatment in medical settings in the past. Amber also knew that many cisgender people assumed that trans women engaged in sex work and was worried that her sexual assault would not be believed or would be dismissed because of these stereotypes. She also experienced gender dysphoria related to her body and was anxious about any physical examination of other areas.

Even though Amber did not disclose information about the sexual assault, the nurse respected Amber's desire not to share more about what happened to her and provided Amber with information about a local sexual assault program known for its TGD-inclusive practices in case Amber needed this information in the future. The nurse knew that Amber was at continued risk for violence while experiencing homelessness and invited the hospital social worker to meet with Amber to discuss a few local resources. The social worker explained that she had researched these programs and knew that their staff were trained in working with TGD people in competent and affirming ways. One of these resources was a homeless shelter specifically for sexual and gender minority individuals. Amber had been unaware of this resource and decided to seek shelter there when she left the hospital the next day.

Discussion

The providers who interacted with Amber took basic steps to indicate their affirmation of TGD people's identities and experiences, such as asking names and pronouns and using the correct ones consistently. These behaviors allowed Amber to be more open with her medical providers. In addition, these providers were trained and aware of the disproportionate rates of violence TGD people experience and other common adverse experiences that TGD people endure, such as discrimination and homelessness. As a result, they viewed Amber in compassionate ways rather than passing judgment on her. Although Amber did not disclose information about her sexual assault due to her worries that the forensic exam may trigger gender dysphoria and her fears about how others may perceive her, the providers respected this boundary and provided her with well-vetted resources in case she might need related care in the future. In addition, the providers were mindful about consent during their interactions with Amber and made sure to talk through all the points of care prior to any contact, answering her questions along the way. The providers also offered her additional resources and supports that could help her after her discharge from the hospital.

Summary

TGD people experience disproportionate rates of violence and are often targeted related to their gender identity or expression. Many service providers are undertrained in working with TGD people and may need additional support to create an affirming experience for these clients. By learning about common life experiences, terminology, and TGD people's health care needs, service providers can take necessary steps to improve their services for TGD people. Ultimately, learning and growing in this area should be viewed as a continual process, with service providers seeking additional ongoing training and tailoring services to the needs of the local TGD community. Providers can also work with local TGD leaders or advocacy groups to learn more about the community's needs in their local context. This will help to ensure that TGD people have better experiences with service providers, creating a greater likelihood that they will obtain care or resources that can aid in their recovery after experiencing gender-based violence.

Additional Resources

— Human Rights Campaign's report on dismantling a culture of violence against transgender people: https://reports.hrc.org/dismantling-a-culture-of-violence#what-leads-to-violence-against-transgender-and-non-binary-people

— Movement Advancement Project's report on hate crime laws: https://www.lgbtmap.org/file/2021-report-hate-crime-laws.pdf

— National Center for Transgender Equality's community resource manual regarding responding to hate crimes: https://transequality.org/sites/default/files/docs/resources/NCTE_Hate_Crimes_Manual.pdf

— National Center for Transgender Equality's remembrance report: https://transequality.org/sites/default/files/docs/resources/TDOR%20Remembrance%20Report%20by%20NCTE_Nov%202022%20%281%29.pdf

— Power and control wheel in LGBTQIA+ relationships: https://www.va.gov/HOMELESS/nchav/resources/docs/trauma/ipv/LGBT-Wheel-508.pdf

— National Coalition of Anti-Violence Programs' report on supporting LGBTQIA+ survivors of violence during the COVID-19 pandemic: https://avp.org/2020-supporting-lgbtq-survivors-covid19/

— National Coalition of Anti-Violence Programs' reports on hate violence and other related topics: https://avp.org/reports/

— National Coalition of Anti-Violence Programs' Training and Technical Assistance Center: https://avp.org/ncavp/tta-center/

— FORGE Forward's safety planning tool for working with transgender clients: https://forge-forward.org/wp-content/uploads/2020/08/FAQ-01-2013-safety-planning.pdf

— FORGE Forward's YouTube channel, which includes trainings related to working with transgender survivors and other resources: https://www.youtube.com/c/FORGEForwardTrans

— Queering Medicine's intake form guidance for providers: https://www.queeringmedicine.com/resources/intake-form-guidance-for-providers

References

1. Brangwin E, Zhao Z, Shramko M, Toomey RB, Syvertsen AK. The association between family physical abuse and suicide attempts among gender minority adolescents: a comparison study. *LGBT Health*. 2023;10(2):99-108. doi:10.1089/lgbt.2021.0415

2. Stults CB, Gao S, Brandt SA, et al. Intimate partner violence and mental health among transgender and gender diverse young adults. *J Fam Violence*. 2023;1-15. doi:10.1007/s10896-023-00579-7

3. Kia H, MacKinnon KR, Coulombe A. Where is the "T"? Centering trans experiences in social work curricula addressing LGBTQ+ issues. *J Soc Work Educ*. 2023;59(1):104-118. doi:10.1080/10437797.2021.1969302

4. Kosman KA, AhnAllen CG, Fromson JA. A call to action: the need for integration of transgender topics in psychiatry education. *Acad Psychiatry*. 2019;43(1):82-88. doi:10.1007/s40596-018-0966-7

5. Mackie G, Patlamazoglou L, Lambert K. School psychologists' perceptions of transgender training and education: an Australian qualitative investigation. *Psychol Sex Orientat Gend Divers*. 2023;10(4):699-710. doi:10.1037/sgd0000579

6. Morris ER, Lindley L, Galupo MP. "Better issues to focus on": transgender microaggressions as ethical violations in therapy. *Couns Psychol*. 2020;48(6):883-915. doi:10.1177/0011000020924391

7. Jones S, Patel T. Inaccessible and stigmatizing: LGBTQ+ youth perspectives of services and sexual violence. *J LGBT Youth*. 2022;20(2):1-26. doi:10.1080/19361653.2022.2134253

8. Carter LM, Goodmon LB, Urs M, Rutledge-Jukes H. The effects of victim gender identity, juror gender, and judicial instructions on victim blaming, crime severity ratings, and verdicts in sexual assault trials. *J Homosex*. 2023;70(6):1187-1224. doi:10.1080/00918369.2021.2018877

9. Stewart M, Ryu H, Blaque E, et al. Cisnormativity as a structural barrier to STI testing for trans masculine, two-spirit, and non-binary people who are

gay, bisexual, or have sex with men. *PLoS One*. 2022;17(11):e0277315. doi:10.1371/journal.pone.0277315

10. Puckett JA, Cleary P, Rossman K, Mustanski B, Newcomb ME. Barriers to gender-affirming care for transgender and gender nonconforming individuals. *Sex Res Soc Policy*. 2018;15(1):48-59. doi:10.1007/s13178-017-0295-8

11. Puckett J, Giffel R, Brown F, et al. Suggestions for improving healthcare for transgender and gender diverse people in the United States. *Int J Transgend Health*. 2022;25(2):233-250. doi:10.1080/26895269.2022.2150736

12. Matsuno E, Webb A, Hashtpari H, Budge S, Krishnan M, Basam K. Nonbinary fact sheet. APA Division 44. https://www.apadivisions.org/division-44/resources/nonbinary-fact-sheet.pdf

13. Barr SM, Snyder KE, Adelson JL, et al. Posttraumatic stress in the trans community: the roles of anti-transgender bias, non-affirmation, and internalized transphobia. *Psychol Sex Orientat Gend Divers*. 2022;9(4):410-421. doi:10.1037/sgd0000500

14. Sherman ADF, Poteat TC, Budhathoki C, Kelly U, Clark KD, Campbell JC. Association of depression and post-traumatic stress with polyvictimization and emotional transgender and gender diverse community connection among Black and Latinx transgender women. *LGBT Health*. 2020;7(7):358-366. doi:10.1089/lgbt.2019.0336

15. Blondeel K, de Vasconcelos S, García-Moreno C, Stephenson R, Temmerman M, Toskin I. Violence motivated by perception of sexual orientation and gender identity: a systematic review. *Bull World Health Organ*. 2018;96(1):29-41L. doi:10.2471/BLT.17.197251

16. Gyamerah AO, Baguso G, Santiago-Rodriguez E, et al. Experiences and factors associated with transphobic hate crimes among transgender women in the San Francisco Bay area: comparisons across race. *BMC Public Health*. 2021;21(1). doi:10.1186/s12889-021-11107-x

17. Drescher CF, Griffin JA, Casanova T, et al. Associations of physical and sexual violence victimization, homelessness, and perceptions of safety with suicidality in a community sample of transgender individuals. *Psychol Sex*. 2021;12(1-2):52-63. doi:10.1080/19419899.2019.1690032

18. Edwards KM, Camp EE, Lim S, Logan TK, Shorey RC, Babchuk W. Stalking among sexual and gender minorities: a systematic literature review. *Aggress Violent Behav*. 2022;66:101777. doi:10.1016/j.avb.2022.101777

19. Peitzmeier SM, Malik M, Kattari SK, et al. Intimate partner violence in transgender populations: systematic review and meta-analysis of prevalence and correlates. *Am J Public Health*. 2020;110(9):e1-e14. doi:10.2105/AJPH.2020.305774

20. Hereth J. "Where is the safe haven?" Transgender women's experiences of victimization and help-seeking across the life course. *Fem Criminol*. 2021;16(4):461-479. doi:10.1177/15570851211010951

21. Marx RA, Maffini CS, Peña FJ. Understanding nonbinary college students' experiences on college campuses: an exploratory study of mental health, campus involvement, victimization, and safety. *J Divers High Educ*. 2022;17(3). doi:10.1037/dhe0000422

22. Arayasirikul S, Turner C, Trujillo D, et al. A global cautionary tale: discrimination and violence against trans women worsen despite investments in public

resources and improvements in health insurance access and utilization of health care. *Int J Equity Health*. 2022;21(1). doi:10.1186/s12939-022-01632-5

23. Jordan S, Mehrotra G, Fujikawa K. Mandating inclusion: critical trans perspectives on domestic and sexual violence advocacy. *Violence Against Women*. 2020;26(6-7):531-554. doi:10.1177/1077801219836728
24. Bochicchio L, Reeder K, Aronson L, McTavish C, Stefancic A. Understanding factors associated with suicidality among transgender and gender-diverse identified youth. *LGBT Health*. 2021;8(4):245-253. doi:10.1089/lgbt.2019.0338
25. Small LA, Godoy SM, Lau C, Franke T. Gender-based violence and suicide among gender-diverse populations in the United States. *Arch Suicide Res*. 2024;28(1):107-122. doi:10.1080/13811118.2022.2136023
26. Restar AJ, Breslow AS, Jin H, et al. Transgender-specific developmental milestones and associated experiences of violence, discrimination, and stigma among Filipinx transgender women who are sexually active with men. *PloS One*. 2021;16(3):e0248248. doi:10.1371/journal.pone.0248248
27. Brooks VR. *Minority Stress and Lesbian Women*. Lexington Books; 1981.
28. Meyer IH. Prejudice, social stress, and mental health in lesbian, gay, and bisexual populations: conceptual issues and research evidence. *Psychol Bull*. 2003;129(5):674-697. doi:10.1037/0033-2909.129.5.674
29. Meyer IH. Minority stress and mental health in gay men. *J Health Soc Behav*. 1995;36:38-56.
30. Testa RJ, Habarth J, Peta J, Balsam K, Bockting W. Development of the Gender Minority Stress and Resilience Measure. *Psychol Sex Orientat Gend Divers*. 2015;2(1):65-77. doi:10.1037/sgd0000081
31. Matsuno E, Bricker NL, Savarese E, Mohr R Jr, Balsam KF. "The default is just going to be getting misgendered": minority stress experiences among nonbinary adults. *Psychol Sex Orientat Gend Divers*. 2022;11(2). doi:10.1037/sgd0000607
32. Lindley L, Galupo MP. Gender dysphoria and minority stress: support for inclusion of gender dysphoria as a proximal stressor. *Psychol Sex Orientat Gend Divers*. 2020;7:265-275. doi:10.1037/sgd0000439
33. Rostosky SS, Richardson MT, McCurry SK, Riggle EDB. LGBTQ individuals' lived experiences of hypervigilance. *Psychol Sex Orientat Gend Divers*. 2022;9(3):358-369. doi:10.1037/sgd0000474
34. Puckett JA, Price SF, Mocarski R, Mustanski B, Newcomb ME. Transgender and gender diverse individuals' daily experiences of rumination. *Am J Orthopsychiatry*. 2022;92(5):540-551. doi:10.1037/ort0000636
35. Puckett JA, Aboussouan AB, Ralston AL, Mustanski B, Newcomb ME. Systems of cissexism and the daily production of stress for transgender and gender diverse people. *Int J Transgend Health*. 2021;24(1):113-126. doi:10.1080/26895269.2021.1937437
36. Gamarel KE, Jadwin-Cakmak L, King WM, et al. Stigma experienced by transgender women of color in their dating and romantic relationships: implications for gender-based violence prevention programs. *J Interpers Violence*. 2022;37(9-10):NP8161-NP8189. doi:10.1177/0886260520976186
37. Salomaa AC, Livingston NA, Bryant WT, et al. A bottom-up approach to developing a unified trauma-minority stress model for transgender and

gender diverse people. *Psychol Trauma.* 2022;15(4):618-627. doi:10.1037/tra0001373

38. Gorman KR, Shipherd JC, Collins KM, et al. Coping, resilience, and social support among transgender and gender diverse individuals experiencing gender-related stress. *Psychol Sex Orientat Gend Divers.* 2022;9(1):37-48. doi:10.1037/sgd0000455
39. Sherman ADF, Balthazar M, Klepper M, et al. Approach and avoidant coping among black transgender women who have experienced violence: a qualitative analysis. *Psychol Serv.* 2022;19(Suppl 1):45-61. doi:10.1037/ser0000581

Chapter 2

Sexism, Misogyny, Transnegativity, and Homonegativity: *Key Contributors to Gender-Based Violence*

David Solomon, PhD, HSP-P
Kasey E. Vigil, MA
Patrick C. Barton, PsyD
Ash Moomaw, MA
Oak Reed, PhD

Key Points

1. *Sexism, misogyny, transnegativity, homonegativity, and other forms of prejudice can cause physical and psychological harm to individuals across the gender and sexual identity spectrums.*
2. *While traditional forms of prejudice are often more overt and recognizable, more modern forms of prejudice can be subtler, even as they cause harm and perpetuate systems of inequity.*
3. *Members of helping professions should assess and address the impact of these prejudices on clients and be aware of how their own biases may impact their work.*

Background and Significance

Various types of prejudices (such as misogyny, sexism, homonegativity, and transnegativity) are all driving forces of gender-based violence and cause harm in and of themselves, even when harbored by individuals who have never participated in direct acts of physical or verbal violence. These attitudes can subtly impact the way a person treats others and feels about themselves (eg, through the internalization of prejudice in members of minority groups). They can influence voting choices, which can in turn lead to the creation of laws and other systemic regulations that cause physical, financial, emotional, and other harm to individuals based on their gender or sexual orientation. In fact, the mere awareness of such prejudices can cause harm to marginalized groups. For example, the well-validated minority stress model, first suggested by Meyer in 2003,[1-3] suggests that in addition to harm through the internalization of stigma and direct experiences of discrimination, sexual minorities (which includes a range of nonheterosexual identities including gay, lesbian, bisexual, and pansexual) are also emotionally harmed by the anticipation of future discrimination. This model has since also been applied to gender minorities[2] and other marginalized groups.[4] Therefore, the presence of prejudice causes harm both directly and indirectly, and helping professionals should be aware of how these prejudices impact clients. Likewise, it is important for members of the helping professions (eg, doctors, nurses, social workers, counselors, psychologists) to understand how they themselves can hold such prejudices in subtle, covert ways. Professionals should realize that these attitudes are continuous constructs and exist in varying levels across individuals, as opposed to an all-or-nothing view that a person either is or is not misogynistic, sexist, homonegative, or transnegative. The ubiquity of these attitudes in our society also means that no one is immune from their influence. As DiAngelo[5] writes in *White Fragility: Why It's So Hard for White People to Talk About Racism*:

> "All humans have prejudice; we cannot avoid it. If I am aware that a social group exists, I will have gained information about that group from the society around me. This information helps me make sense of the group from my cultural framework. People who claim not to be prejudiced are demonstrating a profound lack of self-awareness. Ironically, they are also demonstrating the power of socialization – we have been taught in schools, through movies, and from family members, teachers, and clergy that it is important not to be prejudiced. Unfortunately, this prevailing belief that prejudice is bad causes us to deny its unavoidable reality."

Does the banal nature of prejudice absolve people from the need to challenge its appearance in society and themselves? No, and only by being aware of prejudices and biases can people actively work on the continuous process of reducing these prejudices and their impact on behavior in ways that can cause harm to clients or others. These influences are often subtle, unintentional, or even well-meaning, but this does not mean that the impact of such attitudes and corresponding behaviors are benign. More subtle displays of biases, sometimes referred to as microaggressions, can have negative effects on individuals seeking health care and represent an ethical concern,[6] given that most professional ethical standards indicate that helping professionals limit the negative impact of their biases on their work with clients.

Types of Prejudice and Their Relevance to Gender-Based Violence

While this chapter focuses primarily on specific types of gender-based prejudice (misogyny, sexism, transnegativity, and homonegativity), the influence of other types of prejudice, such as racism, are further explored in other chapters. Note that this chapter uses the words transnegativity and homonegativity instead of the terms transphobia and homophobia since the word "phobia" denotes fear, while these prejudices more likely represent hostility and contempt. Prejudice includes negative attitudes towards groups of people.[7] More traditional or "old-fashioned" forms of prejudice tend to reflect beliefs that a specific group of individuals is inferior to another and may lead to overt hostility towards the perceived inferior group. Modern forms of prejudice, often referred to as symbolic prejudice, include the belief that marginalized groups no longer experience significant discrimination, that they do not work hard enough to get ahead, and that policies supporting marginalized groups are not warranted.[8] Finally, prejudice reflected in policies and laws that perpetuate inequities against groups of people is referred to as systemic or institutional prejudice.[7,9]

Misogyny and Sexism

While misogyny and sexism are similar concepts and are discussed together in this chapter, there are distinct differences between them. While misogyny is the active hatred of women, sexism is the belief that men are superior to women[10] and may even be "benevolent," such as when a man believes women need to be protected by men. Sexism can influence reactions to, and attitudes about, people based on their gender expression. It can also influence the way people are perceived, depending on how their gender expression is congruent or incongruent with existing gender stereotypes.[11] While sexism is traditionally used to describe male attitudes towards women, perceived congruence with traditionally assigned gender norms can impact all genders.[12] For example, benevolent sexism, described above, portrays women as weak and in need of protection by men.[12] In this case, the term benevolent is misleading, as it relegates women to traditionally assigned gender roles and removes many traces of their autonomy. The "benevolence" of protection is also rather limited—only offered to those women that are deemed "worthy" of it through strict adherence to the aforementioned gender roles.[13] Similarly, sexism can result in prejudices towards men who do not fully represent traditional norms related to masculinity. Hostile sexism is, as the name would suggest, an altogether different form of sexism than benevolent sexism. This hostile form, according to Hernandez,[14] is characterized by a paternalistic and heavy-handed approach to maintaining social order.

One way that sexism influences gender-based violence is through its relationship to rape myths and victim blaming. ***Rape myths*** can be defined as "false beliefs about sexual violence that encourage blaming the victim and exonerating the offender."[15] McMahon & Farmer[16] describe several categories of rape myths based on their advanced psychometric analysis of a scale related to rape myth, utilizing a sample of 900 undergraduates in the United States. The first category is "She Asked for It," which includes beliefs that a woman is at fault for her rape if she has been drinking, wearing revealing clothing, or not saying "no" strongly enough. The second category is "He Didn't Mean To," which posits that a man may not be able to control his own behavior, either because his sexual desire is too strong, or because he is intoxicated and committing rape is unintentional. The third category is "It Wasn't Really Rape," which includes the belief that an act is not rape if the woman does not fight back hard enough, does not have marks or bruises, or is not threatened with a weapon. The final category is "She Lied," which includes the idea that a woman is not really raped, but instead has consensual sex and lies because she regrets it, is caught cheating, or simply has emotional problems. It should be noted that the categories described by McMahon & Farmer[16] are based on their research using a measure of heterosexual man-to-woman assault, but rape myths can apply to all genders (eg, the belief that men cannot be raped is itself a rape myth) and sexual orientations.[17]

One study found that hostile sexism had medium to large correlations with the categories of rape myths acceptance described above (range .47 [He Didn't Mean To] to .64 [She Asked for It]), while benevolent sexism had small to medium correlations with the categories of rape myths described above (range .22 [It Wasn't Really Rape] to .37 [He Didn't Mean to]). It is notable that these findings do not apply exclusively to males as this sample was 54.9% female, although females did report lower overall endorsement of rape myths.[15] The finding that sexism is a strong predictor of acceptance of rape myths in men and women has been replicated in multiple other studies as well.[18,19] This is problematic, given that individuals high in rape myth acceptance tend to see rape defendants as less guilty,[20] and a meta-analysis of 28 studies found a significant moderate correlation between rape myth acceptance and the perpetration of sexual coercion.[21]

Research suggests that hostile sexism, along with underlying correlates such as perceptions of power and power imbalance (ie, differences in control and decision-making authority) within relationships, can lead to aggression in heterosexual couples. For example, a systematic review of 15 studies on sub-Saharan Africa children published between 2004 and 2019 found that measures of intimate relationship power equality were associated with experiencing intimate partner violence (IPV) in women and perpetrating IPV in men.[22] Cross and colleagues[23] noted across several studies that interpersonal aggression was the ultimate consequence of perceptions of male power imbalance and hostile sexist attitudes.

Even controlling for such factors as trait dominance and aggression, the power distribution in relationships predicted hostile sexism which, in turn, predicted aggression and violence towards the female partner.[23] The relationship between sexism and misogyny and perpetrating or endorsing physical and psychological IPV has been established by multiple studies in multiple cultures and communities.[24-26]

Sexism, especially hostile sexism when seen through the lens of power imbalance, is not unique to cisgender, heterosexual male-female dyads in impacting hostility and harassment. For example, Glick et al[12] found that men with higher levels of hostile sexism had more negative views towards most "nontraditional" individuals such as masculine women, feminist women, career women, feminine men, feminist men, and stay-at-home fathers. Furthermore, in their review of the literature, DeSouza and colleagues[27] noted that sexual harassment in the workplace can be committed by and directed towards individuals of any gender. Other research has indicated that power imbalance in lesbian relationships was related to instances of interpersonal violence (which in this study included physical IPV, in addition to threats to reveal a partner's sexual orientation).[28] Another study of 272 queer men in China found that hostile sexist attitudes towards both men and women were related to reports of both controlling behavior and psychological, physical, and sexual intimate partner abuse.[29]

Another type of sexism is ***institutional*** or ***systemic sexism***, which can be defined as "gender discrimination reflected in the policies and practices of organizations such as governments, corporations (workplaces), public institutions (schools, health care), and financial institutions."[30] In the workplace, women earn less on average than men,[30] and women's perception of the "glass ceiling" (ie, systemic barriers to women's upward mobility at their jobs) can have a negative impact on their hope and intentions of staying at their jobs.[31] In education, women in graduate science, technology, engineering, and mathematics (STEM) programs report experiencing bias and sexism from male professors and increased stress due to having to work harder than male students to prove their worth.[32] Legal changes, such as the Supreme Court of the United States overturning *Roe v Wade* in June of 2022—a change that has resulted in the reduction or elimination of women's reproductive rights in many states in the United States[33]—can have a direct and negative impact on women's physical and emotional health.

Transnegativity

Transgender and gender diverse (TGD) identities represent a range of marginalized non-cisgender identities, such as transgender, gender nonbinary, and gender nonconforming. However, much of the research focuses on a subset of the TGD community (primarily those who identify specifically as transgender). Because identities within the TGD spectrum should not be treated as interchangeable or assumed to have the same experiences, the discussion of the research below will identify the groups being discussed by each specific source.

Negative attitudes and opinions about the TGD community have existed for a long time. Acts of harassment and violence, while still common in modern times, are the more "traditional" form of transnegativity. While systematic investigation of prejudices against TGD identities has rarely been conducted before the past few decades, a study from data collected in the late 1990s reported that over 1/2 of transgender individuals had experienced some form of harassment and 1/4 had experienced a violent incident.[34] A more recent study from 2020 found that transgender college students continue to be more likely to experience violence than their cisgender peers, particularly when it comes to experiences of sexual violence.[35] Analyzing data collected by the National Crime Victims Survey, the Williams Institute at UCLA School of Law indicated that transgender individuals experience violent crimes, such as sexual assault and physical assault, at rates that are more than 4 times greater than cisgender individuals.[36]

While violence towards transgender individuals continues, other forms of transnegativity have become more common with the increasing visibility of TGD individuals in the last few decades. One of the more common forms of modern transnegativity occurs when the perpetrator invalidates or ignores the identity/experiences of a TGD individual. A few examples of this include incorrect use of pronouns, exoticization (ie, portraying TGD identities as "exotic" as opposed to typical variations of human gender identity), endorsement of the gender binary, and denial of the existence of transnegativity.[37] Experiencing higher levels of microaggressions, similar to experiencing more overt victimization, is associated with higher levels of anxiety and stress and lower levels of self-esteem.[38] For example, in a therapy setting, misuse of pronouns or the use of a deadname (ie, any name previously used by a TGD person that is no longer used) may damage the relationship between client and therapist.[39]

Institutional transnegativity also exists. Individuals within the TGD community have recently been the focus of several pushes in legislation to limit or eliminate their rights. As of September 2022, 140 bills and policies have been proposed that specifically restrict the rights of transgender and nonbinary individuals in the areas of gender-affirming medical care, educational records, sports, housing, bathroom usage, and name change procedures.[40] In a study reported by the Trevor Project in January 2022,[41] 85% of transgender and nonbinary children reported that their mental health was negatively impacted by knowing about or experiencing the changes that came from these laws. Similarly, a study published in 2022 reported that adult LGBTQIA+ individuals have increased symptoms of anxiety and depression due to anti-LGBTQIA+ legislation and those who have experienced discrimination are at even higher risk for increased mental health concerns due to the negative psychological impact of these laws.[42]

In terms of physical and mental health care, gender diverse identities first appeared in the *Diagnostic and Statistical Manual of Mental Disorders* (DSM) or *International Classification of Diseases* (ICD) in the 1960s. Given that many medical providers increasingly required psychological and physical assessments prior to an individual undergoing any medical interventions, the introduction of these terms into the ICD and DSM potentially created a barrier (eg, access, finances) to the pursuance of a physical transition. In the eighth edition of the ICD,[43] gender diverse identities were introduced under the parent category of "Sexual Deviations" and classified as "Transvestitism," and in the second version of the DSM,[44] they were introduced under the category of "Sexual Deviation" and labeled as "Transsexualism." Not only do these terms conflate sexual and gender identity, but they may also insinuate homonegative and transnegative attitudes characteristic of the time that they were introduced. Notably, as both the DSM and ICD have updated throughout the years, neither have reflected a consensus regarding terminology on how TGD identities are conceptualized. These discrepancies illustrate the longstanding separation between psychological and medical services and the ongoing challenges gender diverse individuals face when seeking health care. Research has also shown that many TGD individuals either experience denial of care, outright rejection, or avoidance of seeking health care due to fear of being pathologized, marginalized, or discriminated against.[45] These populations' interactions with the health care system are further harmed by the fact that medical schools often do not require training in treating this population, leaving those in health care underprepared to address the needs of their TGD patients.[46]

Homonegativity

Traditional homonegativity is defined as outward negative attitudes and prejudices towards queer-identified individuals, such as the attitude that nonheterosexual relationships are sinful, unnatural, inferior, a sign of pathology, or related to pedophilia, and that lesbian, gay, or bisexual individuals should be avoided.[47,48] Some examples of traditionally homonegative discrimination include refusal to provide medical or therapeutic services based on sexual orientation, use of derogatory slurs, and perpetration of hate crimes based on sexual identity. Antisexual minority stereotypes are prevalent within traditional homonegativity. Some examples of these harmful stereotypes include beliefs that members of the sexual minority community are melodramatic, aggressive, promiscuous, unwilling to commit to relationships, and sexually deviant. While many of these stereotypes focus on monosexual individuals (ie, individuals attracted to 1 gender), there are similarly harmful stereotypes directed at plurisexual individuals (ie, individuals attracted to 2 or more genders). These stereotypes include that plurisexual individuals are more likely to change their sexual identity, are more promiscuous and sexually irresponsible, are more likely to be involved in noncommitted or nonmonogamous relationships, and that this identity is illegitimate.[49] It should also be noted that plurisexual individuals may also experience monosexist stereotypes from both outside and inside of the LGBTQIA+ community.

As outward prejudice against sexually marginalized populations (ie, traditional homonegativity) has been deemed less socially acceptable over time,[48] more subtle forms of homonegative attitudes have emerged. Modern homonegativity refers to hostile or negative attitudes towards policy change and activism that protects the LGBTQIA+ community, along with denial of the existence of widespread homonegative discrimination.[47] Some examples of modern homonegativity include ideologies that social change leading to greater LGBTQIA+ acceptance is unnecessary, that anti-LGBTQIA+ prejudice and discrimination no longer occurs, and that if LGBTQIA+ people do experience discrimination, it is their fault for centering their sexuality in their identity. For example, someone exhibiting modern homonegativity may see laws promoting marriage equality as "special rights" and not "equal rights." While modern homonegativity is subtler than the more overt traditional homonegativity, the 2 are directly correlated but distinct constructs.[47]

Institutional homonegativity, which encompasses many levels of oppression and discrimination against sexual minority individuals, is defined as a system of social policies and institutions that grant privileges to heterosexual individuals and exclude or discriminate against sexual minority individuals.[48] The history of systemic homonegativity can be traced through the history of the political, legal, medical, and mental health care fields. For example, the DSM listed homosexuality as a pathological diagnosis of sexual deviance until 1973 (although it was maintained in different forms and with different terminology such as "ego-dystonic homosexuality" and "persistent and marked distress about sexual orientation" until the publication of the DSM-5 in 2013). The ICD continued to use homosexuality as a diagnosis through 1990, but terms referring to being upset about one's sexual orientation remained until the ICD-11, written in 2019 and taking effect in 2022.[50,51] Medical researchers are calling for increased efforts to be made for equitable access to health care for LGBTQIA+ patients by avoiding assumptions of a patient's sexual orientation or gender identity, understanding that sexual orientation and gender identity are separate aspects of identity, using gender-neutral language, mitigating the use of microaggressions towards patients, and understanding unique health disparities that impact this community.[52]

Despite the removal of homosexuality as a diagnosis in both the DSM and ICD, there are continued health disparities between sexual minority and heterosexual populations, and there are additional examples of institutional homonegativity within the medical and mental health fields. For instance, as of the writing of this chapter, sexual minority children are not currently protected from the harms of sexual orientation change efforts (SOCE)—sometimes referred to as conversion therapy, reparative therapy, or reorientation therapy—at the federal level. SOCEs are harmful clinical or medical practices that attempt to "cure" an individual's attraction to people of the same gender in an attempt to convert that individual's sexual orientation to heterosexual.[53] This practice has been associated with increased suicidality and depression, among other negative outcomes, in both sexual minority and TGD communities.[53-55] As Hancock and colleagues point out, "half a century of scientific research on a variety of [SOCE] has not demonstrated their effectiveness according to the criteria of consistent positive effects and absence of serious harmful effects."[56] While the American Psychological Association,[57] American Psychiatric Association,[58] and many LGBTQIA+ scholars[53] have issued statements condemning this unethical and harmful practice on the basis of their codes of ethics, as of early 2023, only around 20 states in the United States prohibit conversion therapy completely for minors, with a small number of states disallowing state funding to go towards such "treatments."[59,60] Because of recent increases in public scrutiny related to conversion therapy, some practitioners have elected to change the description of their services to seemingly innocuous labels and goals, such as Sexual Attraction Fluidity Exploration in Therapy (SAFE-T), treating "sexual addiction," and generally offering SOCE and terming it sex therapy.[60] The United States falls behind many countries, such as Brazil, which was the first country to prohibit health professionals from practicing SOCE in 1999, and which followed up with similar laws protecting individuals from gender identity change efforts in 2018; other countries, such as Germany, prohibit SOCE to be used against minors altogether as well as prohibiting the use of force or other coercive methods from being used to pressure adults into SOCE.[61]

Institutional homonegativity has persisted into the 2020s in the United States, despite developments such as the decriminalization of sexual minority sexual activity by striking down anti-sodomy laws (*Lawrence v Texas,* 2003),[62] and the Supreme Court decision to recognize same-sex marriages (*Obergefell v Hodges,* 2015).[63] Several states have proposed[64] or enacted, as in the state of Florida,[65] litigation such as "Don't Say Gay" bills. Laws like these prevent children with sexual minority parents from discussing their family in class assignments, further erasing positive representation for LGBTQIA+ children, and possibly silencing children who are questioning their sexual or gender identities. This prohibition of discussing LGBTQIA+-related issues in schools perpetuates the idea that heterosexuality is considered the norm and that sexual minority identities are ultimately tied to sexual deviance.

Impact of Prejudice and Clinical Implications

Experiencing sexism, homonegativity, and transnegativity have serious implications for the physical, mental, and relational wellbeing for women and LGBTQIA+ individuals. These forms of violence have been associated with increased difficulties accessing care,[66] increased rates of internalizing symptoms (eg, depression or anxiety), suicidality,[67] feelings of not being accepted by others,[68] and lower quality of life.[69] Internalized stigma has been associated with a number of negative outcomes, including substance abuse, depression, anxiety, suicidal ideation, shame, low self-esteem, and guilt.[1,70-72] Internalized stigma is also related to physical health outcomes, such as higher levels of sexual risk behavior[73] and less compliance with COVID-19 preventative behaviors during the pandemic.[74] As previously established, experiences of systemic oppression, such as restricted access to abortion with the overturn of *Roe v Wade* or gender-affirming care for children in several states in the United States, will likely have continuing effects on physical health, mental health, and feelings of autonomy.

It is therefore important for clinicians to be aware of, and assess, the impact of these many forms of prejudices on clients' physical and mental health. Clinicians should be aware that clients may be impacted by both overt and more subtle forms of discrimination and may have internalized societal prejudices, impacting how they see themselves and their identities. Clinicians can assist by engaging in the process of assessing, not assuming, information about their clients. For example, when clinicians directly ask clients about their pronouns, gender identity, and sexual orientation, they show their clients that it is safe to discuss these aspects of themselves in a session, and it allows clients the space to define these labels for themselves and examine the significance that these constructs play in their lives. It can be similarly helpful to not assume the client has experienced rejection, or that any attribute of their identity is their reason for coming to therapy. Over- or under-emphasizing the importance of any of a client's identities could pathologize or invalidate their lived experiences. When clients have experienced prejudice that is clinically relevant, treatment should address this. For example, many authors have pointed out that the reduction of internalized stigma can be an important potential treatment outcome, as it may contribute to mental health difficulties and distress.[75,76] Internalized stigma may be addressed in therapy by addressing associated automatic negative thoughts (eg, "I am unworthy because I am gay"), or displaying unconditional positive regard towards the client.[76,77] Finally, the assessment process should also focus on uncovering strengths and protective factors, such as identifying how the client has coped with discrimination in the past and identifying the client's sources of positive social support. Some clients may also find it helpful to combat institutional prejudice through social and political activism.

While attempting to address and reduce the impact of prejudice, clinicians must aim to avoid the enactment of those prejudices in the therapy room. A social microcosm is created within therapeutic settings; gender-based violence can be recreated within therapeutic spaces unless clinicians are mindful of implicit biases that they may hold. This situation may emerge when the clinician directs microaggressions towards their clients.[78] Perpetration of microaggressions and other discrimination in the therapy room can lead to a weakened therapeutic alliance and rapport, decreased desire to engage in therapy with the current or other therapists, and increased feelings of being ashamed and misunderstood.[77] It is also important to remember that microaggressions may be well-intentioned, and avoiding them may require changes to general therapy practices. For example, while cognitive behavioral techniques are well-supported by research generally, using cognitive restructuring to challenge clients' thoughts about experiencing prejudice (eg, asking what evidence the client has that they were discriminated against) can feel invalidating. As already discussed, deadnaming can also cause harm.[79] This could occur within conversations, or when writing reports or clinical notes which may be accessed by the client or needed for purposes such as receiving gender-affirming care or other resources. Another example might be inadvertently perpetuating rape myths or other types of victim-blaming. While it may be pertinent to discuss safety to prevent future harm, these conversations should not involve what a client "should have" or "could have" done differently, and, barring imminent threat, it may be useful to have such conversations only after any client self-blame has been reduced. Clinicians need to know that for many clients, safety requires additional resources, such as access to domestic violence shelters. There may be further barriers in place when such shelters are not available or may not be available to a client because of their gender. Finally, clinicians must also recognize that while clients' identities and resulting experiences of discrimination can play major roles in their self-concept and experiences of mental health concerns, clinicians should avoid putting their clients in a position to educate them on systems of oppression and the meanings of their identities. Other problematic clinical microaggressions include focusing solely on a client's marginalized identity as a source of distress, avoiding discussion of marginalized identities, making generalizations about identities, structuring therapy to "fix" their identity, further stigmatizing these identities, or focusing on controlling access to gender-affirmative care, if applicable.[80] Furthermore, while clients may want to explore their identities, it is not the clinician's role to "diagnose" or "figure out" what a client's "correct" identity is, but instead to provide a safe space for the client to explore their identity.[81]

Case Study

Case Study 2-1

Jon was a 21-year-old, gender nonbinary, pansexual college student who was assigned male at birth. Jon's pronouns were they/them. Jon was referred by their university's academic support services for an ADHD assessment at the on-campus clinic because of difficulty following lectures and taking notes in their courses. Jon noticed on the intake form that the only options for gender were "male" and "female," so they wrote in "nonbinary" above the option, as there was no write-in option. The intake form had no space to list pronouns or sexual orientation. Jon met with the student clinician, Sandra, who was supervised by a licensed psychologist, Dr. Mills. Sandra expressed confusion to Jon about their nonbinary identity, which Jon explained to her with some discomfort. Sandra later asked if Jon had a current girlfriend, and Jon stated that they were currently single, but had had several partners of several different genders in the past. Later, Sandra went through a list of potentially traumatic experiences. Jon stated they had not had any of the experiences she listed, but they disclosed that they had been sexually assaulted by a man they had gone on several dates with. Sandra asked them about the experience in detail, but did not ask about any trauma symptoms, before moving on to the testing process. Jon received their assessment report several weeks later. The report identified Jon as a "bisexual male who disagrees with gender." The report later described Jon's sexual assault in explicit detail, frequently using the words, "he claims." The report eventually discussed the results of the testing, identifying Jon as having ADHD and providing several recommendations for academic accommodations. While Jon was originally seeking accommodations, they were distressed by the report and shredded it instead of taking it to their university's academic support services.

Discussion

This vignette offers several ways to explore why members of marginalized groups can be reluctant to seek mental and physical health services and may be legitimately harmed by those services when they are performed incorrectly. The vignette also displays many gendered assumptions and conveys the lack of a trauma-informed approach. First, the intake paperwork was not inclusive of Jon's identities and indeed conflated gender with sex assigned at birth by only listing "male" and "female" as genders. This can be seen as an early warning sign by TGD individuals that an organization is not trans-friendly, and also could lead the clinician to engage in microaggressions due to assumptions based on the client's perceived gender and sexual orientation. The student clinician made such a microaggression when asking if Jon had a girlfriend, displaying that she assumed both Jon's gender and sexual orientation. Additional microaggressions include when Jon was misgendered in their assessment report by the use of incorrect pronouns and when their gender was disrespected by being described as "a male who disagrees with gender." The student clinician may also have been displaying the gendered rape myth that men cannot be raped when she, perceiving Jon as a man, asked about various types of trauma, but not sexual assaults. The student clinician perpetuated rape myths further in the assessment report when she used the word "claims," a word that conveys disbelief, multiple times. Additionally, while it can be important to have frank discussions of trauma with clients, the purpose of the assessment was to screen for ADHD. Because the student clinician did not ask further about trauma symptomology (which may have been necessary to rule out other issues that could impact attention), this exploration of the assault seemed like an unnecessary and uncomfortable discussion. Likewise, trauma history should be included in a written report only as necessary and only to the extent necessary, and rarely with explicit details, especially related to sexual assault. The purpose and intended audience of the report (student support services) were not appropriately considered in its execution, and the process did not follow trauma-informed principles. Finally, it appears that not only was the student clinician not well-prepared by her training program to work with diverse clients before she began her direct clinical work, but her supervisor also did not adequately review the report to address sensitivity and inclusive language. As a result, Jon felt unable to share the inaccurate, insulting, and overly personal report with academic support services, resulting in them not receiving proper academic accommodations. Ultimately, the impact of prejudice, which could have been avoided, caused emotional and academic harm to the client, indicating that the clinicians in this case failed to meet their ethical responsibility.

Summary

There is a plethora of research indicating that various forms of gender-based prejudice, including sexism, misogyny, transnegativity, and homonegativity, can lead to instances of gender-based violence and dissuade victims of such violence from seeking help. Even in the absence of overt violence, the existence of these prejudices can lead to distress in members of the targeted groups (eg, through worries about potential discrimination). Furthermore, prejudice can transcend the personal attitudes of individuals and be reflected in institutional policies, which further harm or limit options for women and members of other marginalized groups, such as when biases drive the adoption of laws limiting reproductive rights or legal protections for victims of gender-based violence. Helping professionals should be aware of these types of prejudices and their potential impact on clients. While most individuals can identify more overt, traditional forms of prejudice, more subtle, difficult to recognize forms of prejudice can nonetheless lead to harmful outcomes. For example, unconscious biases may lead clinicians and other helpers to use microaggressions that may discourage victims from help-seeking or cause them further harm. Because these prejudices are ubiquitous in society, helping professionals should not assume that they are immune from such prejudices, and should engage in vigilant self-reflection on their beliefs, attitudes, and actions that may be prejudicial.

References

1. Meyer IH. Prejudice, social stress, and mental health in lesbian, gay, and bisexual populations: conceptual issues and research evidence. *Psychol Bull.* 2003;129(5):674-697. doi:10.1037/0033-2909.129.5.674

2. Helsen V, Enzlin P, Gijs L. Mental health in transgender adults: the role of proximal minority stress, community connectedness, and gender non-conformity. *Psychol Sex Orientat Gend Divers.* 2022;9(4):466-477. doi:10.1037/sgd0000530

3. Mann AM, Naugle AE, Lieberman E. Experiential avoidance and emotion dysregulation as mediators in the LGBTQ minority stress model. *Arch Sex Behav.* 2022;51(7):3443-3456. doi:10.1007/s10508-022-02376-7

4. Buckner JD, Glover NI, Shepherd JM, Zvolensky MJ. Racial discrimination and hazardous drinking among black drinkers: the role of social anxiety in the minority stress model. *Subst Use Misuse.* 2021;57(2):256-262. doi:10.1080/10826084.2021.2002903

5. DiAngelo R. *White Fragility: Why It's So Hard for White People to Talk About Racism.* Beacon Press; 2018.

6. Morris ER, Lindley L, Galupo MP. "Better issues to focus on": transgender microaggressions as ethical violations in therapy. *Couns Psychol.* 2020;48(6):883-915. doi:10.1177/0011000020924391

7. Phelan JC, Link BG, Dovidio JF. Stigma and prejudice: one animal or two? *Soc Sci Med.* 2008;67:358-367. doi:10.1016/j.socscimed.2008.03.022

8. Henry PJ, Sears DO. The symbolic racism 2000 scale. *Political Psychol.* 2002;23(2):253-283. doi:10.1111/0162-895X.00281

9. Payne BK, Vuletich HA, Lundberg KB. The bias of crowds: how implicit bias bridges personal and systemic prejudice. *Psychol Inq*. 2017;28(4):233-248. doi: 10.1080/1047840X.2017.1335568

10. Wolf N, Bindel J, Power N, Gupta R, Cosslett RL, Bidisha. Sexism and misogyny: what's the difference? The Guardian. October 17, 2012. Accessed February 11, 2022. https://www.theguardian.com/commentisfree/2012/oct/17/difference-between-sexism-and-misogyny

11. Zaikman Y, Marks MJ. Ambivalent sexism and the sexual double standard. *Sex Roles J Res*. 2014;71(9-10):333-344. doi:10.1007/s11199-014-0417-1

12. Glick P, Wilkerson M, Cuffe M. Masculine identity, ambivalent sexism, and attitudes towards gender subtypes: favoring masculine men and feminine women. *Soc Psychol*. 2015;46(4):210-217. doi:10.1027/1864-9335/a000228

13. Oswald DL, Baalbaki M, Kirkman M. Experiences with benevolent sexism: scale development and associations with women's wellbeing. *Sex Roles J Res*. 2019;80(5-6):362-380. doi:10.1007/s11199-018-0933-5

14. Hernandez AD. Intersections of feminist identification and hostile sexism. *J Sci Study of Religion*. 2021;60(1):27-45. doi:10.1111/jssr.12694

15. Rollero C, Tartaglia S. The effect of sexism and rape myths on victim blame. *Sex Culture Interdiscip Q*. 2019;23(1):209-219. doi:10.1007/s12119-018-9549-8

16. McMahon S, Farmer GL. An updated measure for assessing subtle rape myths. *Soc Work Res*. 2011;35(2):71-81. doi:10.1093/swr/35.2.71

17. Rape myths. University of Richmond Center for Awareness, Response, and Education. Accessed February 12, 2023. https://prevent.richmond.edu/prevention/education/rape-myths.html

18. Borgogna NC, Lathan EC, McDermott RC. She asked for it: hardcore porn, sexism, and rape myth acceptance. *Violence Against Women*. 2022;28(2):510-531. doi:10.1177/10778012211037378

19. Poerwandari EK, Utami CP, Primasari I. Ambivalent sexism and sexual objectification of women as predictors of rape myth acceptance among male college students in Greater Jakarta. *Curr Psychol*. 2021;40(12):5909-5918. doi:10.1007/s12144-019-00500-w

20. Süssenbach P, Eyssel F, Bohner G. Metacognitive aspects of rape myths: subjective strength of rape myth acceptance moderates its effects on information processing and behavioral intentions. *J Interpers Violence*. 2013;28(11):2250-2272. doi:10.1177/0886260512475317

21. Trottier D, Benbouriche M, Bonneville V. A meta-analysis on the association between rape myth acceptance and sexual coercion perpetration. *J Sex Res*. 2021;58(3):375-382. doi:10.1080/00224499.2019.1704677

22. Closson K, Ndungu J, Beksinska M, et al. Gender, power, and health: measuring and assessing sexual relationship power equity among young sub-Saharan African women and men, a systematic review. *Trauma Violence Abuse*. 2022;23(3):920-937. doi:10.1177/1524838020979676

23. Cross EJ, Overall NC, Low RST, McNulty JK. An interdependence account of sexism and power: men's hostile sexism, biased perceptions of low power, and relationship aggression. *J Personality Soc Psychol*. 2019;117(2):338-363. doi:10.1037/pspi0000167.supp

24. Blake KR, O'Dean SM, Lian J, Denson TF. Misogynistic tweets correlate with violence against women. *Psychol Sci*. 2021;32(3):315 325. doi:10.1177/0956797620968529

25. Juarros-Basterretxea J, Overall N, Herrero J, Rodríguez-Díaz FJ. Considering the effect of sexism on psychological intimate partner violence: a study with imprisoned men. *Eur J Psychol Appl Leg Context.* 2019;11(2):61-69. doi:10.5093/ejpalc2019a1

26. Laslett A, Graham K, Wilson IM, et al. Does drinking modify the relationship between men's gender-inequitable attitudes and their perpetration of intimate partner violence? A meta-analysis of surveys of men from seven countries in the Asia pacific region. *Addiction.* 2021;116(12):3320-3332. doi:10.1111/add.15485

27. DeSouza ER, Solberg J, Elder C. A cross-cultural perspective on judgments of woman-to-woman sexual harassment: does sexual orientation matter? *Sex Roles J Res.* 2007;56(7-8):457-471. doi:10.1007/s11199-007-9184-6

28. Eaton L, Kaufman M, Fuhrel A, et al. Examining factors co-existing with interpersonal violence in lesbian relationships. *J Fam Violence.* 2008;23(8):697-705. doi:10.1007/s10896-008-9194-3

29. Li D, Zheng L. Intimate partner violence and controlling behavior among male same-sex relationships in China: relationship with ambivalent sexism. *J Interpers Violence.* 2021;36(1-2):208-230. doi:10.1177/0886260517724835

30. Capodilupo CM. Institutional sexism. In: Nadal KL, ed. *The SAGE Encyclopedia of Psychology and Gender.* SAGE Publications, Inc.; 2017:941-942.

31. Javadizadeh B, Ross J, Valenzuela MA, Adler TR, Wu B. What's the point in even trying? Women's perception of glass ceiling drains hope. *J Soc Psychol.* 2022;5:1-23. doi:10.1080/00224545.2022.2119121

32. Powless MD, Wilkins-Yel KG, Li Y, et al. "[He] gave me a 30-minute lecture on how I was a shitty grad student": examining how male faculty can eradicate systemic oppression and support women in STEM. *J Divers High Educ.* 2022;17(1):81-95. doi:10.1037/dhe0000393

33. After Roe fell: abortion laws by state. Center for Reproductive Rights. 2022. Accessed February 12, 2023. https://reproductiverights.org/maps/abortion-laws-by-state/

34. Lombardi EL, Wilchins RA, Priessing D, Malouf D. Gender violence: transgender experiences with violence and discrimination. *J Homosex.* 2001;42(1):89-101. doi:10.1300/j082v42n01_05

35. Griner S, Vamos C, Thompson E, Logan R, Vázquez-Otero C, Daley E. The intersection of gender identity and violence: victimization experienced by transgender college students. *J Interpers Violence.* 2017;35(23-24):5704-5725. doi:10.1177/0886260517723743

36. Transgender people over four times more likely than cisgender people to be victims of violent crime. Williams Institute at UCLA School of Law. March 23, 2021. Accessed September 19, 2023. https://williamsinstitute.law.ucla.edu/press/ncvs-trans-press-release/

37. Nadal K, Davidoff K, Davis L, Wong Y. Emotional, behavioral, and cognitive reactions to microaggressions: transgender perspectives. *Psychol Sex Orientat Gend Divers.* 2014;1(1):72-81. doi:10.1037/sgd0000011

38. Seelman KL, Woodford MR, Nicolazzo Z. Victimization and microaggressions targeting LGBTQ college students: gender identity as a moderator of psychological distress. *J Ethn Cult Divers Soc Work.* 2017;26(1-2):112-125. doi:10.1080/15313204.2016.1263816

39. Knutson D, Koch JM, Goldbach C. Recommended terminology, pronouns, and documentation for work with transgender and non-binary populations. *Pract Innov*. 2019;4(4):214-224. doi:10.1037/pri0000098

40. Legislative tracker: anti-transgender legislation filed for the 2022 legislative session. Freedom for All Americans. 2022. Accessed September 8, 2022. https://freedomforallamericans.org/legislative-tracker/anti-transgender-legislation/

41. Issues impacting LGBTQ youth. The Trevor Project. 2022. Accessed September 8, 2022. https://www.thetrevorproject.org/wp-content/uploads/2022/01/TrevorProject_Public1.pdf

42. Horne S, McGinley M, Yel N, Maroney M. The stench of bathroom bills and anti-transgender legislation: anxiety and depression among transgender, nonbinary, and cisgender LGBQ people during a state referendum. *J Couns Psychol*. 2022;69(1):1-13. doi:10.1037/cou0000558

43. *The ICD-8: International Statistical Classification of Diseases and Related Health Problems*. World Health Organization; 1965.

44. *Diagnostic and Statistical Manual of Mental Disorders*. 2nd ed. American Psychiatric Association; 1968.

45. James SE, Herman JL, Rankin S, Keisling M, Mottet L, Anafi M. The report of the 2015 US Transgender Survey. National Center for Transgender Equality. 2016. https://transequality.org/sites/default/files/docs/usts/USTS-Full-Report-Dec17.pdf

46. Dubin S, Nolan I, Streed Jr C, Greene R, Radix A, Morrison S. Transgender health care: improving medical students and residents training and awareness. *Adv Med Educ Pract*. 2018;9:377-391. doi:10.2147/amep.s147183

47. Górska P, Bilewicz M, Winiewski M, Waszkiewicz A. On old-fashioned versus modern homonegativity distinction: evidence from Poland. *J Homosex*. 2017;64(2):256-272. doi:10.1080/00918369.2016.1179029

48. Morrison MA, Morrison TG. Development and validation of a scale measuring modern prejudice towards gay men and lesbian women. *J Homosex*. 2003;43(2):15-37. doi:10.1300/j082v43n02_02

49. Dyar C, Feinstein BA. Binegativity: attitudes towards and stereotypes about bisexual individuals. In: Swan DJ, Habibi S, eds. *Bisexuality*. Springer International Publishing; 2018:95-111.

50. Drescher J. Queer diagnoses revisited: the past and future of homosexuality and gender diagnoses in DSM and ICD. *Int Rev Psychiatry*. 2015;27(5):386-395. doi:10.3109/09540261.2015.1053847

51. *ICD-11: International Classification of Diseases (11th revision)*. World Health Organization; 2019.

52. West-Livingston LN, Dittman JM, Park JA, Pascarella L. Sexual orientation, gender identity, and gender expression: from current state to solutions for the support of lesbian, gay, bisexual, transgender, and queer/questioning patients and colleagues. *J Vasc Surg*. 2021;74(2S):64S-75S. doi:10.1016/j.jvs.2021.03.057

53. Drescher J, Schwartz A, Casoy F, et al. The growing regulation of conversion therapy. *J Med Regul*. 2016;102(7):7-12.

54. Salway T, Ferlatte O, Gesink D, Lachowsky NJ. Prevalence of exposure to sexual orientation change efforts and associated sociodemographic characteristics and

psychosocial health outcomes among Canadian sexual minority men. *Can J Psychiatry*. 2020;65(7):502-509. doi:10.1177/0706743720902629

55. Turban JL, Beckwith N, Reisner SL, Keuroghlian AS. Association between recalled exposure to gender identity conversion efforts and psychological distress and suicide attempts among transgender adults. *JAMA Psychiatry*. 2020;77(1):68-76. doi:10.1001/jamapsychiatry.2019.2285
56. Hancock KA, Gock TS, Haldeman DC. Science meets practice in determining effectiveness of sexual orientation change efforts. *Am Psychol*. 2012;67(6):499-500. doi:10.1037/a0029805
57. Anton BS. Proceedings of the American Psychological Association for the legislative year 2009: minutes of the annual meeting of the Council of Representatives and minutes of the meetings of the Board of Directors. *Am Psychol*. 2010;65(5):385-475. doi:10.1037/a0019553
58. Position statement on conversion therapy and LGBTQ patients. American Psychiatric Association. 2018. https://psychiatry.org/getattachment/3d23f2f4-1497-4537-b4de-fe32fe8761bf/Position-Conversion-Therapy.pdf
59. Conversion Therapy. GLAAD. Accessed August 19, 2022. https://www.glaad.org/conversiontherapy
60. Equality maps: conversion therapy laws. Movement Advancement Project. Accessed February 21, 2023. https://www.lgbtmap.org/equality-maps/conversion_therapy
61. Which countries have already banned conversion therapy? Stonewall UK. April 1, 2022. Accessed February 21, 2023. https://www.stonewall.org.uk/about-us/news/which-countries-have-already-banned-conversion-therapy
62. *Lawrence v Texas*, 539 US 558 (2003).
63. *Obergefell v Hodges*, 576 US 644 (2015).
64. Barbeauld PH. "Don't say Gay" bills and the movement to keep discussion of LGBT issues out of schools. *J Law Educ*. 2014;43:137.
65. Diaz J. Florida's governor signs controversial law opponents dubbed 'Don't Say Gay'. National Public Radio. March 23, 2022. Accessed August 19, 2022. https://www.npr.org/2022/03/28/1089221657/dont-say-gay-florida-desantis
66. Rapp KS, Volpe VV, Hale TL, Quartararo DF. State-level sexism and gender disparities in health care access and quality in the United States. *J Health Soc Behav*. 2022;63(1):2-18. doi:10.1177/00221465211058153
67. Kota KK, Salazar LF, Culbreth RE, Crosby RA, Jones J. Psychosocial mediators of perceived stigma and suicidal ideation among transgender women. *BMC Public Health*. 2020;20(1):125. doi:10.1186/s12889-020-8177-z
68. Fiani CN, Han HJ. Navigating identity: experiences of binary and non-binary transgender and gender non-conforming (TGNC) adults. *Int J Transgend*. 2018;20(2-3):181-194. doi:10.1080/15532739.2018.1426074
69. Thepsourinthone J, Dune T, Liamputtong P, Arora A. Out of the closet, not yet out of the house: gay men's experiences of homonegativity and internalized homonegativity. *Healthcare (Basel)*. 2021;9(11):1479. doi:10.3390/healthcare9111479
70. Allen DJ, Oleson T. Shame and internalized homophobia in gay men. *J Homosex*. 1999;37(3):33-43. doi:10.1300/J082v37n03_03

71. Herek GM, Gillis JR, Cogan JC, Glunt EK. Hate crime victimization among lesbian, gay, and bisexual adults: prevalence, psychological correlates, and methodological issues. *J Interpers Violence.* 1997;12(2):195-215. doi:10.1177/088626097012002003

72. Szymanski DM, Henrichs-Beck C. Exploring sexual minority women's experiences of external and internalized heterosexism and sexism and their links to coping and distress. *Sex Roles J Res.* 2014;70(1-2):28-42. doi:10.1007/s11199-013-0329-5

73. Newcomb ME, Mustanski B. Moderators of the relationship between internalized homophobia and risky sexual behavior in men who have sex with men: a meta-analysis. *Arch Sex Behav.* 2011;40(1):189-199. doi:10.1007/s10508-009-9573-8

74. Solomon DT, Morey KE, Williams CJ, Grist CL, Malesky LA. COVID-19 health behaviors in a sexual minority sample: the impact of internalized stigma. *Psychol Sex Orientat Gend Divers.* 2021;8(2):159-171. doi:10.1037/sgd0000466

75. Frost DM, Meyer IH. Internalized homophobia and relationship quality among lesbians, gay men, and bisexuals. *J Counsel Psychol.* 2009;56(1):97-109. doi:10.1037/a0012844

76. Pachankis JE, Hatzenbuehler ML, Rendina HJ, Safren SA, Parsons JT. LGB-affirmative cognitive-behavioral therapy for young adult gay and bisexual men: a randomized controlled trial of a transdiagnostic minority stress approach. *J Consult Clin Psychol.* 2015;83(5):875-889. doi:10.1037/ccp0000037

77. Solomon DT, Reed OM, Sevecke JR, O'Shaughnessy T, Acevedo-Polakovich ID. Expert consensus on facilitating the coming-out process in sexual minority clients: a Delphi study. *J Gay Lesbian Ment Health.* 2018;22(4):348-371. doi:10.1080/19359705.2018.1476279

78. Spengler ES, Miller DJ, Spengler PM. Microaggressions: clinical errors with sexual minority clients. *Psychother.* 2016;53(3):360-366. doi:10.1037/pst0000073

79. Kassel G. What is deadnaming and why is it so harmful? Plus, exactly how to respond with grace if you accidentally deadname someone. Shape. September 21, 2022. Accessed February 21, 2023. https://www.shape.com/lifestyle/mind-and-body/what-is-deadnaming

80. Mizock L, Lundquist C. Missteps in psychotherapy with transgender clients: promoting gender sensitivity in counseling and psychological practice. *Psychol Sex Orientat Gend Divers.* 2016;3(2):148-155. doi:10.1037/sgd0000177

81. Solomon DT, Heck N, Reed OM, Smith DW. Conducting culturally competent intake interviews with LGBTQ youth. *Psychol Sex Orientat Gend Divers.* 2017;4(4):403-411. doi:10.1037/sgd0000255

Chapter 3

Trauma- and Violence-Informed Care: *Considerations for Providers and Those Who Serve the Community*

Kaleigh Mancha, MS, LMFT, Certified Full Spectrum Doula
Christine Foote-Lucero, MSN, RN, CEN, SANE-A, SANE-P, AFN-C, DF-AFN

Key Points

1. *Trauma is one of the most accurate predictors regarding likelihood of onset for almost all medical and mental health conditions.*[1]
2. *Trauma- and violence-informed care (TVIC) prevents revictimization by utilizing accessible and empowering language, collaborative interventions, and accountability in policy creation, thereby emphasizing the mutual benefits of intentional care at all points of contact between individuals, providers, organizations, and communities.*
3. *Healing centered engagement expands upon TVIC's model of care to incorporate social justice and advocacy, culturally specific assets, and individual strengths as key components to uplifting survivors of institutional, systemic, and interpersonal violence in enacting change within oppressive and violent systems.*

Introduction

Violence in the United States is a community health crisis and has been a pervasive epidemic in society since the country's formation. All violence is traumatic and impactful, so much so that trauma is one of the single greatest predictive risk factors for nearly all behavioral, mental health, and substance use disorders.[1] In a study conducted by the World Mental Health Survey Consortium, researchers found that out of 24 countries surveyed, the United States ranked third highest in its citizens' prevalence of exposure to a traumatic event.[2] More than 82% of the United States' population reported experiencing 1 traumatic event in their lifetime and collectively, more than 30.5% of individuals in the study reported experiencing 4 or more traumatic life events.[2] This survey is consistent with other data that has been collected specifically within the United States, including a study conducted by the World Health Organization (WHO), which found 7.2% of the United States' population met the criteria for post-traumatic stress disorder (PTSD)/complex post-traumatic stress disorder (C-PTSD).[3] When youth exposure to violence is studied, the data highlights a growing need for reformation in parenting philosophies and practices within educational, health care, and criminal justice systems. More than 2/3 of children in the United States reported experiencing at least 1 traumatic event by age 16, and every day, 1300 youth in the United States are treated in emergency departments for violence-related injuries.[1]

Background and Significance

When discussing the significance of TVIC as the standard for providers to operate from, it is not only to acknowledge the violence and trauma experienced in one's community or within intimate relationships, but also an acknowledgement of harm experienced over many generations, in every system of care.

Over the course of United States history, there were many terms coined to describe what is now known as PTSD, including "shell shock," "combat stress reaction," "soldier's heart," "nostalgia," and "railway spine." In 1952, the American Psychological Association (APA) included "gross stress reaction" in its first rendition of the *Diagnostic and Statistical Manual of Mental Disorders* (DSM-1), yet by the second edition had completely removed any nod to PTSD-related ailments or conditions resulting from trauma and violence exposure.[3] By the 1980s, after years of research which integrated the voices and lived experiences of those impacted by trauma, such as the first-hand accounts and experiences of veterans, Holocaust survivors, and survivors of sexual violence, the APA declared PTSD a formal diagnosis. This standardization in language laid the groundwork for the recognition of the impact trauma has on individuals and society, as well as offered a distinction between symptoms related to traumatic events and stressful situations. In 1994, the Substance Abuse and Mental Health Services Administration (SAMHSA) held the Dare to Vision Conference.[4] This was the first national conference that intentionally brought trauma to the forefront of mainstream mental health conversations. By amplifying the voices of female-identified trauma survivors who expressed being retraumatized in their experiences with standard care practices in hospitals, medical professionals began to consider and explore how to implement what is now known as trauma-informed care practices. In 1998, the landmark Adverse Childhood Experiences (ACEs) Study, which is still the largest and most comprehensive study of its kind, was concluded after multiple years of data collection. These combined events led to a booming interest in the study of trauma and care practices, all of which ultimately shaped the Four R's and the Six Guiding Principles of Trauma- and Violence-Informed Care, written by SAMHSA in collaboration with the Centers for Disease Control and Prevention (CDC). In the 2010s, Canadian researchers and providers introduced the concept of TVIC to expand on how health care providers address, treat, and honor survivors of violence.

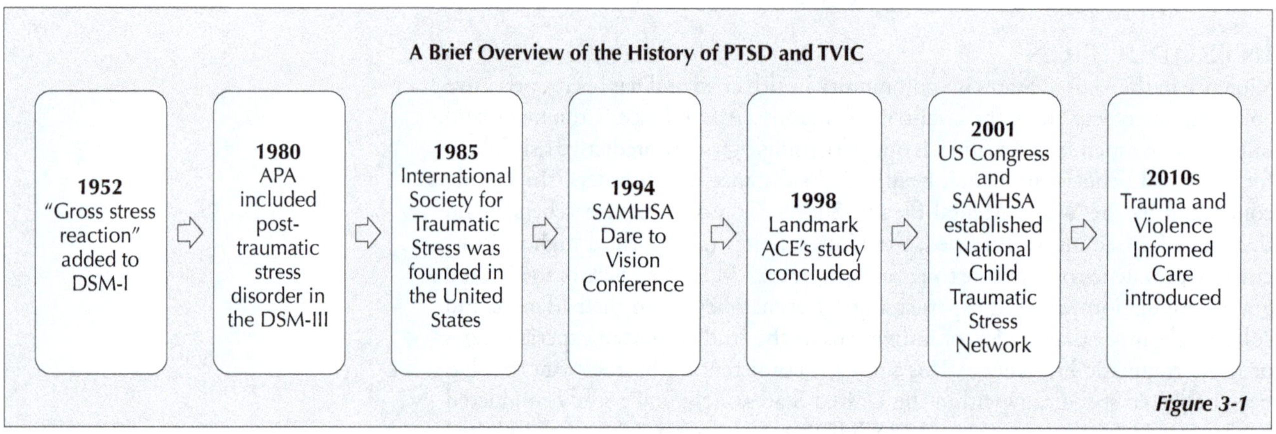

Figure 3-1. *A brief overview of the history of PTSD and TVIC.*

What is Trauma?

> "Trauma in a person, decontextualized over time, looks like personality. Trauma in a family, decontextualized over time, looks like family traits. Trauma in a people, decontextualized over time, looks like culture."
>
> — Resmma Menakem, author of *My Grandmother's Hands: Racialized Trauma and the Pathway to Mending our Hearts and Bodies*

For the sake of a shared definition, this chapter will define trauma as an event, series of events, chronic conditions, or circumstances that an individual or group of individuals experience, in which there is a real or perceived threat of physical or emotional harm to oneself or others. Events can be human-directed (eg, a mechanical error that causes a disaster, war, terrorism), physical in nature (eg, sexual abuse or violence), or of the natural world (eg, unpredictable natural hazards, flooding, hurricanes, and tornadoes).[4] The event(s) overwhelms the individual/group's ability to utilize resources to cope, resulting in a fight, flight, freeze, or fawn response. For some, this response is temporary, whereas others may have prolonged reactions that vary in acuity, severity, and expression (eg, manifestations in mental health may include post-traumatic stress and other anxiety disorders, substance use, or mood disorders, whereas manifestations in medical health may include arthritis, headaches, or chronic pain).[4] Individuals, families, groups, and communities, regardless of socioeconomic factors, age, or developmental stage, are vulnerable to the impact of trauma. It is important, though, to recognize that all individuals have cultivated varying degrees of resilience to fortify themselves in order to move forward. This recognition of resilience is necessary and powerful.

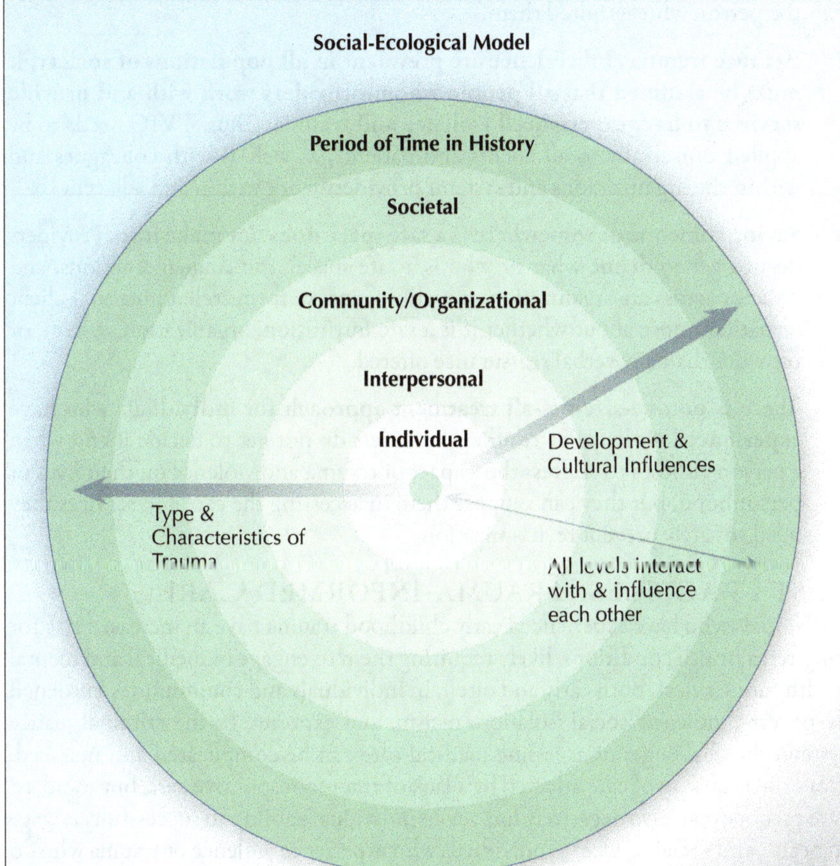

Figure 3-2

Figure 3-2. *SAMHSA: a social-ecological model for understanding trauma and its effects.*[4]

Violence and trauma are not isolated to the inter- and intrapersonal; notably, these personal violations are influenced and normalized by the frequency and duration of violence occurring in institutions and organizations. Medical and mental health services, as well as the Unites States' legal system, have historically been complicit in upholding and maintaining systems of oppression and violence through power imbalances that have traumatized, victimized, and perpetuated violence against vulnerable individuals. Science and laws have weaponized medicine and limited access to basic needs and services, all guided by and rooted in the beliefs and fears stemming from "-isms," "-phobias," and implicit biases. The eugenics movement, legal until 1979, is an example of medically endorsed, state-sanctioned violence in which over 60 000 people in the United States were forcibly sterilized in 32 states throughout the 20th century.[5] Eugenics is a grossly underreported practice and still occurs today in immigration detention centers across the southwestern United States. A historical example of systemic violence that has reverberating effects in the present can be seen in the Code of Indian Offences of 1883 that prevented access to and engagement in Native American rituals and traditions until 1978 when Congress passed the American Indian Religious Freedom Act (AIRFA).[6] A society is only as violent as the oppressive laws, health care, and educational systems that are perpetuated against its people.

This chapter makes the following assertions about TVIC:

1. **Providers do <u>not</u> need to know someone's trauma history or exposure to violence to provide TVIC.** The process of disclosing one's experience with sexual violence, for example, is a personal and often complicated process. Around 25% of female-identified sexual assault survivors do not disclose their experience, particularly those that are involved in an intimate relationship with the person who assaulted them.[7]
2. **Because trauma and violence are prevalent in all populations of society, it must be assumed that all people whom providers work with and provide services to have experienced violence and trauma.** Thus, TVIC needs to be applied universally to all clients and patients, as well as with colleagues and within the organizations and systems providers work within and adjacent to.
3. **Saying someone or somewhere is a safe space does not make it so.** Providers do not get to define what or who is a safe space. The language, actions, and policies across an organization or a clinic's intake forms tell a potential client or patient more about whether it is a safe institution, organization, system, or provider than any verbal reassurance offered.
4. **There is no one-size-fits-all treatment approach for individuals who have experienced violence or trauma.** Providers do not get to decide if and when a person chooses to address the impact of trauma and violence on their lives or personhood, but they can support them in accessing the care and services they need to safely prevent revictimization.

Best Practices: Trauma-Informed Care

Individuals who have experienced early childhood trauma have an increased risk for long-term health conditions, likely requiring them to engage in medical and mental health care services, both early and often. In individuals and communities burdened by poverty, violence, social isolation, racism, and exposure to the criminal justice system, the challenges of accessing medical care can be complicated and nuanced. Not only is quality of care affected by a lack of trauma-responsive care, but standard care practices can also negatively impact an individual's ability to successfully engage in health and social services.[8] Individuals who experience violence or trauma who do not receive trauma-informed care (TIC) tend to pursue anonymized, transactional care from emergency departments and urgent care centers, rather than establish relationships with primary care providers.[8] This disengagement from resources prevents individuals from cultivating trusting relationships with care providers, limits their ability to receive and engage in community resources, and hinders their participation in follow-up care.

While a lack of TIC directly impacts the quality of care and overall health for individuals interacting with medical and mental health systems, the maladaptive behaviors developed by persons who have experienced trauma because of trauma-related neurodevelopmental changes, systemic discrimination, disenfranchisement, and ongoing life stressors result in providers experiencing increased rates of burnout and vicarious trauma.[8] TIC is a cyclical and interactive relationship between provider and clients/patients that enhances the therapeutic relationship and overall wellbeing of all involved.

TIC is not an intervention; it is a philosophy that guides how providers interact with others through empathy and understanding.

The Four R's: Key Assumptions in a Trauma-Informed Approach

The Four R's is a framework that SAMHSA[9] regards as essential to caring for communities, clients, and practitioners alike. How health care providers understand, address, and implement treatment is highly influential in the outcomes of those who are impacted by trauma. **Table 3-1** details the Four R's framework.

Table 3-1. The Four R's Philosophy and Implementation

	Philosophy	Systemic Interventions
Realize	Coping strategies learned as a direct result of trauma, designed to aid individuals in surviving adversity, are contextualized to understand a person's lived experiences and behaviors. Whether a person has had experiences with trauma/violence in the past (eg, client processing childhood abuse), present (eg, a staff member is living with a person who commits violence towards the staff member), or has developed coping skills as a result of vicarious or secondary trauma (eg, clinician having a secondary stress response from hearing a traumatic story of another), it is realized that trauma has the ability to affect outcomes for individuals and ripples outward within systems.	Trauma impacts all arenas of care: — Mental health — Medical/primary health care — Child welfare — Criminal justice — Peer-run/community organizations
Recog-nize	Providers must be able to recognize the signs and symptoms of trauma. These symptoms can manifest in those providing or receiving services. There is a recognition of factors and variables that increase the risk of trauma and violence exposure.	— Trauma screening and assessment is a part of all services — Workforce development — Employee assistance programs — Supervision practices
Respond	The system and its providers respond by implementing a TIC approach with the knowledge that traumatic events impact all people involved, including those who have experienced, witnessed, or hold/held space for the processing of said experiences.	Organization-wide policies: — The impact of language, behaviors, and policies are regularly examined to consider the experiences of trauma on clients/patients/staff — Promote an organizational culture based on beliefs about resilience, recovery, and healing from trauma — Provide a physically, culturally, and psychologically safe environment

(continued)

Table 3-1. The Four R's Philosophy and Implementation *(continued)*

	Philosophy	Systemic Interventions
(Resist) Retraumatization	This consideration is extended to clients, patients, and staff. Special care is taken to identify organizational practices that trigger and retraumatize individuals engaging in services and then replaces those practices with more responsive and client-centered care practices. This is an ongoing process of re-evaluation that requires regular feedback from community members, staff, and invested parties.	— Analyze and review existing policies continually — Invite feedback from individuals receiving and providing services about ways to increase safety and positive interactions — Be accountable and transparent when harm was caused in order to repair and restore trust and safety

Better Practices: Trauma- and Violence-Informed Care

The expanded model of TIC is TVIC. TVIC is an evidence-based, theoretical framework designed to improve how service providers and organizations serve clients and patients who have experienced traumatic life events. TVIC does not focus on encouraging clients to disclose details of their trauma or on treating their trauma symptoms. Instead, TVIC fosters an environment wherein all clients feel safe, and there is less possibility that they will be traumatized again. TVIC recognizes the connections between violence, trauma, negative health outcomes, and behaviors. It accounts for the intersecting impacts of broader structural and social conditions, such as inequities based on gender, ethnicity, or income that are embedded in the political and economic organization of the world, as well as ongoing violence and institutional violence.[10] TVIC takes into account the systemic sources of violence and inequalities and how those can affect health outcomes. Inherently, TVIC has an awareness of the impact that trauma can have across settings, services, and populations while anticipating and avoiding institutional processes and individual practices that are likely to retraumatize patients who already have histories of trauma. While a provider implementing TIC only considers traumatic experiences before recommending treatment, a provider implementing TVIC may consider and ask about a patient's structural barriers to accessing services, such as experiences with health care discrimination, lack of money for transportation, or inability to find childcare, before recommending treatment. A narrow definition of trauma may be inadequate to best understand and address the needs of diverse clients/patients whose vulnerabilities to and experiences with violence and trauma are different.[11] However, the TVIC approach considers all aspects of a patient's life, and emerging research suggests that using a TVIC approach may be better for both those seeking and providing care.[10]

Six Guiding Principles to Trauma- and Violence-Informed Care

The goal of TVIC is not to treat trauma, but to minimize harm.[12] The following core TVIC principles were developed to guide multidisciplinary professionals through the process of applying core values to care that promote resilience, healing, and recovery for those impacted by trauma.[9]

1. Safety

From the macro to micro level of care and for every individual engaged in and impacted by the system, safety must be the foundation of all care. Safety in a physical space is considered one that is free of threats or harm; has messaging and services that are designed to prevent or reduce psychological harm; has interpersonal interactions that facilitate a sense of trust and respect; and provides cultural safety that recognizes the historical oppression and harm that communities and groups have experienced so as not to continue to perpetuate unsafe environments of care. A high priority is placed on understanding safety as it is defined by those who are being served. Providers and staff are also considered within a TVIC approach when they actively work to prevent compassion fatigue, burnout, and secondary trauma. Examples of establishing safety are staff education, ensuring the physical space is American Disabilities Act (ADA) accessible for individuals of varying abilities, requiring informed consent in every interaction, creating crisis plans guided by the patient/client, and staying consistent in how, when, and where services are provided.[13]

2. Trustworthiness and Transparency

To operate in a transparent and trustworthy way, organizations must have practices in place that measure the effectiveness of services provided, take accountability for decisions made, and be able to outline the progress they are making towards goals established through collaborative processes. Creating an environment that builds and maintains trust with clients, patients, community members, staff, and providers is at the core of this principle. Examples of trustworthiness and transparency are an organization publishing reader-friendly and accessible information to the public, outlining their pathways for community feedback, and planning strategies to ensure their policies and services are meeting the needs of those they serve.

3. Peer Support

Peers are individuals who have lived experiences with trauma or who are supporting individuals who have experienced traumatic events and are guiding those individuals through recovery and healing (eg, a parent supporting a child who lived through trauma). Hope and trust are established through shared lived experiences and histories that promote a space of collaboration and safety. Trauma survivors offer a unique perspective of the journey through and towards healing. An example of peer support would be the National Alliance for Mental Illness's (NAMI) Warmline Hotline, which offers callers emotional support and is peer-led and staffed by volunteers who are in recovery.

4. Collaboration and Mutuality

All individuals in an organization—from the CEO, to the clinician, to the medical biller, to the housekeeping staff—can offer restorative TVIC to each other and clients/patients. With an acknowledgment of power imbalances inherent in a hierarchical and historically oppressive system, great care is placed on shared power and decision making. Healing occurs in collaborative relationships wherein both parties share a common goal. Effective models of communication lean on shared decision making to facilitate relationships between providers and clients/patients to engage in joint decisions about necessary interventions or next steps of care.[14] An example of collaboration and mutuality is when a receptionist who is trained in TVIC practices patient and compassionate support to a person in distress who is inquiring about how to schedule an appointment, understanding that every point of contact can be therapeutic.

5. Empowerment, Voice, and Choice

Every person has unique strengths and experiences. Trauma-informed organizations strive to recognize and build upon these factors, both for individuals seeking services and providers, in order to foster an environment that promotes self-determination, dignity, autonomy, and resiliency. Providers, clients/patients, and communities may have intersecting, shared experiences with trauma and the organization considers this in every aspect of care to ensure providers and clients/patients feel empowered and supported. There is a recognition of the historical impact on individuals and communities who have been unable to assert their autonomy, excluded from decision making regarding their care, and subjected to coercive treatments. Self-advocacy is encouraged, and the client/patient is seen as the expert on themselves. An example of empowerment, voice, and choice would be the formation of an advisory council or public forum that invites individuals to provide feedback regarding service design, users' rights, and grievances.[13]

6. Cultural, Historical, and Gender Issues

Organizations and providers must consider not only the unique histories and experiences of individuals, but also structural violence that has permeated health care spaces and its impact historically on decreasing access to quality of care. There is a specific emphasis on identifying and addressing biases and stereotypes that reduce care outcomes and prevent culturally- or gender-responsive care from occurring. By integrating the traditional cultural practices of a community, the policies, protocols, and processes to meet the cultural, ethnic, and racial needs of staff and clients/patients are shaped. An example of cultural, historical, and gender-affirming care would be ensuring space on all intake forms and during each introduction to include an acknowledgement of pronouns and to model and normalize diversity in gender identity and expression.

Preventing Retraumatization

How can providers and community members intervene to reduce rates of violence and trauma or prevent retraumatization within their communities? They must first prepare to implement TVIC at the personal level through self-awareness and self-compassion, then at the clinical level via direct care services, and lastly, at the organizational level.

Notably, as health care and human services professionals across disciplines, providers are often tasked with bearing witness to humanity's greatest challenges and atrocities while also holding space for the immense capacity that humankind has for growth and resilience. This is a sacred task.

Cultural awareness is imperative in understanding how trauma responses may be expressed and shared within communities and groups. How are providers connecting to the communities they are serving? Being open to learning about and having interactions with groups other than the ones that the provider belongs to, cross-collaborations with diverse communities and community members, and welcoming feedback are actionable tasks of culturally-responsive care.

Trauma-informed organizations have cultures that exemplify "democratic, nonviolent (safe), and emotionally intelligent" practices to facilitate the expectation that staff and those receiving services will thrive.[13]

A TVIC approach at the organizational level proactively addresses the needs of providers by creating a culture of reflection and safe debriefing regarding client/patient interactions. It is the engagement in resiliency-building practices, alongside system-wide self-care policies, that help to protect against compassion fatigue and burnout. Compassion fatigue or burnout in a provider could result from an imbalanced or excessive case load with little to no organizational support, providing care in a (perceived or actual) dangerous environment, chronic exposure to trauma (firsthand or secondary), or providing care in specialties related to death, suicide, and trauma exposure. This erosion of compassion or capacity for providing responsive care could result in an inability to feel or offer empathy and compassion to others, resulting in poor patient-provider relations and increased negative health outcomes for both parties. Burnout is centered around the stressors and demands present in the workplace, while compassion fatigue revolves around the impact of helping others. Burnout can be harder to recover from and may necessitate a career pause, while recovery from compassion fatigue can be experienced more immediately if managed early. **Table 3-2** provides symptoms of burnout and compassion fatigue.

Table 3-2. Compassion Fatigue vs Burnout Symptoms

Compassion Fatigue	Burnout
— Sudden, acute onset	— Gradual, over time
— Life dissatisfaction	— Work dissatisfaction
— Feels out of control	— Feels overwhelmed and under pressure
— Lacks motivation	— Withdrawal
— Physical symptoms (headaches, insomnia, etc)	— Exhaustion (emotional/mental)
— Mood swings, hopelessness	— Diminished morale
— Imbalance of objectivity and empathy	— Depression, anger
	— Decreased empathy or apathy

Resilience-building practices within an organization involve offering resources that address staff wellbeing, having flexible and responsive workplace policies (eg, paid parental leave, no mandatory debriefings, etc), clear communication of expectations and needs, opportunities for professional development and learning, and a commitment to healthy workplace culture.[13] Dr. Sandra Bloom's "Sanctuary Model" identifies 7 commitments that trauma-informed organizations can subscribe to in order to enhance engagement and positive outcomes. This model has been shown to foster an environment of cultural humility with providers and staff to improve service delivery with individuals who are (or who have historically been) part of a marginalized community.[15] The following commitments are based upon the philosophy of TVIC practices:

1. Nonviolence: helping to build safety skills and a commitment to a higher purpose
2. Emotional intelligence: helping to teach emotional management skills
3. Social learning: helping to build cognitive skills
4. Open communication: helping to overcome barriers to healthy communication, learning conflict management, reducing acting out, enhancing self-protective and self-correcting skills, and teaching healthy boundaries
5. Social responsibility: helping to build social connection skills, establish healthy attachment relationships, and establish a sense of fair play and justice
6. Democracy: helping to create civic skills of self-control, self-discipline, and administration of a healthy authority
7. Growth and change: helping to work through loss and prepare for the future

Trauma-Informed Language

Trauma-informed language is the intentional use of language to shape thoughts, statements, and questions in ways that empower individuals offering, seeking out, and receiving support. This shift in language considers the pervasive nature of trauma and serves to see all points of contact and connections as an opportunity to be a restorative experience. By using trauma-informed language, there is an increase in providers' abilities to identify and respond empathetically to traumatized individuals and communities. Providers can nurture relationships within the community by creating space for accountability and acknowledgement when harm has been caused.[16] The use of trauma-informed language also promotes increased engagement in community-based initiatives, programs, and services. There is a greater opportunity to address the consequences and challenges individuals have faced in navigating health care services when TVIC providers are guided by this awareness. Mayra Gomez, with The Trauma-Informed Legal Advocacy (TILA) Project, in association with the National Center of Domestic Violence, Trauma and Mental Health (NCDVTMH) stated that in order for "...advocates to take a trauma-informed approach to their work with trauma survivors, they must have a basic understanding of how trauma can affect the ways that survivors think, feel, and interact with other people and the world."[17]

Person-First Language

"Person-first language" means using descriptors of someone's experience rather than emphasizing their experience as a noun. Instead of "disabled," say "person with a disability" or instead of "drug addict," say "person who is struggling with addiction." In reference to violence and trauma work, the newest trends in language suggest replacing "offender" and "perpetrator" with "person/people who commit violence" in recognition that someone's behavior is not their identity and those who perpetuate or commit violence have also been victimized by violence. The TVIC model replaces labels about individuals being sick or uncooperative with language about how the individual has been affected by an injury. Normalizing trauma as an injury moves the conversation from "what is wrong with you?" to "what happened to you?"[13]

A provider asking someone who has experienced violence how they identify with their experience(s) can be a chance for processing and integration. Likewise, it offers an opportunity for individuals to reclaim their voice and reflect upon their narratives with intention. How individuals conceptualize their journey through trauma and violence and who they are in relation to those experiences will evolve over time. Consider the distinctions between the terms "victimization," "victimized," and "victim." A person's experiences and personhood can be validated with the acknowledgement that a victimization happened or they were victimized by a person who commits violence, regardless of whether they identify as a victim or a survivor. It is considered best practice to ask each person which language they prefer or research the agreed-upon (if there is a unanimous term) identifying language for specific communities. Identity-first language can be powerful for some who feel their condition or proximity to a condition is core to their identity.

Further, using language rooted in deficits is disempowering to individuals and cultivates an environment of shame and guilt; it centers individuals' identities as their challenges and decreases feelings of safety and validation. Trauma-informed language, on the other hand, emphasizes a person-first approach which pulls upon a strengths-based perspective to create an environment of understanding, care, and curiosity.

The following table provides phrases and words that are used to describe a person who has experienced trauma from a deficit perspective, then poses the preferred strengths-based perspective (**Table 3-3**).

Table 3-3. Deficit Perspective vs Strengths-based Perspective

Deficit Perspective (Disempowering)	Strengths-based Perspective (Empowering)
What is wrong with you? What is your problem? Why are you acting like that?	What happened to you? What is happening right now? How can I support you?
Symptoms Problems Issues Disorders	Responses Adaptations Adjusting to Attempt to acclimate to new norms
Attention-seeking Dramatic	This person is communicating the best way they know how. What am I not hearing, seeing, or understanding that this person wants me to know?
Borderline personality disorder Narcissistic	This person is doing the best they can to navigate relationships given their early experiences. How can I practice curiosity with this person about what they are experiencing?
Oppositional Defiant Malingering Treatment resistant Non-compliant	This person is communicating that something in this interaction of help or support is not safe to engage in. How can I support this person in feeling safe? What barriers exist for this person that prevents them from engaging in this experience?
Manipulative	This person is having difficulty expressing and asking directly for what they need. Which need is this behavior trying to meet right now?
Controlling Rigid Difficult Demanding	This person appears to be trying to assert their power. This person has learned to self-advocate. How can I create space for opportunities that respect this person's autonomy and wisdom?

Future Considerations: Healing Centered Engagement

The healing centered engagement (HCE) model operates from a broad framework that is led by communities rather than providers and combines social work, social justice movement strategies, restorative justice practices, the fields of community and positive psychology, youth and contemporary culture, and the celebration of spiritual, cultural, and ritual resources within communities of color.[18] Pulling from positive psychology philosophies, HCE focuses on an individual's desire and quest towards wellbeing, while also taking TVIC's reflection on "what happened to you?" a step further by asking "what is right with you?" This approach puts culture, spirituality, civic action, and collective healing at the forefront of healing and continued wellness.[18] There is no question this form of care is political in nature as it demands participation in changing the root causes of harm within systems and cultivating interdependence through collective liberation and engagement. HCE is a salutogenic approach, asserting that individuals are more than the worst things that have happened to them. Rather, there is an emphasis on experiences, knowledge, and skills as things to be enhanced in order to foster wellbeing, strong identity formation, and a sense of belonging.[18] The Urban Peace Movement's Conceptual Map to Healing Centered Youth Organizing: Building a Case for Healing Justice[19] states, "healing is understood as a regenerative process that is inclusive of the mind, body, and spirit and that aims to restore and renew the individual and collective emotional and spiritual wellbeing of youth, families, and the broader community." According to research, cultivating a sense of power and control in individuals who have experienced trauma is one of the most impactful components of restoring holistic wellbeing. By offering traumatized individuals the ability to participate in anti-violence movements or social activism, they can reclaim their power and utilize their voices. When people are involved in holistic healing and collective activism simultaneously, they: experience an increased understanding of themselves and their experiences with violence/trauma; cultivate new coping strategies; improve self-confidence and strengthen relationships; amplify their ability to speak out against rape culture; create a community of support, validation, and connection; and provide a sense of fulfillment and meaning to their journeys.[20]

Case Studies

Case Study 3-1

This patient was a 19-year-old Latinx, trans male who presented to the emergency department (ED) with abdominal pain and had inquired about receiving a testosterone prescription refill. The intake nurse noticed the patient arrived with someone who the patient appeared to be tense around. He had communicated that he felt anxious about receiving care and had felt dismissed by his primary care physician (PCP), so he had not returned to see him. The patient had been admitted to the ED 4 times in the last 6 months. He was evasive in his responses to questions surrounding his living situation but did indicate a history of sexual abuse, unemployment, and no permanent address on the intake forms.

Discussion

Table 3-4. Case Study 3-1 Discussion

Standard Care Approach	TVIC Approach
"You are back again?" Begins intake and asks questions in front of the person accompanying the patient "I cannot help you if you are not honest." "You will need to go to your PCP for that prescription; we do not do that here. For your stomach pain, it seems to have gone away with fluids, so I think you are good to go."	"My name is Cristine. My pronouns are she/her, and I'll be asking some questions for your intake. To protect your privacy, let us go to a separate room; the person you came with can wait there. You can choose how and if you would like to answer any question I ask or if you would like the person you came with to join us." "I know that people who have had hard life experiences often have difficulty trusting people and often deal with chronic pain. Can you tell me more about what you are experiencing right now?" "I would like to help you get your medication needs met consistently. Would you be open to sharing the experiences you have had with your PCP with me so I can refer you to a provider who is more responsive?"

(continued)

Table 3-4. Discussion *(continued)*

STANDARD CARE APPROACH	TVIC APPROACH
Does not assess current needs or barriers to accessing follow-up care	"It looks like you have had some challenges with accessing your medications and securing a safe place to stay. Can I connect you with the hospital social worker? Their role is to provide patients with resources they need."

Case Study 3-2

This client was a 28-year-old Black, heterosexual, and cisgender female who presented at a family services agency that provides group and individual counseling for individuals who are court mandated for therapeutic services. The client had her 2 children, ages 2 and 5 years, removed from her custody after multiple house calls were made to police with reports of intimate partner violence between herself and her partner. Criminal charges were filed against the client. Child protective services had been involved for the past month. The client was meeting with a licensed clinical social worker, per the requirement of the courts and her case manager, for an initial intake to begin mandated therapy, but she arrived 20 minutes late due to transportation issues.

Discussion

Table 3-5. Case Study 3-2 Discussion

STANDARD CARE APPROACH	TVIC APPROACH
Greets client in lobby where other clients are waiting, and says, "please complete these forms in their entirety. If you have any forms for me to sign, please leave them with the receptionist." "This could be a long process for you to get your kids back. I must report when you are non-compliant to your case manager, so make sure you arrive early for all your appointments and attend the required parenting classes." "Why did you not leave the relationship after the first incident?" "You do not seem to want to talk much. Your participation is needed for this to work."	"Welcome. Today is our chance to get to know each other and better understand what to expect of this process. Would you prefer to complete the intake forms in the lobby or for us to go over them together in my office?" "This must be a very difficult and stressful time for you. I am sorry that we are meeting under these circumstances. I will do my best to make this process smooth and accessible. Did you have any challenges getting here today?" "That sounds like a horrible experience. You have survived a lot. What has helped you get through this experience?" "If bringing a family member, friend, or someone you trust would help you feel more comfortable at our next meeting, you are more than welcome to do so."

Case Study 3-3

This client was a 49-year-old Caucasian, homosexual, cisgender male returning to a local nonprofit community center for a follow-up visit to obtain his STI testing results. The client had been diagnosed previously with chronic depression that often presented with symptoms of suicidal ideations and self-harm behaviors, such as cutting and unprotected sexual encounters. The client arrived at his appointment in which the nurse at the center would be informing him he is HIV-positive.

Discussion

Table 3-6. Case Study 3-3 Discussion

Standard Care Approach	TVIC Approach
"We're going to go over your test results today. Go ahead and sit over there so we can get started. You're my last appointment of the day."	"I understand you are here to go over some test results. I want to make sure we have some privacy and uninterrupted time for your appointment. Let's sit in this room here."
"You're HIV-positive. I'm going to give you some brochures that you can look over and you can let me know if you have any questions."	"Unfortunately, your labs came back positive. I understand this may be overwhelming news to receive. I'll do my best to answer any questions you may have regarding next steps and your treatment options, but I imagine you may need a moment to process this."
"You will get a call from the health district about your positive status sometime this week."	"As discussed in our initial appointment, all positive test results are reported to the health district by the lab that runs the blood work. Let's revisit what information is shared and how it's used so that you understand your rights and limitations to privacy."
Does not ask questions about mental health	"I want to help you stay safe. Does this information trigger any feelings of self-harm or suicidal ideation?"
"Here's a brochure with numbers to therapists in town that work with HIV-positive clients."	"It's okay if you feel angry, shocked, ashamed, or scared. Anything you feel right now is normal. I want to make sure you have support when you leave here. I'm not a therapist, but I'd like to help you connect with someone who is. In the meantime, is there anyone you'd like to call who can pick you up or stay with you this evening?"

Summary

Reflecting on this chapter and moving forward through subsequent chapters, observe any internal beliefs and perceptions that change or shift. How can one utilize TVIC/HCE care in practice or when serving diverse communities? Consider medical or mental health care services that utilize TVIC practices. What can provider(s) say or do to help patients feel safe and heard? How do providers acknowledge lived experiences and wisdom or integrate patient voices into treatment and care? Consider how exchanges or interventions influence patient outcomes when the provider or health care center utilizes TVIC practices.

References

1. Walsh L. Understanding child trauma. Substance Abuse and Mental Health Services Administration. 2015. https://www.samhsa.gov/child-trauma/understanding-child-trauma

2. Benjet C, Bromet E, Karam EG, et al. The epidemiology of traumatic event exposure worldwide: results from the World Mental Health Survey Consortium. *Psychol Med.* 2016;46(2):327-343. doi:10.1017/S0033291715001981

3. Friedman MJ. PTSD history and overview. PTSD: National Center for PTSD, US Department of Veterans Affairs. 2007. https://www.ptsd.va.gov/professional/treat/essentials/history_ptsd.asp

4. Center for Substance Abuse Treatment (US). Trauma-informed care: a sociocultural perspective. In: Substance Abuse and Mental Health Services Administration, ed. *Trauma-Informed Care in Behavioral Health Settings.* Substance Abuse and Mental Health Services Administration; 2014. https://www.ncbi.nlm.nih.gov/books/NBK207195/

5. Stern A. Forced sterilization policies in the US targeted minorities and those with disabilities – and lasted into the 21st century. University of Michigan Institute for Healthcare Policy & Innovation. 2020. https://ihpi.umich.edu/news/forced-sterilization-policies-us-targeted-minorities-and-those-disabilities-and-lasted-21st

6. *Richard E. Lying, Secretary of Agriculture, et al, Petitioners v Northwest Indian Cemetery Protective Association, et al,* 485 US 439, 86-1013 (1988). https://www.law.cornell.edu/supremecourt/text/485/439

7. Carson KW, Babad S, Kosuri M, et al. Sexual victimization disclosure: a cluster analysis approach to understanding victimization experiences in disclosers and non-disclosers. *Int J Environ Res Public Health.* 2021;18(22):11919. doi:10.3390/ijerph182211919

8. Chaudhri S, Zweig KC, Hebbar P, Angell S, Vasan A. Trauma-informed care: a strategy to improve primary healthcare engagement for persons with criminal justice system involvement. *J Gen Intern Med.* 2019;34(6):1048-1052. doi:10.1007/s11606-018-4783-1

9. Substance Abuse and Mental Health Services Administration. *SAMHSA's Concept of Trauma and Guidance for a Trauma-Informed Approach.* Substance Abuse and Mental Health Services Administration; 2014.

10. Wathen CN, MacGregor JCD, Beyrem S. Impacts of trauma-and violence-informed care education: a mixed method follow-up evaluation with health & social service professionals. *Public Health Nurs.* 2021;38(4):645-654. doi:10.1111/phn.12883

11. Befus DR, Kumodzi T, Schminkey D, St Ivany A. Advancing health equity and social justice in forensic nursing research, education, practice and policy: introducing structural violence and trauma- and violence-informed care. *J Forensic Nurs.* 2019;15(4):199-205. doi:10.1097/JFN.0000000000000264

12. Trauma and violence-informed approaches to policy and practice. Public Health Agency of Canada. 2018. https://www.canada.ca/en/public-health/services/publications/health-risks-safety/trauma-violence-informed-approaches-policy-practice.html

13. Poole N, Urquhart C, Jasiura F, Smilie D. Trauma-informed practice guide. 2013. https://www.researchgate.net/publication/280626594_Trauma_Informed_Practice_Guide

14. Weiss P, Redlich-Amirav D, Daass-Iraqi S, Hadas-Lidor N. Aspects of shared decision making in a cognitive-educational intervention for family members of persons coping with severe mental illness. *Front Psychiatry.* 2021;12:681118. doi:10.3389/fpsyt.2021.681118

15. Esaki N, Reddy M, Bishop CT. Next steps: applying a trauma-informed model to create an anti-racist organizational culture. *Behav Sci.* 2022;12(2):41. doi:10.3390/bs12020041

16. Parker S, Johnson-Lawrence V. Addressing trauma-informed principles in public health through training and practice. *Int J Environ Res Public Health.* 2022;19(14):8437. doi:10.3390/ijerph19148437

17. Radcliffe S, Pollack D. In plain language, what is "trauma-informed care"? Daily Business Review. April 18, 2022. https://repository.yu.edu/server/api/core/bitstreams/a1f047ad-c41b-4a27-85e0-2b18064fa9d6/content

18. Ginwright S. The future of healing: shifting from trauma informed care to healing centered engagement. Medium. 2020. https://ginwright.medium.

com/the-future-of-healing-shifting-from-trauma-informed-care-to-healing-centered-engagement-634f557ce69c

19. Chavez-Diaz M, Lee N. A conceptual mapping of healing centered youth organizing: building a case for healing justice. For Urban Peace Movement. 2015. https://urbanpeacemovement.org/wp-content/uploads/2014/02/Healing Mapping_FINALVERSION.pdf

20. Strauss Swanson C, Szymanski DM. From pain to power: an exploration of activism, the #Metoo movement, and healing from sexual assault trauma. *J Couns Psychol.* 2020;67(6):653-668. doi:10.1037/cou0000429

Chapter 4

Transgender and Gender Non-Conforming Health Care

Kimberly Fuller, PhD, LISW-S, CST

Key Points

1. *The history of health care for transgender and gender non-conforming (TGNC) people has been, and continues to be, contemptuous for transgender youth and those living in more conservative areas of the United States.*
2. *The World Professional Association for Transgender Health (WPATH) standards were developed to give guidance, but often create a gatekeeping issue for access to care.*
3. *Transgender health care is a right, and current legislation to prevent gender-affirming treatment is harmful and leads to poorer physical and mental health outcomes.*

Background and Significance

Health care has been an inaccessible system for TGNC people across the United States. Many TGNC people are concerned about having quality and safe health care options from even primary care providers and often experience discrimination and harassment from those that are uninformed and transphobic. There are no systems in place to ensure that a provider is TGNC-friendly or competent, and while many people market themselves as such, the quality of the services is quite variable. Many TGNC people feel uncomfortable receiving care and may even hide their gender identity from their health care provider to prevent discrimination or maltreatment.

Access to gender-affirming treatment has been a challenge.[1] Historically, TGNC people were seen as mentally ill and in need of mental health care to treat the "disease" of transsexualism.[1] Only a few providers over the course of the early 1900s felt that affirming trans* people was the right treatment protocol. Research and time have shifted the cultural perspective to greater affirmation of TGNC people.[1] WPATH was developed in 1979 as the first organizing body to support gender dysphoria, or the feeling of one's gender identity feeling incongruent with their sex assigned at birth. Over the course of several decades, WPATH began creating standards of care (SOC) for gender-affirming treatment of TGNC people.[1] While these standards have given a good framework, they can often lead to gatekeeping services to only those who can afford to receive care and have the knowledge of how to navigate the medical system.

TGNC youth experience additional barriers to gender-affirming health care. Between 2021 and 2022, 19 states introduced health care bills banning TGNC youth from accessing any gender affirmation care.[2] These bills inaccurately portray gender-affirming care and make broad generalizations about the extent to which youth can transform their bodies and at what age. For example, many opponents of gender-affirming care discuss the perceived problematic impact of starting hormone replacement therapy (HRT) at a young age. However, doctors closely follow the youth's prepubescent period to monitor when starting hormones would align with their natural development. These same legislators often discuss the implications of detransitioning and the problematic impact of managing the residual side effects of taking HRT, which may not be reversable. Research shows that approximately 97.5% of youth who identify as trans* continue to identify this way 5 years later.[3] Several bills have also been presented attempting to limit providers' treatment options by allowing the state to take legal recourse if the provider is found to be aiding a TGNC youth in transitioning. Many legislators believe that trans* youth are undergoing invasive surgeries at a young age without knowing the implications of their decisions. However, most transgender youth do not complete surgeries until after the age of 18. By attempting to pass such legislation, politicians are attempting to enact laws that will limit or block TGNC youth from being able to access life-affirming care. This constitutes a human rights issue, as no one should be barred from health care.

History of TGNC Health Care

Health care for TGNC people began in 1918, with Magnus Hirschfield at his Institute for Sexual Science (ISS) in Berlin, Germany.[4] Hirschfield was a leader in the field, and he first coined the term *transvestite*, which originally described people who experienced their gender identity as different from their sex assigned at birth.[4] While many of the scholars and medical providers at the time felt that transgender people should be cured, Hirschfield believed that the best treatment for TGNC people was to support them wanting to live in their gender identity instead of forcing them to maintain a role aligning with their sex assigned at birth.[4] Hirschfield and colleagues at ISS were the first to begin offering gender-affirming treatment through hormone treatments and surgical procedures. There is evidence indicating that Hirschfield performed castration on Dora Richter in 1922, followed by subsequent surgeries of penectomies and vaginoplasties throughout the 1930s.[4] Unfortunately, much of the origin story of gender-affirming care at ISS has been erased from history, as Nazis destroyed the institute and its records.[4]

In America, Alfred Kinsey began his pivotal work on sexuality and gender in the 1940s.[1] Though much of his research emphasized sexual minorities (ie, lesbian women and gay men), Kinsey was the first person in the United States to create language regarding medical transitioning. Kinsey was the first to coin the term transsexual, as used in its current form, to represent someone who has had surgery to align with their gender identity.[3] Kinsey's work in sexuality only touched on gender identity but played a part in the building dialogue around transgender lives and health care.

In 1952, Christine Jorgensen made a New York Times headline by being the first American patient to undergo gender-affirming surgery.[5] At this time, the United States was not performing gender-affirming surgeries, which resulted in Jorgensen traveling to Denmark. Jorgensen's story of transitioning and traveling was one of the first of its kind to enter the public sphere. Jorgensen's surgeon recommended a rising professional in the area of transgender surgical medicine located in the United States, Henry Benjamin, who wrote *The Transsexual Phenomenon*.[6] This book became the foundation for the modern treatment of gender dysphoria. A 1979 study by Meyer & Reter[7] claimed that the psychosocial outcomes of transgender patients who underwent gender affirmation surgery were no better than those who did not. Although this article drew criticism and had methodological flaws, the outcomes led to the closure of the John Hopkin's Gender Identity Clinic, one of the few hospitals of its time performing gender affirmation surgeries. The stigma and shunning of services related to transgender health care is not surprising at this time—transgender people were very misunderstood and discriminated against, and any efforts to support transgender people were met with harsh criticism from the public and medical community. In an effort to produce contradictory research findings, Benjamin and colleagues founded WPATH, developing the first SOC for the treatment of transgender people.[1]

Around this same time, the American Psychiatric Association published Gender Identity Disorder in the third iteration of the *Diagnostic and Statistical Manual of Mental Disorders* (DSM-III).[1] While this may have felt like a backstep by once again pathologizing transgender people, it was the addition of this diagnosis that provided the rationale that TGNC persons need to be treated with affirmation and support. The more recent shift in the DSM-5 to gender identity dysphoria also emphasizes that the person is not ill and therefore needs to be treated, to address their dysphoria.[1,4] Gradually, the health care landscape appears to be changing for TGNC adults. In 2014, a government appeals board ruled that Medicare must cover surgery for gender transitions, a significant policy change from the 1980s, which ruled that surgery would not be covered.[8] Steady improvement in the quality of gender-affirming care available to TGNC people is likely due to the work of WPATH, as well as multiple research studies stating gender-affirming health care is beneficial to trans* people.[9,10]

While there has been a significant change in health care access and quality over the course of the last 100 years, TGNC people continue to experience discrimination in health care and still must confront many hurdles to access gender-affirming care.[11] Both primary care professionals and specialists continue to harm trans* patients, and even those who practice in good faith may continue to create barriers for trans* people to access health care needed to reduce dysphoria and the feelings of depression, anxiety, and suicidality that may sometimes accompany it.

WPATH

The WPATH SOC, last updated in 2022, provides the framework medical and mental health professionals working with TGNC people should utilize to provide gender-affirming assessment and treatment.[12] The SOC are organized based on age (ie, adult, adolescent, child) and label (ie, transgender, nonbinary, eunuch, intersex), which allows clinicians to appropriately apply criteria for diagnosis, referrals, and treatment. Many major hospital systems, especially those who provide medical care to TGNC people, require that medical providers closely follow the SOC for treatment provision.

WPATH Criteria for Adults

The WPATH SOC requires TGNC adults who are interested in hormonal and surgical interventions to meet certain criteria.[12] Across most states, TGNC adults seeking medical and surgical interventions can receive gender-affirming services by a competent provider. Several areas should be assessed prior to providing medical care.

- Gender incongruence cannot be explained by any other reasons, such as a brief psychotic episode or dissociative identity disorder.
- Gender incongruence does not originate from a medical condition, mental health condition, or neurodiversity, if these conditions do not explain the origin of gender incongruence or may interfere with the outcome of treatment.[13]

Providers are required to provide psychoeducation about potential contraindications to care, and should counsel their clients on their substance use and its potential impact on surgical outcomes or complications. Long-term side effects should also be discussed with patients, including increased risks for breast and cervical cancer and changes to bone health and reproductive capacity.[14]

WPATH Criteria for Youth

Like adults, adolescents and children have WPATH SOC that provides medical guidance on best practices. The SOC separate youth as prepubescent (children) and pubescent (adolescents) and utilizes separate criteria based on age, maturity, and developmental appropriateness.

Adolescents

During adolescence, transgender youth have some autonomy over their body and medical choices, though this is location dependent.[12] Depending on their country of residence, youth have varying levels of access to puberty suppressors that can be started around the time puberty begins, as well as hormones, which can be started in later adolescence. Puberty suppressants may be provided and utilized at a younger age to manage gender incongruence, while surgical interventions are often not available until later adolescence or young adulthood, and may take even more time to be approved by medical professionals or insurance providers.[12] According to the SOC, youth are often good candidates for gender-affirming hormones, and occasionally, transgender boys who have gone through puberty and grown chest buds are given the opportunity to have a gender-aligning mastectomy. SOC also indicate transgender youth should be given the opportunity to take menstrual suppressants when applicable, especially trans-masculine youth who are not currently on testosterone.[15] Adolescents also need assessment to ensure they meet the criteria for care and are at a developmentally-appropriate age where they can consent to treatment as well as understand the full range of outcomes for engaging in partially reversible or non-reversible medical procedures.[12] They must have the emotional and cognitive maturity to provide assent for medical transitioning by acknowledging what the treatment is, why it would be provided, and acknowledge the long-term consequences of this decision.[16] This is not necessarily determined by age, but instead is often a collaborative effort between the patient, parent(s), and their medical team.

Children

Prepubescent gender diverse children are treated using a significantly different set of SOC.[12] Regardless of which state they reside in, children are unable to receive any medical or surgical treatments until they reach adolescence; however, children in this age range may engage in social experimentation and begin the process of changing school and state documents to incorporate new names and pronouns that align with their gender identity. Gender diversity in this age range is considered an expected element of human development and should be embraced and explored. During this stage, acceptance and nurturance of gender diverse youth is key and can set the foundation for being well-adjusted.[16] As a child nears puberty, this is the time to begin conversations about the development of secondary sex characteristics and the potential implications of gender-related treatments on puberty and future adult fertility.[17]

Criticism of WPATH

Many providers of TGNC health care find that the SOC gatekeep many people from being able to receive the health care that would help them to align with their gender identity.[18] Historically, TGNC people seeking gender-affirming medical and surgical treatments needed to see 2 qualified mental health professionals prior to receiving interventions.[12] However, the new SOC recognize the benefit of only having 1 person write a recommendation letter. A study by Jones et al[19] found similarities between the 2 opinions, making the need for a second letter redundant. Having 2 assessors also seemed to question the autonomy of people in making choices for their own body and care.[20] Changing this criterion can benefit TGNC people who have low and no income, who may not be able to afford a consult from 2 professionals. Although this is an improvement, requiring any letters still means that a professional must make the decision that a person is of sound mind to consent to treatment. There is no other surgery, except bariatric surgery, where this is a requirement to receive medical treatment. The practice of requiring letters can lend itself towards being discriminatory and harmful for the health of LGBTQIA+ people and creates an often unnecessary barrier to care.

Barriers to Health Care Access

TGNC people are often reluctant to enter care due to the real or perceived discrimination they experience within the medical field.[21] Even when they enter medical treatment, they may not engage with the appropriate professionals or ones providing affirming care. Many TGNC people report a lack of providers with expertise in trans* health.[22] Medical education can be blamed for most of these barriers as it typically includes less than 5 hours of course content allocated to all areas of sexuality—a small percentage of this time is spent on LGBTQIA+ competencies, which means that an even smaller amount of time focused on this subject area is specifically about trans* health needs.[23] Some mental health providers feel uncomfortable helping TGNC people transition or may be reluctant to provide letters of support.[23] That can exacerbate mental health symptoms and may damage the provider-client relationship.

Even when TGNC people are willing to seek services, there are other systemic barriers to care. Many TGNC people are un(der)employed due to discrimination from potential employers and may have trouble obtaining health insurance.[24] Although the Affordable Care Act has helped facilitate access to medical insurance, it can still be a financial barrier when underemployed, or with the large deductible plans, it may be impossible for TGNC individuals to pay for hormones and surgeries.[25] Electronic health records can present additional problems—if a person has not legally changed their name, their health record may show their deadname (ie, their legal name that is no longer used and is "dead" to them) and former pronouns.[26] Old health records prior to transition may also carry their legal name, making it difficult to not have to out oneself to providers where one's gender identity is unimportant to their treatment plan.

TGNC people with insurance may not always have access to equitable health care and may be discriminated against for both sex assigned at birth and their gender identity. It is currently illegal for health insurance providers to discriminate against transition-related care or even specific transition-related procedures (eg, facial feminization surgeries or setting age minimums for surgeries).[8] Insurance companies also cannot discriminate based on a person's status as a trans* person—all persons should be able to receive the same equitable care regardless of gender or congruency with sex assigned at birth.[8] For example, breast reconstruction for cancer treatment must be available for all genders, and trans* women should have access to women's health care. However, many health insurance companies still discriminate against transgender health care.[8] TGNC people who face these barriers may lack the knowledge or capability to advocate with their insurance carrier to fully cover their health care, and thus, may not receive the care they need. Although TGNC adults and youth may experience these barriers equally, TGNC adults who have the resources to gain access to gender-affirming care have the autonomy to follow through with any procedures that allow them to express their gender. This is significant because access to affirming care removes barriers for TGNC people to be able to live authentic lives and improves the likelihood that a person is more likely to engage in health care, including primary care treatment. Provider discrimination perpetuates the health disparities experienced by TGNC people.[27]

Health Disparities for TGNC Adults

Transgender women, especially transgender women of color, experience HIV diagnoses disproportionate to the rest of the population. Worldwide, they make up 20% of all HIV cases.[28] TGNC people also experience higher rates of depression, anxiety, suicidality, and somatic symptomology than the general population.[29] They also report substance use at higher rates than the general population—TGNC people smoke at 1.5 times the rate of the general population and over 1/4 of all TGNC persons use alcohol and drugs to cope.[30] Although these health disparities exist, multiple studies have shown reduction in these disparities if TGNC people are able to transition.

Social and medical transitioning has been shown to significantly decrease mental health problems.[31] For many people, the benefits of transitioning significantly outweigh the potential side effects of the medication or surgery, as well as the loss of social support from family or friends and the financial burden of medical treatment.[32] Socially and medically transitioning to conform one's gender expression with their gender identity is the best predictor of positive mental health outcomes and quality of life.[33] This has also been shown to increase feelings of safety in public settings.[34] Consequently, having access to medical and social transitions can be life-changing for TGNC adults.

Outcomes for Youth Seeking Health Care Treatment

Like TGNC adults, youth also face significant health disparities compared to peers.[35,36] Experiences of discrimination, harassment, and victimization have been linked to higher levels of depressive symptomology, including self-harm, suicidal ideation and attempts, disordered eating, and post-traumatic stress disorder.[37] TGNC individuals are also more likely to report physical health disparities—they are more likely to report issues with mobility, higher levels of pain or discomfort, and barriers to enjoying and investing in activities of daily living.[36] More than 1/2 of TGNC youth in one study[38] reported their health as poor, fair, or good compared to very good or excellent, which is twice the rate cisgender youth report. These same youth identified increased mental health problems than cisgender youth, including disproportionately more physical ailments leading to missing school or going to the nurse's office. TGNC youth were also less likely to seek preventative medical and dental care, and when they attempted to do so, they experienced difficulty accessing affordable, competent, and affirming health care providers, resulting in treatment delays and increased negative health outcomes.[35]

One consistent argument from opponents of gender-affirming care focuses on the unknown long-term negative health outcomes of allowing medical transitions in adolescence. However, the consequences to mental health and the need for further surgical interventions (eg, growth of chest buds, growth of penis, hair growth) due to the delaying of care cannot be ignored.[39] TGNC people who are interested in transitioning are often well aware of the decisions they are making and the impact of those decisions. Research has shown when youth were supported in receiving treatment, their mental health significantly improved, as did their body image and treatment satisfaction from 3 months to 2 years from the initiation of treatment.[40] Multiple studies indicate youth who reported gender dysphoria and were allowed to receive puberty suppression drugs or hormones found that well into adulthood, none of them reported regretting the decisions they made during adolescence.[41]

Current Landscape of Gender-Affirming Care for Youth

After a change in federal leadership in 2020, several states put forward health care ban bills that would prohibit TGNC youth from accessing any trans-affirming health care until after age 18.[2] Over 60 000 youth and young adults across 15 states were at risk of losing gender-affirming care. In 2021, Arkansas enacted a ban on gender-affirming care for TGNC people younger than 18. This law also bans insurance from covering gender affirmation care for minors, including Medicaid and Medicare policies. Medical providers who fail to follow these laws can be sued or sanctioned. In February 2022, another anti-transgender bill passed in the state of Texas. This bill classified gender-affirming treatment as child abuse and was therefore reportable to child protective services. Two additional bills, 1 in Alabama and another in Arizona, have been passed into law.[5] Alabama's bill disallows any type of medication or surgery for the purpose of altering or affirming a minor's gender identity, including hormones and puberty blockers/hormone suppressants. Arizona's bill is a bit narrower in scope, prohibiting minors from receiving irreversible gender affirmation surgeries, which occur infrequently for TGNC youth. A fifth bill, from Ohio, is still in committee as of the writing of this chapter. If passed, it will prevent all TGNC-affirming health care, including puberty blockers, hormones, and surgeries for TGNC youth.

Case Studies

Case Study 4-1

Cassie was a trans* woman who was taking a testosterone suppressant and estrogen, and she underwent laser hair removal on her face, legs, and arms, had received breast implants, a vaginoplasty (ie, a surgery that creates both the inner and outer vagina using the flesh of the penis), a vulvoplasty (ie, the surgery that creates the labia minora and majora), and an oriectomy (ie, a surgery to remove the testicles) over the course of the last 5 years. She presented as feminine in nature, had long hair, and had legally changed her name and gender marker on her driver's license. She received competent surgical care from her plastic surgeon and felt supported and affirmed throughout the process. She had no issues finding mental health providers to write her WPATH approved letters, and still had an ongoing therapeutic relationship with one of the therapists to discuss ongoing stress issues with her job and her romantic relationship. Cassie's job required her to relocate to a rural part of Kansas 6 months ago, resulting in a need to obtain new service providers for all her medical care. She had been experiencing issues with her blood pressure and needed to get a new primary care doctor to adjust her current blood pressure medications.

Cassie looked online to find available primary care providers who would be trans-competent and affirming. She searched her local hospital system and found 1 provider that stated he was LGBTQIA+ friendly. Cassie shared in her intake paper that she was assigned male at birth, and some relevant medical history about her transition. At the appointment, Cassie's doctor stated that he did not know anything about the kind of surgeries she had and made her be the educator of her experiences. He used the phrase "when you used to be a man" to talk about her life pre-transition. When Cassie asked about needing to have chest exams or pap smears, he stated that he did not know what a "transgendered person needs for their sexual health." When she brought up her concerns regarding her blood pressure, he wondered if it could be her testosterone suppressant and estrogen that caused the elevated blood pressure. While he was not rejecting of her identity or intentionally harassing her, he was incredibly unsupportive and utilized multiple microaggressions (ie, negative comments) to describe her identity.

Discussion

Cassie's case fits a very stereotypical experience for a TGNC person seeking care from hospital systems without designated competent and affirming providers. While Cassie's experience was not one of abuse or violence, Cassie was still made to feel unsafe and discriminated against by her provider. Many clinicians label themselves as LGBTQIA+ friendly—which often means that they are not transphobic or homophobic. This does not necessarily indicate a foundational knowledge of LGBTQIA+ identities or any additional training tailored to the unique needs of LGBTQIA+ people. Sometimes when this label is used, providers are LGB-affirming and knowledgeable but are not transgender-competent or friendly. The acronym of

LGBTQIA+ often gets lumped together without regard for the nuanced differences of these identities.

Cassie's case is also quite typical of TGNC people working with a general provider who is not knowledgeable of her experiences as a trans* woman. Cassie becomes the educator of her needs, health care, and identities, which can often interfere with or distract a provider from providing competent care. Although the doctor's questions may come from a place of good intention, it can still be harmful and depressing to have to spend time educating instead of receiving basic health care.

Case Study 4-2

Alex was an 11-year-old trans boy living in Texas. As far back as his parents can recall, Alex had always been a boy. He was always interested in stereotypical boy toys like trucks and balls, and was often outside rough and tumbling with his older brothers. When he was 4, he told his parents he wanted short spiky hair like his brothers, and when they said no because he was a girl and girls had long hair, he yelled back saying he was a boy. Alex refused to go by an elongated version of his name that was gendered, and stated he was Alex. At age 8, after a fight with his parents about not wanting to wear a dress, Alex stated that he would rather die than be a girl. Alex's parents sought out mental health counseling. They began supporting his gender and advocated for him to be treated like a boy by his family, friends, and teachers. Despite any teasing he received from peers growing up, he continued to insist he was a boy.

Alex was at an age where puberty suppressants needed to be considered to prevent the onset of puberty. His family had started to see signs that he was nearing the onset of puberty, and it was in his best interest that he began taking medication to delay this. Under Texas law, Alex's parents could be turned in to child protective services for maltreatment if they allowed him to begin taking these medications. Alex would also have significant difficulty finding a provider in the state of Texas who would prescribe the medication. Consequently, Alex's parents must choose between moving to gain access to appropriate medical care, staying and facing legal repercussions, or delaying care for Alex. By staying in Texas, Alex would begin to grow chest buds, develop fatty deposits in his hips, and begin menstruation, which would likely increase his gender dysphoria and exacerbate his mental health symptoms.

Discussion

Current legislation aimed at preventing TGNC youth from undergoing medical care is incredibly harmful and potentially life-threatening. Alex's experiences are all too common for youth in states with such restrictive laws. Alex and his parents are forced to choose between staying in Texas and delaying care, staying and continuing to advocate for his needs despite the legal implications, or moving to a state where he would be able to access the developmentally-appropriate medical care he is seeking. As noted earlier in this chapter, LGBTQIA+ people are at higher risk for suicidal ideation and attempts. This sort of situation is exactly the kind of circumstances that may lead to higher levels of mental health concerns.

Summary

Although medical care for TGNC people has transformed over the last 100 years, there is still room for growth in 2 key areas—accessing competent medical providers and receiving gender-affirming care. In order to address these issues, it is essential that medical schools implement curriculum and training on how to assess and treat the needs of TGNC people in all medical settings. Offering or requiring medical providers to obtain continuing education on these topics would also go a long way to improving medical services for TGNC individuals. At present, when TGNC people seek out health care, it is the responsibility of the medical professional to determine whether the presenting problem is related to their gender identity, or if it is entirely unrelated. Continued advocacy is necessary for TGNC people to have the autonomy to access medical and surgical care that has shown to be successful for reducing gender dysphoria and increasing psychological wellbeing. As such, continued advocacy efforts at the state and federal level are needed to protect the rights of transgender people seeking health care, especially transgender youth.

References

1. Naz Khan F. A history of transgender health care. Scientific American. November 16, 2016. https://blogs.scientificamerican.com/guest-blog/a-history-of-transgender-health-care/
2. Legislative tracker: youth healthcare bans. Freedom for All Americans. 2022. https://freedomforallamericans.org/legislative-tracker/medical-care-bans/
3. Olson J. Gender identity 5 years after social transition. *Pediatrics.* 2022; 150(2):e2021056082. doi:10.1542/peds.2021-056082
4. Keuroghlian AS, Potter J, Reisner SL. *Transgender and Gender Diverse Health Care: The Fenway Guide.* McGraw Hill; 2022.
5. Meyerowitz J. Transforming sex: Christine Jorgensen in the postwar US. *OAH Mag Hist.* 2006;20(2):16-20. doi:10.1093/maghis/20.2.16
6. Benjamin H. The transsexual phenomenon. *Trans N Y Acad Sci.* 1967;29(4):428-430. doi:10.1111/j.2164-0947.1967.tb02273.x
7. Meyer JK, Reter DJ. Sex reassignment follow-up. *Arch Gen Psychiatr.* 1979;36(9):1010-1015. doi:10.1001/archpsyc.1979.01780090096010
8. Crocq MA. How gender dysphoria and incongruence became medical diagnoses–a historical review. *Dialogues Clin Neurosci.* 2022;23(1):44-51. doi: 10.1080/19585969.2022.2042166
9. Know your rights: healthcare. Advocates for Trans Equality. 2021. https://transequality.org/resources/know-your-rights-healthcare
10. Aldridge Z, Patel S, Guo B, et al. Long-term effect of gender-affirming hormone treatment on depression and anxiety symptoms in transgender people: a prospective cohort study. *Andrology.* 2021;9(6):1808-1816. doi:10.1111/andr.12884
11. Hughto JM, Gunn HA, Rood BA, Pantalone DW. Social and medical gender affirmation experiences are inversely associated with mental health problems in a US non-probability sample of transgender adults. *Arch Sex Behav.* 2020; 49(7):2635-2647. doi:10.1007/s10508-020-01655-5
12. Owen Smith AA, Gerth J, Sineath RC, et al. Association between gender confirmation treatments and perceived gender congruence, body image satisfaction, and mental health in a cohort of transgender individuals. *J Sex Med.* 2018;15(4):591-600. doi:10.1016/j.jsxm.2018.01.017
13. Coleman E, Radix AE, Bouman WP, et al. Standards of care for the health of transgender and gender diverse people, version 8. *Int J Transgend Health.* 2022;23(Suppl 1):S1-S259. doi:10.1080/26895269.2022.2100644
14. Rosen HN, Hamnvik OP, Jaisamrarn U, et al. Bone densitometry in transgender and gender non-conforming (TGNC) individuals: 2019 ISCD official position. *J Clin Densitom.* 2019;22(4):544-553. doi:10.1016/j.jocd.2019.07.004
15. Defreyne J, Van Schuylenbergh J, Motmans J, Tilleman K, T'Sjoen G. Parental desire and fertility preservation in assigned male at birth transgender people living in Belgium. *Int J Transgend Health.* 2020;21(1):45-57. doi:10.1080/15532739.2019.1692750
16. Grootens-Wiegers P, Hein IM, van den Broek JM, de Vries MC. Medical decision-making in children and adolescents: developmental and neuroscientific aspects. *BMC Pediatr.* 2017;17(1):120. doi:10.1186/s12887-017-0869-x

17. Malpas J, Glaeser E, Giammattei SV. Building resilience in transgender and gender expansive children, families, and communities: a multidimensional family approach. In: Keo-Meier C, Ehrensaft D, eds. *The Gender Affirmative Model: An Interdisciplinary Approach to Supporting Transgender and Gender Expansive Children*. American Psychological Association; 2018:141-156.

18. Jones BA, Brewin N, Richards C, Van Eijk M, Stephenson-Allen A, Arcelus J. Investigating the outcome of the initial assessment at a national transgender health service: time to review the process? *Int J Transgend*. 2017;18(4):427-432. doi:10.1080/15532739.2017.1372838

19. Verbeek W, Baici W, MacKinnon KR, Zaheer J, Lam JS. "Mental Readiness" and gatekeeping in trans healthcare. *Can J Psychiatry*. 2022;67(11):828-830. doi:10.1177/07067437221102725

20. Spencer KG, Berg DR, Bradford NJ, Vencill JA, Tellawi G, Rider G. The gender-affirmative life span approach: a developmental model for clinical work with transgender and gender-diverse children, adolescents, and adults. *Psychotherapy*. 2021;58(1):37-49. doi:10.1037/pst0000363

21. Conron KJ, O'Neill KK, Vasquez LA, Mallory C. Prohibiting gender affirming medical care for youth. 2020. UCLA Williams Institute. March 2022. https://williamsinstitute.law.ucla.edu/wp-content/uploads/Trans-Youth-Health-Bans-Mar-2022.pdf

22. Cobos DG, Jones J. Moving forward: transgender persons as change agents in health care access and human rights. *J Assoc Nurses AIDS Care*. 2009;20(5):341-347. doi:10.1016/j.jana.2009.06.004

23. Sanchez NF, Sanchez JP, Danoff A. Health care utilization, barriers to care, and hormone usage among male-to-female transgender persons in New York City. *Am J Public Health*. 2009;99(4):713-719. doi:10.2105/AJPH.2007.132035

24. Koch JM, McLachlan CT, Victor CJ, Westcott J, Yager C. The cost of being transgender: where socio-economic status, global health care systems, and gender identity intersect. *Psychol Sexual*. 2020;11(1-2):103-119. doi:10.1080/19419899.2019.1660705

25. Defreyne J, Motmans J, T'sjoen G. Healthcare costs and quality of life outcomes following gender affirming surgery in trans men: a review. *Expert Rev Pharmacoecon Outcomes Res*. 2017;17(6):543-556. doi:10.1080/14737167.2017.1388164

26. Jaffee KD, Shires DA, Stroumsa D. Discrimination and delayed health care among transgender women and men. *Med Care*. 2016;54(11):1010-1016. doi:10.1097/MLR.0000000000000583

27. Lombardi E. Transgender health: a review and guidance for future research—proceedings from the summer institute at the Center for Research on Health and Sexual Orientation, University of Pittsburgh. *Int J Transgend*. 2011;12(4):211-229. doi:10.1080/15532739.2010.544232

28. Baral SD, Poteat T, Stromdahl S, Wirtz AL, Guadamuz TE, Beyrer C. Worldwide burden of HIV in transgender women: a systematic review and meta-analysis. *Lancet Infect Dis*. 2013;13(3):214-222. doi:10.1016/S1473-3099(12)70315-8

29. Bouman WP, Claes L, Brewin N, et al. Transgender and anxiety: a comparative study between transgender people and the general population. *Int J Transgend*. 2017;18(1):16-26. doi:10.1080/15532739.2016.1258352

30. Grant JM, Mottet LA, Tanis J, Harrison J, Herman JL, Keisling M. *Injustice at Every Turn: A Report of the National Transgender Discrimination Survey.* National Center for Transgender Equality and National Gay and Lesbian Task Force; 2011.

31. Witcomb GL, Bouman WP, Claes L, Brewin N, Crawford JR, Arcelus J. Levels of depression in transgender people and its predictors: results of a large matched control study with transgender people accessing clinical services. *J Affect Disord.* 2018;235:308-315. doi:10.1016/j.jad.2018.02.051

32. Austin A, Goodman R. The impact of social connectedness and internalized transphobic stigma on self-esteem among transgender and gender non-conforming adults. *J Homosex.* 2017;64(6):825-841. doi:10.1080/00918369.2016.1236587

33. Rood BA, Reisner SL, Puckett JA, Surace FI, Berman AK, Pantalone DW. Internalized transphobia: exploring perceptions of social messages in transgender and gender-nonconforming adults. *Int J Transgend.* 2017;18(4):411-426. doi:10.1080/15532739.2017.1329048

34. Toomey RB, Ryan C, Diaz RM, Card NA, Russell ST. Gender-nonconforming lesbian, gay, bisexual, and transgender youth: school victimization and young adult psychosocial adjustment. *Psychol Sex Orientat Gend Divers.* 2013;1(s):71-80. doi:10.1037/2329-0382.1.S.71

35. de Vries AL, Richards C, Tishelman AC, et al. Bell v Tavistock and Portman NHS Foundation Trust [2020] EWHC 3274: weighing current knowledge and uncertainties in decisions about gender-related treatment for transgender adolescents. *Int J Transgend Health.* 2021;22(3):217-224. doi:10.1080/26895269.2021.1904330

36. Rider GN, McMorris BJ, Gower AL, Coleman E, Eisenberg ME. Health and care utilization of transgender and gender nonconforming youth: a population-based study. *Pediatrics.* 2018;141(3):e20171683. doi:10.1542/peds.2017-1683

37. Chodzen G, Hidalgo MA, Chen D, Garofalo R. Minority stress factors associated with depression and anxiety among transgender and gender-nonconforming youth. *J Adolesc Health.* 2019;64(4):467-471. doi:10.1016/j.jadohealth.2018.07.006

38. Maragh Bass AC, Torain M, Adler R, et al. Is it okay to ask: transgender patient perspectives on sexual orientation and gender identity collection in healthcare. *Acad Emerg Med.* 2017;24(6):655-667. doi:10.1111/acem.13182

39. Achille C, Taggart T, Eaton NR, et al. Longitudinal impact of gender-affirming endocrine intervention on the mental health and wellbeing of transgender youths: preliminary results. *Int J Pediatr Endocrinol.* 2020;2020:8. doi:10.1186/s13633-020-00078-2

40. Becker-Hebly I, Fahrenkrug S, Campion F, Richter-Appelt H, Schulte-Markwort M, Barkmann C. Psychosocial health in adolescents and young adults with gender dysphoria before and after gender-affirming medical interventions: a descriptive study from the Hamburg Gender Identity Service. *Eur Child Adolesc Psychiatry.* 2021;30(11):1755-1767. doi:10.1007/s00787-020-01640-2

41. de Vries AL, McGuire JK, Steensma TD, Wagenaar EC, Doreleijers TA, Cohen-Kettenis PT. Young adult psychological outcome after puberty suppression and gender reassignment. *Pediatrics.* 2014;134(4):696-704. doi:10.1542/peds.2013-2958

Chapter 5

Intersectional Identities, Marginalization, & Violence

Kaleigh Mancha, MS, LMFT, Certified Full Spectrum Doula
Mitzy D. Flores, PhDc, MSN, RN, AHN-BC, CHSE, COI, Caritas Coach®, Introspective Hypnosis Practitioner

Key Points

1. *Comprehend the impact social, political, and cultural beliefs have on how language can be weaponized against individuals or used to facilitate empowering exchanges within health care settings.*
2. *Be able to acknowledge the intersectionality of disability, intimate partner violence (IPV), and power and privilege, specifically during COVID-19.*
3. *Understand how body size and anti-fat bias influences health care treatment and social/cultural ideologies around body size as an indication of morality.*

Background and Significance

Language helps us make sense of the world, including how we build and maintain relationships with the people around us and form meaning from our experiences. "Language can offer a means to understand and change underlying power structures."[1] Therefore, shifting language can help providers confront their own implicit biases and offer insight into the power dynamics that shape individual's identities and the care they do or do not receive as a result.

Below are key terms necessary to developing a deeper understanding of violence and the significance of language throughout this text.

Key Terms

The terms outlined in **Table 5-1** are written as defined by the National Association of Counties (NACo) for Diversity, Equity, and Inclusion.[2]

Table 5-1. Key Terms

Term	Definition	Example of Health Care Response(s)
Ableism	A belief or set of discriminatory actions against individuals with physical or intellectual disabilities or psychiatric disorders.	Provider does not include an autistic client in treatment planning due to perceiving client as having limitations that prevent them from engaging meaningfully in their own care.

(continued)

Table 5-1. Key Terms *(continued)*

Term	Definition	Example of Health Care Response(s)
Accessibility	The intentional design or redesign of physical spaces, technology, policies, system, entity products, and services (to name a few) that increase one's ability to use, access, and obtain the respective element.	Social worker ensures there is always a third-party translator that has no prior relationship with the client present during appointments for a client that speaks a different language than the social worker.
Acculturation	The process of learning and incorporating the language, values, beliefs, and behaviors that make up a distinct culture. This concept is not to be confused with assimilation, where an individual or group may give up certain aspects of its culture to adapt to that of the prevailing culture. Under the process of acculturation, an individual will adopt new practices while still retaining their distinct culture.	A treatment facility recognizes the significance of spirituality in healing and treatment when serving Indigenous people, so they hold a listening session within the community to understand how to respectfully integrate Indigenous medicine and practices into treatment programs.
Ageism	Prejudiced thoughts and discriminatory actions based on differences in age; usually that of younger persons against older.	Hospitals rationing and prioritizing medical care for younger patients before older patients.
Ally	Someone who makes the commitment and effort to recognize their privilege (based on gender, class, race, sexual identity, etc) and work in solidarity with oppressed groups in the struggle for justice. An ally recognizes that though they are not a member of the marginalized group(s) they support, they make a concentrated effort to better understand the struggle of another's circumstances. An ally may have more privilege and recognizes that privilege.	A perinatal professional who takes annual implicit bias trainings to combat preventable maternal and infant injuries and deaths that disproportionately impact Black pregnant persons and infants due to systemic racism and implicit bias in medical care systems.
Assimilation	The process by which an individual of a minority group gradually adopts characteristics of the majority culture, thereby becoming a member of that culture. This can include the adoption of language, culinary tastes, interpersonal communication, gender roles, and style of dress. Assimilation can be voluntary or forced.	A receptionist at a health care facility asking a client who speaks both English and their native language which language they would prefer to receive correspondence and information in.
Bias (Prejudice)	An inclination or preference, especially one that interferes with impartial judgment. A form of prejudice that results from the universal tendency and need of individuals to classify others into categories.	Non-White patients receive fewer cardiovascular interventions and fewer renal transplants; are less likely to be prescribed pain medications (non-narcotic and narcotic); and are more likely to be blamed for being too passive about their health care.[3]
Classism	The institutional, cultural, and individual set of actions and beliefs that assign differential value to people according to their socioeconomic status.	Providers not providing timely detection of illnesses for people from lower socioeconomic classes or discharging patients from care due to prejudiced attitudes.[4]

(continued)

Table 5-1. Key Terms *(continued)*

Term	Definition	Example of Health Care Response(s)
Cultural Competence	The ability of an individual or organization to understand how inequity can be (and has been) perpetuated through socialized behaviors and using that knowledge to disrupt inequitable practices; the ability to function effectively and empathetically as an individual and/or as an organization within the context of the cultural beliefs, behaviors, and needs presented by another's culture.	— Recruit and retain minority staff. — Provide training to increase cultural awareness, knowledge, and skills. — Incorporate culture-specific attitudes and values into health promotion tools. — Locate clinics in geographic areas that are easily accessible for certain populations. — Provide linguistic competency that extends beyond the clinical encounter to the appointment desk, advice lines, medical billing, and other written materials.[5]
Cultural Humility	An interpersonal stance that is open to individuals and different cultural communities and experiences in relation to aspects of one's own cultural identity. Maintaining cultural humility requires learning and understanding the complexity of identities and how they evolve over time.	An oncologist informing a family that their loved one is dying of cancer, but the family is reluctant to use the word cancer so the provider seeks to understand what belief exists regarding the terminology being used from a place of curiosity rather than shame or dismissiveness.
Disability	The physical or mental condition, the perception of a physical or mental impairment, or a history of having had a physical or mental impairment that can affect an individual's life in 1 or more ways.	An organization provides notices and information in alternate formats for individuals with visual impairments because inaccessible formats are a critical barrier to equally effective program participation.
Discrimination	The unequal and unfair treatment of individuals or groups based on race, gender, social class, sexual orientation, physical ability, religion, national origin, age, intellectual or mental abilities, and other categories that may result in differences. It also describes the act of making unjustified distinctions between certain social or racial groups or classes.	Providers dismissing a patient's symptoms or health concerns based on the patient's presenting identities, or offering different treatments based on a patient's type of insurance.
Distributional Equity	Programs, policies, and practices that result in a fair distribution of benefits and burdens across all segments of a community, prioritizing those with highest need.	A health care center charging people based on their ability to pay, rather than the same rate for all patients without regard to economic status or household income.
Health Equity	Everyone has a fair and just opportunity to be as healthy as possible. This requires removing obstacles to health such as poverty, discrimination, and their consequences, including powerlessness and lack of access to good jobs with fair pay, quality education and housing, safe environments, and health care.	A provider offering and participating in mobile health screenings to help those who may not have access to transportation.

(continued)

Table 5-1. Key Terms *(continued)*

Term	Definition	Example of Health Care Response(s)
Health Disparity Populations	As defined by the National Institutes of Health (NIH), include Blacks/African Americans, Hispanics/ Latinos/ Latinx(e), Indigenous Peoples/Alaska Natives, Asian Americans, Native Hawaiians and other Pacific Islanders, socioeconomically disadvantaged populations, underserved rural populations, and sexual and gender minorities.	Proper funding for the Indian Health Service[6] to reduce disparities in the disproportionate rates of chronic liver disease and cirrhosis, diabetes mellitus, unintentional injuries, assault/ homicide, intentional self-harm/suicide, and chronic lower respiratory diseases.
Implicit Bias (Hidden or Unconscious Bias)	The unconscious attitudes or stereotypes that affect a person's understanding, actions, or decisions as they relate to people from different groups.	Documented high levels of "anti-fat" bias in health care providers, resulting in patients with obesity receiving poorer care and having worse outcomes.[7]
Institutional Racism	Unfair or biased institutional or organizational practices and policies that create different (or inequitable) outcomes for different racial groups. These policies may not specifically target any racial group but may create advantages for some groups and oppression or disadvantages for others. Examples can include policies within the criminal justice system that punish people of color more than their White counterparts, or within the workforce system in which hiring practices can significantly disadvantage workers of color.	A medical textbook publisher using images and diagrams showing Black human forms to highlight variations as the example, instead of exclusively using only White human forms.
Intersectionality	The intertwining of social identities such as gender, race, ethnicity, social class, religion, sexual orientation, or gender identity, which result in unique experiences, opportunities, barriers or social inequality.	Being conscious that a Black male-identified survivor of abuse may struggle to seek help due to stigmatizing gender norms, distrust of medical systems, and/or socioeconomic status.
Marginalization	The process that occurs when members of a dominant group relegate a particular group (minority groups and cultures) to the edge of society by not allowing them an active voice, identity, or place for the purpose of maintaining power. Marginalized groups have restricted access to resources like education and health care for achieving their aims.	Not including minority groups in community discussions and advisory boards, or not soliciting feedback about care practices, policies, and treatment options that directly impacts their health care.
Microaggression	Commonplace daily verbal, behavioral or environmental indignities, whether intentional or unintentional, which communicate hostile, derogatory slights toward culturally marginalized groups.	Health campaigns aimed at increasing healthy food choices amongst lactating individuals, that shame breast/chest feeding parents for drinking sodas or eating fast food even though human milk remains nutritionally dense regardless of lactating parents' food choices.

(continued)

Table 5-1. Key Terms *(continued)*

Term	Definition	Example of Health Care Response(s)
Minority Group	Any group of people who, because of their physical, neurological, or cultural characteristics, are singled out from others in society through differential and unequal treatment, and who therefore regard themselves as objects of collective discrimination. Being a numerical minority is not a characteristic of being in a minority group; it is the lack of power that is the predominant characteristic of a minority group.	The Association of American Medical Colleges, in 2014, developed a set of competency guidelines to improve health care for people who are lesbian, gay, bisexual, transgender (LGBT), gender non-conforming, or born with disorders of sex development (DSD).[8]
Misogyny (Gender Bias)	Hatred, aversion, or prejudice against women or female presenting individuals. Misogyny can be manifested in numerous ways, including sexual discrimination, denigration of women, violence against women, and sexual objectification of women.	Providers are trained to recognize the signs and symptoms of how a heart attack manifests in females vs males.
Misogynoir	An extreme form of sexism rooted in racism. The term describes contempt for or ingrained prejudice toward Black women. The unique oppression experienced by Black women due to the intersectional identities of gender, race, class, and sexual orientation combined with discrimination. Misogynoir utilizes and reinforces stereotypes of Black women.	In 2021, California passed Senate Bill 464, known as the California Dignity in Pregnancy and Childbirth Act, requiring implicit bias training for all health care professionals working in perinatal services to address pregnancy-related mortality rates for Black pregnant and postpartum people, which are 3 times higher than the rate for White pregnant and postpartum people in the US.[9]
Neurodiversity	The presence of neurological differences that present in the way individuals act, think, hear, and communicate. These differences in neurological conditions can include Dyspraxia, Dyslexia, Attention Deficit Hyperactivity Disorder, Dyscalculia, Autism Spectrum Disorder, and more.	A doctor's office offers a patient multiple options to choose from for receiving appointment confirmations (ie, phone call, text message, or email) and outlines the check-in process clearly, checking if clarification is needed.
Oppression	A system of supremacy and discrimination for the benefit of a limited dominant group perpetuated through differential or unjust treatment, ideology, and institutional control.	To understand the historical and current impact of oppressive policies and beliefs on health outcomes, medical schools can incorporate antiracism lectures into their curricula, and health care settings can provide training opportunities to providers, facilitated by experts trained in addressing institutional racism in health care and medical education.
Power	The ability to exercise one's will over others. Power occurs when some individuals or groups wield a greater advantage over others, thereby allowing them greater access to and control over resources. Wealth, whiteness, citizenship, patriarchy, heterosexism, and education are a few key social mechanisms through which power operates.	Providers not engaging in sexual relationships with their patients due to inherent power dynamics that prevent patients from consenting.

(continued)

Table 5-1. Key Terms *(continued)*

Term	Definition	Example of Health Care Response(s)
Prejudice	An inclination or preference, especially one that interferes with impartial judgment and can be rooted in stereotypes that deny the right of individual members of certain groups to be recognized and treated as individuals with unique characteristics.	Patients or clients who are incarcerated being denied or delayed treatment due to provider beliefs about whether or not they deserve care based on the crime(s) they committed.
Privilege	An unearned, sustained advantage afforded to some over others based on group identities related to race, gender, sexuality, ability, socioeconomic status, age and/or other identities.	Higher socioeconomic status individuals being more likely to secure an organ transplant.[10]
Racial Disparity	The imbalances and incongruities between the treatment of racial groups, including economic status, income, housing options, societal treatment, safety, and many other aspects of life and society. Contemporary and past discrimination in the United States, and globally, has profoundly impacted the inequalities seen in society today.	In March 2021, the NIH launched the UNITE Initiative to address structural racism and racial inequities in biomedical research.[11]
Racism	The systematic subjugation of members of targeted racial groups, generally non-White groups, who hold less socio-political power. It involves actions correlated with or resulting from bigotry or the thinking that one's racial differences produce an inherent inferiority of a particular race, mainly the dominant race. Racism differs from prejudice, hatred or discrimination because it requires one racial group to have systematic power and superiority over other groups in society.	Auditing medical school curricula for erroneous references to race or reviewing clinical algorithms that erroneously rely on race.
Structural Inequality	Systemic disadvantage(s) of 1 social group compared to other groups, rooted and perpetuated through discriminatory practices (conscious or unconscious) and reinforced through institutions, ideologies, representations, policies/laws, and practices. Structural inequality thus refers to the system of privilege and inequality created, designed, and maintained by interlocking societal institutions.	Routinely screening for food and housing insecurity or exposure to violence can decrease misdiagnoses and increase access to resources that impact health outcomes.
Structural Racism	The overarching system of racial bias across institutions and society. It is a system in which public policies, institutional practices, cultural representations, and other norms work in various, often reinforcing ways to perpetuate racial inequities. It encompasses dimensions of our history and culture that have allowed privileges associated with "whiteness" and disadvantages associated with "color" to endure and adapt over time.	In 2020, the Centers for Disease Control and Prevention launched the Partnering for Vaccine Equity (P4VE) program, which serves to increase equity in adult immunization, with a particular focus on racial and ethnic communities that have historically had inequitable access to vaccinations.[12]

(continued)

Table 5-1. Key Terms *(continued)*

Term	Definition	Example of Health Care Response(s)
Systemic Racism	An interlocking and reciprocal relationship between the individual, institutional, and structural levels which function as a system of racism. These various levels of racism operate together in a lockstep model and function together as a whole system. These levels are: (1) Individual (within interactions between people), (2) Institutional (within institutions and systems of power) and (3) Structural or societal (among institutions and across society). In many ways "systemic racism" and "structural racism" are synonymous.	Health care providers advocating at the systemic (within their organizations) and legislative level for policy changes that increase access to services and/or help guide decision-making around the allocation of resources to meet the needs of communities that have experienced barriers to health care due to systemic racism.
Under-represented Groups	Groups who traditionally (or historically) have not had equal access to economic opportunities because of discrimination or other societal barriers. This may vary by context and geography but can include race, gender, ethnicity, sexual orientation, disability, or low-income status.	Patients are more likely to report a high patient experience score for a physician of the same race than one outside of their own race, resulting in better patient-provider communication, care, and health outcomes.[13]

Types Of Violence

There are various overlapping and complex experiences with violence a person or group can and will encounter throughout their lifetime. In discussing IPV, it is crucial to acknowledge the intersectional and comorbid nature of all forms of violence on coping, belief formation, decision making, normalization, perpetration, perpetuation, and victimization. **Table 5-2** has just a few examples of possible sources of violence; not included in this list are economic, social, and political violence.

Table 5-2. Types of Violence

Types of Violence	Definition	Example(s)
Direct Violence	An act of force, which 1 party uses to impart or inflict physical harms or injuries on another party	— Gun violence — IPV — Hate crimes — Child maltreatment
Structural Violence	A permanent state of violence embedded in the social, political, and economic structures that make up a society, often referred to as indirect violence. These are social norms resulting from hierarchical relationships between historically oppressed and dominant members of society.	— Economic exploitation — Marginalization and fragmentation of oppressed people — Racism — Militarism

(continued)

Table 5-2. Types of Violence *(continued)*

Types of Violence	Definition	Example(s)
Cultural Violence	Aspects of culture, exemplified by religion and ideology, language and art, and empirical and formal science, that can be used to justify or legitimate direct or structural violence. The fundamental inequality of differential access to power and resources is justified through the normalization of cultural or ideological beliefs.	— Female genital mutilation or circumcision — Authoritarian parenting styles — Eugenics — Segregation
Systemic Violence	The harm racialized or marginalized people suffer from the social structures and institutions sustaining and reproducing violent policies and actions. This type of violence prevents its victims from satisfying their basic needs and is an avoidable impairment to the fundamental means necessary for human existence.[14]	— Excessive legal prosecution, sentencing, and imprisonment of people of color — Redlining in real estate — Preschool to prison pipeline
Institutional Violence	Abuses or assaults, much like those of direct personal violence, that are practiced by groups, organizations, or even a single individual on behalf of others—including forms of violence that over time have become "institutionalized," towards 1 individual or a group of individuals in a marginalized or oppressed group.	— Medical racism — Forced sterilizations — Police violence — Genocide

Intersectional Identities

In discussing the impact of trauma and violence on individuals, their family systems, and communities, it is important to first contextualize how exposure to IPV, ability, culture, race, and ethnicity play a role in an individual's ability to frame their experiences, then interpret and make meaning of traumatic events. When discussing risk factors or an individual's vulnerability to experiencing poor health outcomes, how providers conceptualize the issue and solutions at hand is a direct result of prevailing societal and personal beliefs and cultural norms. There is a substantial and meaningful difference between race being a risk factor for a medical condition versus racism creating disparities in health outcomes for specific populations. Intersectionality[15] was a term coined in the 1990s by Kimberlé Williams Crenshaw, a Black woman highlighting the ways Black American women have been excluded from women's rights equality struggles, especially those related to violence against women. Intersectionality has come to represent the ways in which individuals, communities, systems, and historical events have shaped one's predisposition to experiencing various life events and health outcomes, as well as distinguishing the ways individuals embody power and privilege. In the context of intersectionality, it is pertinent to stay cognizant that at all times every individual exists at the intersection of their privileged and marginalized identities, regardless of the circumstances or experiences they are part of.

Much of the literature around intersectionality permeating medical and mental health care systems are from Black, often queer-identified, intersectional feminists such as: Patricia Hill Collins, Alice Walker, Bell Hooks, Toni Morrison, Audre

Lorde, and Dr. Lisa Bowleg. Other leading activists contributing to this literature include: Valdecir Nascimento, Gloria Anzaldúa, and Alice Wong, just to name a few. Black feminist theorist Patricia Hill Collins, inspired by the works of Hooks and Crenshaw, "demonstrated that cultural patterns of oppression are bound together and influenced by race, gender, class, and ethnicity to form intersectional systems in society or 'interlocking oppressions'."[16] Interlocking oppressions is a term coined by the Combahee River Collective (CRC) in 1977, a Black, lesbian, feminist, socialist organization from Boston that served to challenge political systems and influence political theory and practice.[17] Interlocking oppressions highlight that as it is recognized that each oppressive identity does not exist on its own, these identities also form and compound one's relationship to domination and subordination within the systems they live in. Patients and clients may struggle to request what they need or to communicate their health experiences within systems of oppression because a person's needs are filtered through each of the -isms and marginalizing experiences they encounter.

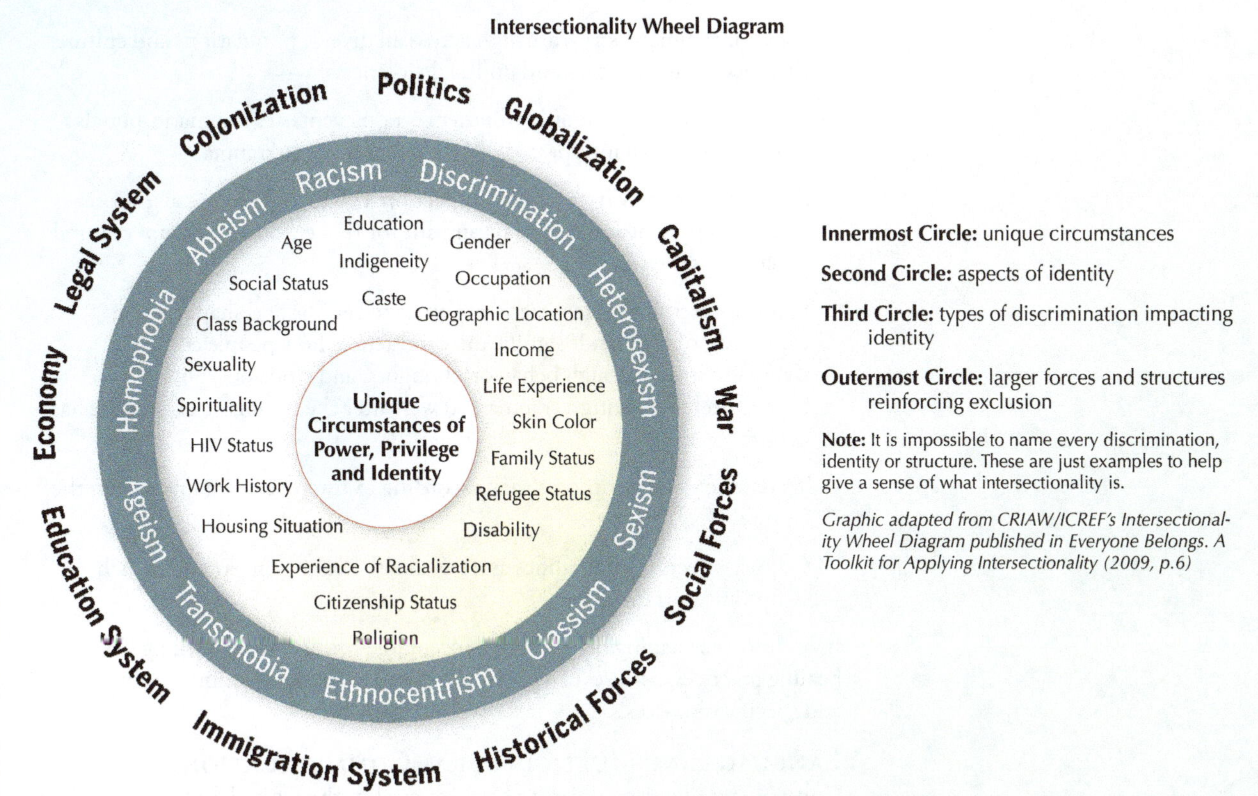

Figure 5-1

Figure 5-1. *Intersectionality wheel diagram.*[15]

Examples of interlocking oppressions include:

— Health campaigns that desire to increase lactation rates marginalize sexual gender minorities by not acknowledging or featuring queer-identified or gestational parents' experiences. By utilizing inclusive language in lactation education and interventions (ie, breast/chestfeeding, human milk), it is possible to reduce homophobia, transphobia, and stigma around lactation due to racism and socioeconomic status that negatively influence efforts to increase lactation rates.

— In 2021, the highest increase in trans individuals being murdered in the United States ever recorded was documented with a total of 57 murders (double the number of anti-trans murders in 2020). The correlation between the passing of anti-trans legislation, racism, and misogynoir influences higher rates of violence towards Black trans women.[18]

— Teen parents are more likely to experience violence in their relationships[19] and are most likely of all parents to experience perinatal mental health conditions (60%).[20] Due to economic, social, and physical barriers in accessing care and social stigmas around young people having babies, they are not likely to seek out or receive mental health care.

Culture and Trauma

Culture shapes how individuals and communities respond to events; beliefs about individual responsibility for the trauma experienced and subsequent responses; and acceptability of symptoms, support, and help-seeking behaviors. The Substance Abuse and Mental Health Services Administration (SAMHSA) identified the following points about culture and trauma[21]:

— Some populations and cultures are more likely than others to experience a specific traumatic event or type of trauma.

— Rates of traumatic stress are high across all diverse populations and cultures that face military action and political violence.

— Culture influences not only whether certain events are traumatic, but also how an individual interprets and assigns meaning to trauma.

— Some traumas may have greater impact on a given culture because those traumas represent something significant for that culture or disrupt cultural practices or ways of life.

— Culture determines acceptable responses to trauma and shapes the expression of distress. It significantly influences how people convey traumatic stress through behavior, thoughts, and emotions, both immediately following a trauma and well after the traumatic experience has ceased.

— Traumatic stress symptoms vary according to the type of trauma within the culture.

— Culture affects what qualifies as a legitimate health concern and which symptoms warrant help.

In addition to shaping beliefs about acceptable forms of help-seeking behavior and healing practices, cultures can provide a source of strength, unique coping strategies, and specific resources.

Language and Multicultural Communication

Cultural and linguistic diversity has increased in the United States within the past century, creating significant communication challenges in both health care and social service fields.[22,23] As such, the creation of Culturally and Linguistically Appropriate Services (CLAS) was conceptualized in the early 2000s, and the US Department of Health and Human Services Office of Minority Health (HHS OMH) has advocated for CLAS in health care since its establishment.[23] Furthermore, in 2013, the HHS OMH revised the standards of CLAS to account for ever-growing diversity.[23] The revision accounted for expansions in cultural and linguistic competency fields, as well as incorporating new national policies and legislation, at the time known as the Affordable Care Act (ACA).[23] The goals of these standards are to help increase awareness and activities related to the need for culturally and linguistically appropriate services in health and social sectors.

Yet, what about language is vital to the communication process? What positionality does one take when trying to understand the importance and significance it plays in health care? According to Greenaway et al,[24] the ability to communicate with others is one of the most important human social functions, yet communication is not always investigated from a social perspective. They note that previous research has taken an individual focus that identifies personal skills, traits, psychological biases, or cognitive capacity limitations as the basis for communication success or failure.[24] Research shows that people speak, hear, and process information differently depending on their group's membership.[24] Consequently, intergroup communication is often laden with challenges that make conversations with others from different cultures, gender or sexual orientations, age groups, or different work groups, evermore complex.[24]

Whether conscious or unconscious, language choices have a profound influence on how one perceives, evaluates, and treats other persons.[25] Research on the social evaluation of speech styles, or language attitudes, shows that the use of certain languages, accents, and dialects can have significant communicative, as well as other social, consequences for users of those forms.[26] For example, standard-accented speakers usually have greater power and influence in society than their nonstandard-accented speaker counterparts.[26] Consequently, standard-accented speakers tend to be members of dominant socioeconomic and ethnic groups and further reinforce societal acceptance of the standard language ideology.[25] Dragojevic[25] notes that standard accents are associated with symbolic and economic value, affording standard speakers a form of linguistic capital that nonstandard speakers lack. The latter findings are supported by the principles of social identity theory, which states that internalized group membership provides a sense of social identity that is fundamental in their view of perceptions and behavior.[26,27] As a result, *ingroup* members—those with whom one shares social identity—are more trusted, respected, and influential than *outgroup* members—those with whom one does not share identity.[24] So, what of foreign-accented English speakers? According to the literature, this population tends to be rated less favorably on various traits based on social categorization and stereotyping.[23] Hence, Americans' negative evaluations of certain foreign-accented speakers reflect their negative stereotypes toward those target groups.[28,29] The psychological distinction between "us" and "them" has unmistakable negative

Table 5-3. Considerations When Dealing with Communication in Health Care [30,31]

Barriers to clear communication in health care settings	— Health care/medical visits are typically emotionally charged and can be accompanied by fear, anxiety, pain, and denial, by either the patient or their family members. These emotions may necessitate a limited-English speaker to express themselves in their native language. — Emotions of vulnerability along with confusion may cause further confusion and limit comprehensive understanding of the situation. — Miscommunication between health care providers and patients can have dangerous consequences, potentially compromising the safety of the patient and the liability of the provider. — The language of health care can be taxing and technical. Some of the terms have no equivalent in other languages.
Legal framework for language access in health care[31]	— Document patients' language needs in the patients' medical records. — Have signage and written materials advising patients of their right to have an interpreter at no cost if they may need one. — Create an appropriate medical plan that meets patients' language needs including but not limited to interpretation and translation needs. — Avoid using patients' family, friends, or minors as interpreters.

implications for conversations.[24] This is no different when the "other" is the health care practitioner. Lee[30] notes that in health care, patients' perceptual biases with certain speech styles (ie, linguistic cues) can influence their assessment of their providers. Therefore, it is essential to acknowledge the coexistence between language and culture to improve health organizations.[31] Understanding the role of linguistic biases in health care can help combat racial stereotypes that contribute to underrepresentation in a given population (see **Table 5-3**).[30]

Visible and Non-Visible Disabilities

Persons with disabilities (see **Table 5-4**) in the United States experience significant health disparities. Reports demonstrate that persons with disabilities have worse health outcomes and greater difficulty accessing care than their nondisabled counterparts.[32-37] These disparities have persisted despite broad federal disability rights protections, including Section 504 of the Rehabilitation Act and the Americans with Disabilities Act.[33,35,36] Consequently, in 2010, Congress added a prohibition on disability discrimination specifically identifying health care, Section 1557 of the ACA.[38] Moreover, disability and mental health research has demonstrated that there is higher prevalence of depression or depressive symptoms among people with disabilities.[38] Reasons for the latter derive from social marginalization, varied interactions, and social stressors.[38] Additionally, people with disabilities have been more likely than people without disabilities to experience difficulties at work and home; in personal, family, and social relationships; and in their health and health care access.[38]

COVID-19 has certainly added to the difficulties experienced by this population. Unfortunately, there is no research to date that highlights if pandemic-related strains have also increased discrimination toward people with disabilities.[38] Public opinion research provides evidence of the dismissive treatment rooted in common prejudicial beliefs of persons with disabilities. For example, a United States national opinion poll conducted in 2004[39] found that 60% of persons surveyed felt that persons with physical disabilities have little influence in society, and 65% of those surveyed said there is some or a lot of prejudice and discrimination against persons with physical disabilities. Additionally, participants in another national opinion poll regarding the Americans with Disabilities Act indicated that they oppose workplace accommodations for people with any form of disability.[40] The noted 2004 publication regarding public opinion on disability has not changed much. In a 2022 publication from Health Affair,[41] it was noted that public support for deprioritizing disabled people with diminished life expectancy is not distinguishable from general bias against patients with disabilities, including those with normal life expectancy. The study conducted was related to medical equipment allotment during the pandemic. Additionally, the findings support the long-standing concerns regarding disability bias in health care resource allocation. Per the research findings, the bias identified was against people with disabilities, older patients, and transgender patients, which inevitably provides empirical evidence that will help inform civil rights enforcement efforts and highlights the importance of expanding bias mitigation efforts in health policy making (see **Table 5-5**).[41]

Table 5-4. Disability Questions

Definition of Any Disability[42]	
The ACS definition of disability is based on 6 questions. A person is coded as having a disability if they or a proxy respondent answers affirmatively for 1 or more of these 6 categories.	— **Hearing Disability** (asked of all ages): Is this person deaf or do they have serious difficulty hearing? — **Visual Disability** (asked of all ages): Is this person blind or do they have serious difficulty seeing even when wearing glasses?

(continued)

Table 5-4. Disability Questions *(continued)*

Definition of Any Disability[42] The ACS definition of disability is based on 6 questions. A person is coded as having a disability if they or a proxy respondent answers affirmatively for 1 or more of these 6 categories.	— **Cognitive Disability** (asked of persons aged 5 years or older): Because of a physical, mental, or emotional condition, does this person have serious difficulty concentrating, remembering, or making decisions? — **Ambulatory Disability** (asked of persons aged 5 years or older): Does this person have serious difficulty walking or climbing stairs? — **Self-care Disability** (asked of persons aged 5 years or older): Does this person have difficulty dressing or bathing? — **Independent Living Disability** (asked of persons aged 15 years or older): Because of a physical, mental, or emotional condition, does this person have difficulty doing errands alone such as visiting a doctor's office or shopping?

Table 5-5. Disability Impacts All of Us[42]

Up to 1 in 4 (26%) adults in the United States have some type of disability

Percentage of adults with functional disability types:

- — 11.1% of US adults have a mobility disability with serious difficulty walking or climbing stairs.
- — 10.9% of US adults have a cognition disability with serious difficulty concentrating, remembering, or making decisions.
- — 6.4% of US adults have an independent living disability with difficulty doing errands alone.
- — 5.7% of US adults are deaf or have serious difficulty hearing.
- — 4.9% of US adults have a vision disability with blindness or serious difficulty seeing even when wearing glasses.
- — 3.0% of US adults have a self-care disability with difficulty dressing or bathing.

Disability and health:

Adults living with disabilities are more likely to be obese, smoke, have heart disease and diabetes:

- — 40.5% of adults with a disability are obese while 28.9% of adults without a disability are obese.
- — 24.4% of adults with a disability smoke while 11.7% of adults without a disability smoke.
- — 10.3% of adults with a disability have heart disease while 3.7% of adults without a disability have heart disease.
- — 16.2% of adults with a disability have diabetes while 7.5% of adults without a disability have diabetes.

Disability and health care access:

Health care access barriers for working-age adults include:

- — One in 4 adults with disabilities aged 18 to 44 years do not have a usual health care provider.
- — One in 5 adults with disabilities aged 18 to 44 years have an unmet health care need because of cost in the past year.
- — One in 4 adults with disabilities aged 45 to 64 years did not have a routine checkup in the past year.

Fatphobia and Anti-Fat Bias

Fatphobia, also known as anti-fatness, is defined by Boston Medical Center as, "the implicit and explicit bias of overweight individuals that is rooted in a sense of blame and presumed moral failing."[43] Additionally, fatphobia contributes to a multitude of health care deterrents for patients that include weight-related structural limitations (eg, blood pressure cuffs, wheelchairs, hospital beds, weight scales), assumptions of unhealthiness, and lack of experience by medical professionals caring for diverse bodies.[43]

Consequently, the American Medical Association (AMA) has recently taken steps that will help bridge the current gap in health care equity as it relates to fat bodies. In June 2023, the AMA created a new policy that acknowledged the rampant misuse of the body max index (BMI) as a measurement tool.[44] They recognized the BMI's historical harm, and its use for racist exclusion.[44] The recommendation the association has for clinicians is to use the tool in conjunction with other valid measures of risk that include "measurements of visceral fat, body adiposity index, body composition, relative fat mass, waist circumference and genetic/metabolic factors."[44] The most significant statement made by the association was their recognition that relative body shape and composition differs across race/ethnic groups, sexes, genders, and age span, and BMI data should not be used as a sole criterion to deny appropriate insurance reimbursement.[44]

Other examples of institutions assisting in creating more inclusive environments and decreasing weight discrimination can be seen in legislation. For example, new policies, laws, and protocols designed to decrease weight discrimination at work[45] include:

- Six cities across the United States have prohibited weight bias at work, with Urbana, IL, Madison, WI, and Washington, DC prohibiting discrimination on the basis of "physical appearance," while the other cities and Michigan specify "weight."[46]
- Michigan is the only state that has passed a law to declare weight as a category protected from discrimination.[47]
- In Washington state, obesity is covered by the state anti-discrimination law.[48]
- State legislatures in Massachusetts, New York, New Jersey, and Vermont are considering their own legislation to prohibit weight discrimination.[49]
- New York passed a bill that prohibits discrimination based on height or weight in employment, housing, and access to public accommodations.[50]

Organizations such as the Association for Size Diversity and Health (ASDAH) partner with service providers, educators, and advocates to dismantle weight-centered health policies and practices by using Health At Every Size® Principles (HAES).[51] The HAES approach notes that "while extremes of weight and health problems are correlated, evidence for the role of factors other than weight in people's health is stronger."[52] Additionally, it is important to acknowledge that weight loss research has historically been and currently is problematic partially because data is erroneous, there are high rates of attrition in studies, and the short length of time of the studies being conducted.[52] Hence, it is crucial to cite weight bias in research to conduct and produce more inclusive and holistically accurate data. Finally, focusing solely on weight disregards the impact of systemic injustices such as the United States' food systems being built on forcibly seized Indigenous land, resulting in the colonization of Indigenous diets, and the reliance on exploited labor from Black, Latinx, and Indigenous peoples. This in turn, has created food apartheid, as well as systemic and cultural traumas.[52]

Table 5-6. Weight Stigma is Harmful to Health (and not Controlled for in Research)[52]
Weight stigma is the discrimination or stereotyping based on a person's weight. It is reported at rates comparable to racism and is one of the last types of discrimination still condoned and carried out by public health and medical experts. The incidence of weight stigma has increased by 66% with the rise of public health campaigns to end the "obesity epidemic." Examples of weight stigma include: — Receiving negative comments or "health concerns" about weight from anyone, including health care professionals — Complimenting someone on their weight loss — Receiving poor treatment or being denied treatment because of one's size or being required to lose weight because of one's size in order to receive a medical treatment — Not having comfortable chairs, airplane seats, or other amenities Weight stigma is a risk factor for: — Inflammation, stress, and high blood pressure — Increased blood sugar and risk of Type 2 Diabetes — Depression, anxiety, lower self-esteem, and higher body image dissatisfaction — Disordered eating behaviors, eating disorder symptoms, and weight gain Experiencing weight stigma not only increases one's risk for negative health outcomes, it also leads to health care avoidance by people in larger bodies, increasing the chances that they do not receive preventative care services (eg, cancer screenings).

Power and Privilege

All people have unique internal resources, individual capacities for resilience, as well as cultural, religious, and racially specific protective factors that facilitate and promote wellbeing, even thriving, despite and in spite of adversity. These individual and communal strengths lead to collective power, unifying identities, and powerful movements for change. Providers are responsible for having an awareness not only of core concepts that inform equitable, trauma-informed, and culturally responsive care practices, but also a desire to continue to seek out information, resources, consultations, and continuing education to enhance care practices. Additionally, there is a dire need for health professionals to identify social determinants of health (SDOH) and understand the role they play in patients' health.[53] Subsequently, privilege in SDOH is a meaningful concept because privilege can positively impact all SDOH. The concept can break down negative connotations of privilege, increase awareness of privilege, and promote those with more privilege to help the less privileged.[53] Finally, the recommendation for United States-based providers is to acknowledge and implement the World Health Organization's (WHO) Commission on Social Determinants of Health (CSDH) conceptual framework.[54] The WHO CSDH framework essentially identifies factors or SDOH (eg, policies, cultural values, socioeconomic status, and psychosocial factors) that impact an individual's health, wellbeing, and quality of life. By acknowledging these factors and better understanding them, policies can be improved (eg, health insurance and protected sick time for all Americans) to promote health equity.[54] In order to promote health equity, health care providers must consider how their and their patients' lived experiences and intersectional identities are influenced by the systems, beliefs, and values they collectively operate within.

Case Study

Case Study 5-1

Irene was a 73-year-old female who arrived at a primary care facility for her new patient appointment. She was accompanied by her son as Irene no longer drove since she was legally blind. Irene had recently moved in with her elder son Dimitri and his family because she was getting older and was struggling with diabetic management.

Irene migrated to the United States from Russia when she was 44 years old. She had a heavy accent and often preferred to speak her native language. She was proficient at reading, writing, and speaking English. In Russia, she had worked at her family's local convenience store. She married at 21 years of age and gave birth to 5 children, 3 males and 2 females. Irene was married for 22 years, and only relocated once her spouse passed away suddenly of a tragic work accident. Irene smoked in her early years but stopped in her 30s. She socially drank but was finding the taste less and less pleasing with age. When Irene was 62 years old, she fell on an ice patch and fractured her hip. She used a cane as an assistive device in her daily life, both for mobility and as a support to aid her in navigating spaces that she had difficulty seeing in.

Upon arrival, Irene made her way to the reception area accompanied by her son Dimitri. She advised the staff of her name, and the receptionist provided the intake documents to her son for completion. They were then advised to have a seat and told the medical assistant would call them back when the provider was ready.

During the waiting time, Irene felt uncomfortable. Her leg was bothering her, and she was increasingly feeling uneasy. The medical assistant finally called them back after a 26-minute wait. The male medical assistant took her weight and escorted them back for completion of vitals in an exam room.

The medical assistant noted that Irene's accent was heavy, and he automatically directed his attention to the son for medical and historical collection. Irene felt overlooked, but felt unable to say this. During the collection of data, no assessment for mental health was directed at the patient. Safety and abuse questions were directed at the son rather than Irene. Pain assessment was asked, and Irene answered with "some discomfort," but "okay." No follow-up or request for elaboration was initiated. The medical assistant advised the mother and son that the nurse practitioner would be in shortly.

Discussion

- Consider the patient's native language (especially when utilizing English colloquialisms and metaphors to convey a point).
- Explore implicit bias around the patient's sex (female-identified) and direct communication at the client.
- Directly ask the client/patient what their preferred spoken language is.
- Provide a medical interpreter when possible.
- Consider the patient's age, background, and life experience as well as accessibility to resources when offering information and making referrals.
- Explore subjective answers, particularly pain assessment.
- Screen all patients for mental health concerns annually at minimum, but especially at new patient intakes.

Concepts to Explore:

- Identify at minimum 1 seen and unseen disability.
- Given the understanding of empowerment language, cultural awareness, and competency, discuss what other factors are important to address in the case study.
- How could the client's intersectional identities influence how she vocalizes (or does not) her experiences with mental health and pain?

— What assumptions or biases did the medical assistant make or have about Irene that prevented them from providing trauma-informed, patient-centered care?

Table 5-7. Care Approach

Standard Care Approach	Trauma-Informed Care Approach
Hi there, if you could please sit on the examination chair, we can begin.	Good afternoon, my name is Anita, and I will be your provider today. Who do we have here today?
I'm going to order some lab work to get a baseline of where you are now, and that way we can establish care.	It is very nice meeting you. Irene, how would you like to be addressed? Ms. Ivanov, or Irene or is there another name you feel comfortable with?
Dimitri, if you can make sure that you get all her medication, that would be very helpful.	Great, Irene it is. Irene, is it okay if your son is here in the room with you or do you prefer he wait outside?
Irene, how is your pain today from 0-10 with 0 being no pain, and 10 being the worst pain possible?	Dimitri, there will be some assessments that will require you to step outside. You can go back to the waiting room during this time, and I will have the medical assistant call you back when you can return.
Irene, you seem like you are doing well. You are lucky to have your son taking care of you.	Irene, I noticed that you speak Russian, would you like to speak Russian or is English acceptable?
Let's go ahead and get you scheduled for a follow-up after your lab work is completed, and your medication is updated.	Irene, can you tell me more about your discomfort?
Do you need any medication refilled at this time?	Irene, can you tell me how your cane helps you during the day?
On your way out I'll have the medical assistant give you some brochures about diabetes and bring any questions you have during our next visit.	Irene, I noticed your eyesight has been declining, can you tell me how this impacts your daily life?
	What have you learned about diabetes and what would you like to know more about?

Summary

There is an ethical imperative for providers to intentionally challenge organizational and individual barriers prohibiting or reducing equitable access to care and to responsibly serve community members in health care settings. Implicit bias trainings, listening sessions, and participating in the critical analysis of current procedures and processes of health care systems are only a few ways in which professionals can collectively realign with more person-centered, healing engaged care. On average, it takes 17 years for research-based best practices to reach clinical practice.[55] This means that meaningful, life-affirming, and impactful medical and mental health research is struggling to be translated and implemented into health care settings in a timely manner. Providers and clinicians have a duty to seek out and implement the most current best practices for their fields, which includes eliminating barriers to providers and community members from accessing that information. There is much work to be done to create equitability in health care access and utilization. Providers must collectively examine how what they believe, learn, teach, and practice impact societal wellbeing.

References

1. Nordgren L. Language and power. Stockholm University. 2017. https://www.hum.su.se/english/education/doctoral-level/research-school/research-school/themes/language-and-power-1.333547

2. Diversity, equity and inclusion: key terms and definitions. National Association of Counties. November 29, 2021. https://www.naco.org/sites/default/files/documents/2022-DEI_KeyTerms_V11.pdf

3. Quick safety 23: implicit bias in health care. The Joint Commission. https://www.jointcommission.org/resources/news-and-multimedia/newsletters/newsletters/quick-safety/quick-safety-issue-23-implicit-bias-in-health-care/implicit-bias-in-health-care/#.Y359ay-B2RY

4. Simons AM, Koster A, Groffen DA, Bosma H. Perceived classism and its relation with socioeconomic status, health, health behaviors, and perceived inferiority: The Dutch Longitudinal Internet Studies for the Social Sciences (LISS) panel. *Int J Pub Health.* 2017;62(4):433-440. doi:10.1007/s00038-016-0880-2

5. Cultural competence in health care: is it important for people with chronic conditions? Health Policy Institute. 2018. https://hpi.georgetown.edu/cultural/

6. About IHS. Indian Health Service. https://www.ihs.gov/aboutihs/

7. Tomiyama A, Carr D, Granberg E, et al. How and why weight stigma drives the obesity 'epidemic' and harms health. *BMC Med.* 2018;16:123. doi:10.1186/s12916-018-1116-5

8. Implementing curricular and institutional climate changes to improve health care for individuals who are LGBT, gender nonconforming, or born with DSD: a resource for medical educators. Association of American Medical Colleges. 2014. https://store.aamc.org/implementing-curricular-and-institutional-climate changes-to-improve-health-care-for-individuals-who-are-lgbt-gender-nonconforming-or-born-with-dsd-a-resource-for-medical-educators.html

9. Hoyert DL. Maternal mortality rates in the United States, 2020. National Center for Health Statistics Health E-Stats. 2022. https://www.cdc.gov/nchs/data/hestat/maternal-mortality/2020/e-stat-maternal-mortality-rates-2022.pdf

10. Zehner A, et al. Socioeconomic status disparities in kidney waitlist outcomes and access to kidney transplantation in the United States. Paper presented at: APHA's 2020 Virtual Annual Meeting and Expo; October 24-28, 2020.

11. Green E. NIH Unite Program aims to end structural racism in biomedical research. Genome.gov. April 1, 2021. https://www.genome.gov/about-nhgri/Director/genomics-landscape/April-1-2021-NIH-UNITE-program-aims-to-end-structural-racism-in-biomedical-research

12. National Center for Immunization and Respiratory Diseases. Equity in vaccination. Centers for Disease Control and Prevention. Updated April 5, 2024. https://www.cdc.gov/vaccines/health-equity/index.html

13. Takeshita J, Wang S, Loren AW, et al. Association of racial/ethnic and gender concordance between patients and physicians with patient experience ratings. *JAMA Netw Open.* 2020;3(11):e2024583. doi:10.1001/jamanetworkopen.2020.24583.

14. Ruggiero V. *Visions of Political Violence*. Routledge; 2019.

15. Simpson J. Everyone belongs: a toolkit for applying intersectionality. CRIAW/ICREF. 2009. http://also-chicago.org/also_site/wp-content/uploads/2017/03/Everyone_Belongs-A-toolkit-for-applying-intersectionality.pdf

16. Rosser SV. Intersectionality and ADVANCE. *Adv J.* 2018;1(1). doi:10.5399/osu/ADVJRNL1.1.3

17. Taylor KY, Harcourt BE. 4/13 the Combahee River Collective Statement. Revolution 13/13. November 10, 2021. https://blogs.law.columbia.edu/revolution1313/4-13/

18. Sosin K. For years, Black trans women have been told their life expectancy is 35 years. That's false. The 19th. August 17, 2022. https://19thnews.org/2022/08/black-trans-women-life-expectancy-false/

19. Herrman JW, Palen LA, Kan M, et al. Young mothers' and fathers' perceptions of relationship violence: a focus group study. *Violence Against Women.* 2019;25(3):274-296. doi:10.1177/1077801218780356

20. Hodgkinson S, Beers L, Southammakosane C, Lewin A. Addressing the mental health needs of pregnant and parenting adolescents. *Pediatrics.* 2014; 133(1):114-122. doi:10.1542/peds.2013-0927

21. Center for Substance Abuse Treatment. *Trauma-Informed Care in Behavioral Health Services.* Substance Abuse and Mental Health Services Administration; 2014. Treatment Improvement Protocol Series No. 57. https://www.ncbi.nlm.nih.gov/books/NBK207195/

22. Marquine MJ, Jimenez D. Cultural and linguistic proficiency in mental health care: a crucial aspect of professional competence. *Int Psychogeriatr.* 2020;32(1):1. doi:10.1017/S1041610219000541

23. Lee S. Evaluation of the National CLAS standards: tips and resources evaluation of the National CLAS standards: tips and resources, by Malcolm V. Williams, Laurie T. Martin, Lois M. Davis, Linnea Warren May and Alice Kim, The US Department of Health and Human Services (HHS) Office of Minority Health (OMH), 2018. *J Gerontol Soc Work.* 2021;64(4):442-445. doi:10.1080/01634372.2021.1882638

24. Greenaway K, Peters K, Haslam A, et al. Shared identity and the intergroup dynamics. In: Giles H, Maas A, eds. *Advances in Intergroup Communication.* Peter Lang Inc.; 2016:19-34.

25. Dragojevic M, Mastro D, Giles H, Sink A. Silencing nonstandard speakers: a content analysis of accent portrayals on American primetime television. *Lang Soc.* 2016;45(1):59-85. doi:10.1017/S0047404515000743

26. Giles H, Watson B. *The Social Meanings of Language, Dialect and Accent: International Perspectives on Speech Styles.* Peter Lang Inc.; 2013.

27. Tajfel H, Turner JC. An integrative theory of intergroup conflict. In: Austin WG, Worchel S, eds. *The Social Psychology of Intergroup Relations.* Brooks/Cole; 1979:33-37.

28. Turner JC, Hogg MA, Oakes PJ, Reicher SD, Wetherell MS. *Rediscovering the Social Group: A Self-Categorization Theory.* Blackwell; 1987.

29. Dragojevic M, Giles H, Beck AC, Tatum NT. The fluency principle: why foreign accent strength negatively biases language attitudes. *Commun Monogr.* 2017;84(3):385-405. doi:10.1080/03637751.2017.1322213

30. Lee DN, Hutchens MJ, George TJ, Wilson-Howard D, Cooks EJ, Krieger JL. Do they speak like me? Exploring how perceptions of linguistic difference may influence patient perceptions of healthcare providers. *Med Educ Online.* 2022;27(1):2107470. doi:10.1080/10872981.2022.2107470

31. Rosa J, Flores N. Unsettling race and language: toward a raciolinguistic perspective. *Lang Soc.* 2017;46(5):621-647. doi:10.1017/S0047404517000562

32. Schyve PM. Language differences as a barrier to quality and safety in health care: the Joint Commission perspective. *J Gen Intern Med.* 2007;22(suppl 2):360-361. doi:10.1007/s11606-007-0365-3
33. Chen AH, Youdelman MK, Brooks J. The legal framework for language access in healthcare settings: Title VI and beyond. *J Gen Intern Med.* 2007;22(Suppl 2):362-367. doi:10.1007/s11606-007-0366-2
34. Roberts JL, Eichner H. Disability rights in health care dodge a bullet. *JAMA Health Forum.* 2022;3(6):e221353-e221353. doi:10.1001/jamahealthforum.2022.1353
35. Health equity framework for people with disabilities. National Council on Disability. Updated August 2022. https://www.ncd.gov/assets/uploads/reports/2022/ncd_health_equity_framework.pdf
36. Roberts JL. Health law as disability rights law. *Minn Law Rev.* 2013;97(6):1963-2035.
37. Nondiscrimination, 42 USC §18116 (2010). https://www.govinfo.gov/content/pkg/USCODE-2015-title42/pdf/USCODE-2015-title42-chap157-subchapVI-sec18116.pdf
38. Brown RL, Ciciurkaite G. Disability, discrimination, and mental health during the COVID-19 pandemic: a stress process model. *Soc Ment Health.* 2022;12(3):215-229. doi:10.1177/21568693221115347
39. Kaiser Public Opinion Spotlight. *Americans' Views of Disability.* San Francisco, CA: Kaiser Family Foundation; 2004.
40. Lake C. Public opinion on disability issues. The Arc. 2016. https://thearc.org/wp-content/uploads/forchapters/Tues%20-%201115am%20What%20Do%20the%20Polls%20Tell%20Us%20About%20Our%20Policy%20Priorities.pdf
41. Ne'eman A, Bell E, Schneider MC, Strolovitch D. Identifying and exploring bias in public opinion on scarce resource allocation during the COVID-19 pandemic. *Health Aff.* 2022;41(10):1513-1522. doi:10.1377/hlthaff.2022.00504
42. Disability and Health Data System (DHDS). Centers for Disease Control and Prevention. Updated May 2022. Accessed December 12, 2022. http://dhds.cdc.gov
43. Fatphobia. Boston Medical Center. 2021. https://www.bmc.org/glossary-culture-transformation/fatphobia
44. AMA adopts new policy clarifying role of BMI as a measure in medicine. American Medical Association. June 14, 2023. https://www.ama-assn.org/press-center/press-releases/ama-adopts-new-policy-clarifying-role-bmi-measure-medicine
45. Gonzales M. Laws, policies can counter weight discrimination at work. Society of Human Resource Management. May 9, 2023. https://www.shrm.org/topics-tools/news/inclusion-diversity/laws-policies-can-counter-weight-discrimination-work
46. Two cities offer model to fight weight discrimination: Vanderbilt study. Vanderbilt University Research News. June 21, 2012. https://news.vanderbilt.edu/2012/06/21/weight-discrimination/
47. For victims of unlawful discrimination. Michigan Department of Civil Rights. https://www.michigan.gov/mdcr/for-victims-of-unlawful-discrimination

48. La Corte R. Washington court: obesity covered by antidiscrimination law. The Seattle Times. June 11, 2019. https://www.seattletimes.com/seattle-news/washington-court-obesity-covered-by-antidiscrimination-law/

49. Kaur A. Size discrimination may limit job prospects. Washington Post. March 22, 2023. https://www.washingtonpost.com/politics/2023/03/22/weight-discrimination-ban/

50. Brauner LM. Employment law update: NYC employers weight/height discrimination law takes effect on November 22. Whiteford, Taylor & Preston LLP. November 8, 2023. https://www.whitefordlaw.com/news-events/employment-law-update-nyc-employers-weight-height-discrimination-law

51. About the association for size diversity and health (ASDAH). Association for Size Diversity and Health (ASDAH). 2020. https://www.sizediversityandhealth.org/about-asdah/

52. Montgomery A. Public health needs to decouple weight and health. University Library, University of Illinois at Chicago. October 28, 2021. https://indigo.uic.edu/articles/educational_resource/Public_Health_Needs_to_Decouple_Weight_and_Health/16823341/1

53. Brown EA, White BM. Recognizing privilege as a social determinant of health during COVID-19. *Health Equity*. 2020;4(1):1-4. doi:10.1089/heq.2020.0038

54. A conceptual framework for action on the social determinants of health. World Health Organization. 2010. Accessed November 28, 2020. https://www.afro.who.int/sites/default/files/2017-06/SDH_conceptual_framework_for_action.pdf

55. Morris ZS, Wooding S, Grant J. The answer is 17 years, what is the question: understanding time lags in translational research. *J R Soc Med*. 2011;104(12):510-520. doi:10.1258/jrsm.2011.110180

Chapter 6

Media Influence on Gender-Based Violence

Paul Thomas Clements, PhD, RN, AFN-C™, ANEF, DF-IAFN, DF-AFN
David Solomon, PhD, HSP-P

Key Points

1. *Media can have a negative influence on gender-based violence (GBV) by perpetuating harmful beliefs, biases, and stereotypes.*
2. *In other contexts, media can have a positive influence, such as by reducing prejudices through parasocial contact with sexual and gender minority individuals.*
3. *Social media can have mixed influence, such as raising awareness of GBV, but also provides a platform for individuals to reinforce their and others' problematic beliefs.*

Background and Significance

The media industry, including entertainment such as movies and television shows, news media, and even social media, has an important sphere of influence on how people shape their perceptions of and responses to gender norms. Research shows that news media reporting has a strong role in perpetuating discriminatory gender norms and stereotypes, as well as the normalization of violence.[1] On the other hand, media reporting also has the potential to shed light on the root causes of violence, promote positive social and gender norms, and help in risk mitigation through the provision of essential information to survivors and victims of violence and those who wish to support them.[1,2]

Gender stereotypes are generalized views or preconceived ideas, according to which individuals are categorized into particular gender groups—typically defined as "women" and "men"—and are arbitrarily assigned characteristics and roles determined and limited by their sex.[3] Stereotypes are both descriptive, in that members of a certain group are perceived to have the same attributes regardless of individual differences, and prescriptive, as they set the parameters for what societies deem to be acceptable behavior. Stereotyping becomes problematic when it is used as a vehicle to degrade and discriminate.[4]

Intimate partner violence and sexist attitudes continue to be normalized through their often comedic portrayal in news outlets, magazines, advertisements, and television shows, and such humor may reinforce hostile sexist views and even increase self-reported rape proclivity.[5] Although research on this inter-relationship remains limited, it is suggested that using sexist humor, offensive and prejudicial humor, jokes promoting degradation to victims of intimate partner violence, and language in connection with such behaviors allow society to view this type of violence as more acceptable.[5-7] A prime example would be using the term "wife beater" to describe an undershirt worn by boyfriends and husbands. "Wife beater" is officially a term in the Merriam-Webster dictionary,[8] and the newer Urban Dictionary[9] not only defines "wife beater" as: "a very tight, white tank top that is ribbed in texture. This style of shirt is usually found on overweight white guys hailing from the trailer courts," but also provides an example of how to use the word in a sentence: "Virgil's got his wife beater on, looks like Helen's gonna get taught a lesson tonight!" Similar to the influence of social media discussed below, it is important to note that the Urban Dictionary[9] is written by users and thus can be a reflection of problematic societal views as well as a way through propagating those views by sharing them with others.

The media can play a significant role in either perpetuating or challenging social norms and behaviors that condone violence.[6] Media can be a platform for the objectification of women and girls, as well as a contributor to everyday hyper-sexualization, one-dimensional images of anyone along the gender expression and sexual orientation continuums, and, ultimately, to overt violence.[1,6] Media portrayals of crime also help shape public perceptions of victims and the demographic groups to which they belong.[10,11] For transgender people, who already face heightened disparities and stigma, mainstream news coverage may reinforce negative stereotypes and minimize the wider context of transphobic violence. For example, media coverage on transgender individuals murdered in the United States often focuses on victims' past criminal activities or participation in sex work, employing victim blaming to suggest the deaths were the result of a voluntary involvement in dangerous activities.[12,13]

Examining the various forms, incidence, and levels of severity of exposure to—or experience of—violence has fueled a debate as to whether the impact of viewing images of shootings, bombings, and rapes, and the direct witnessing or experiencing of interpersonal violence, will promote desensitization. In turn, it could also suggest such acts as valid responses to life stress, thereby perpetuating intergenerational transmission of the "cycle of violence."[14] Further, evidence is highly supportive of the parasocial contact hypothesis, which suggests that indirect contact with minority group members such as queer and transgender individuals can reduce viewers' prejudices towards those groups' positive media portrayals of group members[15,16]; however, this can only occur when positive portrayals exist in a substantial way.

Media Permeation of Risk Factors for Violence

Initial studies of the intersection of media and violence in society largely focused on television as the prevailing form of media and entertainment in the United States. As the landscape of media changed throughout the intervening decades to include other forms of digital media and entertainment, the portrayals of violence in various forms of media have become a topic of intense scrutiny. While multiple factors can lead to violent actions, a growing body of literature shows a strong association between the perpetration of violence and exposure to violence in media, digital media, and entertainment through which violence is normalized and desensitized in the public's eye.[11,17] The mechanisms driving this relationship include news media coverage of violence, social and cultural perspectives, intergenerational abuse, and even humor used in advertisements and TV shows. Moreover, these mechanisms present themselves differently according to culture.[5,10,18] This is a serious public health issue that should concern all clinicians, particularly since children, adolescents, and young adults consume digital media from a variety of sources, many of which are mobile, accessible 24 hours a day, and offer both passive and active engagement. Many of these media platforms feature entertainment that contains significant doses of violence and portrays sexual and interpersonal aggression.[11,17]

Multiple studies have shown either a strong association or a suspicion or suggestion of causality between exposure to violence in media and aggressive or violent thoughts, emotions, and behavior in those exposed.[11,17-20] However, it should be noted that this research remains somewhat controversial as much of it is correlational, limiting the certainty of causal effects. For example, while it could be that exposure to violent media can lead to aggressive behavior, it could also be that more aggressive people seek out more violent media, or that a third variable (eg, exposure to violence) leads to both aggressive behavior and seeking out violent media. Even in experimental studies, which yield more confident assertions of causal relationships, aggression is often necessarily measured indirectly or through nonphysical aggression. This has led some to question the validity of such results as they relate to real-world physical aggression. For example, one study measured participant aggression after playing a violent video game using the intensity of noise blasts the participant later administered to a supposed other participant in another room who did not actually exist.[21] Similar studies have measured participant aggression using the amount of hot sauce the participant chose to give to a nonexistent other participant who ostensibly did not like spicy food.[22] However, despite these limitations, the association between violent media and aggression has been consistently established, with meta-analyses tending to find the strongest association between these variables in experimental studies and weaker but still significant associations in cross-sectional or longitudinal (correlational) studies. One study specifically looking at relational aggression (defined in the study as relationship manipulation or attempting to harm another person socially) found that while the overall relationship between exposure to aggressive media had a small correlation with relational aggression overall ($r = 0.15$), the relationship was stronger when examining exposure to media that specifically depicted relational aggression ($r = 0.21$).[23]

For these reasons, whether viewing violent media is a cause of aggression or may simply be a marker for aggression (ie, if the relationship is due to aggressive individuals consuming more aggressive media), clinicians and policy makers may be more effective in prevention and intervention efforts by considering individual and community consumption of aggressive media. It is furthermore incumbent on clinicians to recognize the intersectionality of risk factors for exposure to violence in media, digital media, and entertainment, particularly for vulnerable populations. For instance, research indicates that risk factors for violent movie exposure "include male [sex assigned at birth], racial or ethnic minority status, low socioeconomic status, and poor school performance."[17] Additional researchers have examined individual factors that influence how individual differences may influence the impact of exposure to violent media. For example, Ridge and colleagues[21] examined how individuals' beliefs about their susceptibility to being influenced by playing a violent video game predicted the actual impact of playing such games. Interestingly, while participants who did not think they would be influenced by the violent game were accurate in that they did not show increases in aggression following the game, participants who thought they would be vulnerable to influence were *less* aggressive after playing a violent game. The authors speculated that "it is possible that being mindful of one's vulnerability to violent media might have promoted a motivation to be vigilant in the face of violence, [leading these] individuals to engage in enhanced self-awareness and self-control."[21]

Media portrayals can impact other factors that are related to violence perpetration, especially surrounding the intersection of gender expression and sexual orientation. These risk factors include a perpetrator's feelings of entitlement to use violence to control a victim, gendered stereotypes asserting that men should be aggressive and women should be passive, and victim-blaming rape myths that portray women as either "wanting it" or deserving it.[24]

Portrayals of Transgender Individuals and Violence in the Media

Transgender people are increasingly depicted in both offline and online media. These representations inform the general public about transgender communities and have a significant impact on transgender young peoples' identity development and lived experiences.[25] However, despite increasing awareness of this representation, a lack of research persists on the perspectives of LGBTQIA+ persons regarding their depictions in contemporary media.[25]

Ekins & King[26] argued that "the most significant change in the telling of [transgender] ... stories ... [has been] the rise of the internet." Transgender people are increasingly becoming visible in online media (eg, websites, social media) resulting in a wealth of diverse, real-life, and increasingly positive representations.[27] However, along with this increased visibility has come insight into a significant public health issue. A study analyzing data from the 2017 and 2018 National Crime Victims Survey (one of the first nationally representative surveys to investigate both sex assigned at birth and gender identity) found that transgender people are over 4 times as likely to experience physical and sexual violence compared to cisgender individuals.[28] In another study conducted in 2019,[13] 545 transgender adults completed an online survey assessing demographics, negative transgender-related media messages, violence, and mental health. The findings indicated that 97.6% of the sample reported exposure to negative media depictions of transgender people across a range of mediums. Further, analysis reflected that more frequent exposure to negative depictions of transgender people in the media was significantly associated with clinically significant symptoms of depression, anxiety, post-traumatic stress disorder, and global psychological distress.

While there have been increasing efforts to showcase positive, gender-affirming images of transgender individuals on television and major motion pictures, stigmatizing depictions and messaging related to transgender people persist in the media. Some scripted TV and movies rely on negative stereotypes of transgender people as criminals, villains, or sexual predators, whereas others present narrow depictions of transgender people that fail to capture the diversity of the transgender community.[29-31] For example, TV crime dramas routinely portray transgender women as victims of sexual assault or murder and, in many cases, transgender victims in films are portrayed as being responsible for their own mistreatment due to promiscuity or fetishism.[29-31] Another harmful, common theme of transgender stories in the media is that their gender-affirming treatment is causing them harm, such as their hormone therapy resulting in cancer or increased aggression.[32] As transgender actor Laverne Cox pointed out in the 2020 documentary *Disclosure: Trans Lives on Screen*, which describes media representations of transgender individuals through the eyes of transgender actors, these depictions are all the more harmful given that most Americans do not personally know someone who identifies as transgender. Thus, for many people, their only knowledge of transgender individuals comes from these limited and problematic media depictions.

The news is another medium through which negative messages about transgender people are routinely disseminated. Indeed, a content analysis of the news coverage of the 23 transgender women of color murdered in the United States in 2016 found that in many cases, transgender victims were misgendered and their murders were often trivialized.[33] Several talk news personalities also regularly demonize transgender individuals and have a long history of using dehumanizing language to refer to transgender individuals. Similarly, fearmongering (and in some cases, confrontational acts of violence) regarding transgender individuals' use of public restrooms became a national phenomenon in the United States, repeatedly fueled by inaccurate or politicized media coverage and interviews.[12,33]

Interpreting and Influencing Media Representations

Although it is not realistic to think that clinicians can have a direct impact on what is portrayed in the media, it is possible to promote a more balanced and risk-reducing interpretation of what is viewed and how it relates to the potential for violence. Clinicians being interviewed by the media or who are participating in policy-recommending activities in professional organizations or legislative arms can use the following suggestions to promote a balanced understanding of reporting incidents of GBV[2]:

— Developing awareness of biases that may result from the identifying details of the victim (such as age/occupation), location of the incident (such as abandoned buildings, old warehouses), photograph of the location, description of the steps involved in the crime (such as lured the victim on pretext) and judgmental language (regarding survivor's history, clothes, whereabouts at the time of the event). Mention of these details in the interview may contribute to victim shaming.

— Focusing on providing support service details such as hotlines, shelters and crisis centers, and drawing attention towards any portions of the situation that depict resilience and empowerment as survivors often act as agents of change.

— Prioritizing the importance of the identified survivor's safety, right to dignity, confidentiality, and protection from retribution or harm, and considering how a media story could potentially violate any of these core principles.[34]

— Discussing the consequences to the offenders of violence–highlighting the legal and social consequences of the act on the offender(s) and their family members. These include the impact of punishment mandated by the law for perpetrators of GBV and the legitimate risk of their family being ostracized by the community.

Although secondary and tertiary levels of research are of significant importance in promoting care and understanding in the aftermath of GBV, there is an ongoing lack of research regarding effective primary prevention methods and programs.

Social Media

Social media sites have the potential to serve as a resource for reducing instances of GBV as well as aiding in the healing process. For example, social media could serve to disseminate consciousness-raising information, or to connect survivors with resources and the larger community. For instance, the recent #MeToo movement, which began with a post made by activist Tarana Burke on Myspace in 2006, seemed to grow exponentially in 2017 following a post on twitter (the social media site renamed X in 2023) by actor Alyssa Milano related to allegations of sexual harassment and assault in the entertainment industry.[35] This movement increased visibility of instances of sexual assault and likely helped to reduce stigma towards survivors. The movement also likely led to individuals actively seeking information on sexual assault, with Google searches of relevant terms growing substantially after Milano's post for a period of time.[35]

Despite the positive impact of the #MeToo movement for many, there has also been resistance and negative reactions. A qualitative analysis of thousands of tweets (as posts were called on the social media website known as Twitter at the time) referencing #MeToo over a 4-day period found that about 10% of the tweets were negative reactions towards the movement. These negative reactions included questioning the accuracy of the claims and placing skepticism on motivations behind those that came forward during the movement or on the movement as a whole.[36] Thus, individuals who share their stories on social media may also be subjected to the same doubt and hostility that can accompany real-life disclosures. Comparing the United States with Norway (a country high in egalitarian attitudes), researchers found that in both countries, men reported more negativity towards the #MeToo movement than women, and these differences seemed to be driven by higher levels of rape myth acceptance and sexism and lower levels of identifying with feminism in men.[37] Unfortunately, some researchers found unintended psychological reactance in men who, after reading tweets intended to challenge rape myths, were more likely to believe rape myths.[38] Another study analyzed twitter posts containing #HowIWillChange, a hashtag that was designed to encourage men to consider how their beliefs and behaviors may perpetuate rape culture. The authors found that some posters were resistant to the message of #HowIWillChange (eg, "I didn't do anything to y'all. Most, yes *most*, men respect women. #HowIWillChange"),[40] and others were overtly hostile (eg, "#HowIWillChange there is no rape culture fuck off").[39] Finally, a 2019 study found that exposure to sexual objectification and exposure to sexually explicit material was related to adolescents having more negative attitudes towards the #MeToo movement.[40]

Social media can also perpetuate negative beliefs, such as the belief that people who are assaulted "deserve it" due to their behavior or how they dress.[41] Indeed, one study of twitter posts found that users who tweeted victim-blaming content were more likely to be shared and had more followers than those posting supportive content.[41] It is also not uncommon for postings of news stories about sexual assault to receive uncivil reactions, having comments containing profanity, insults, and threats, although such reactions may be influenced by the tone of the article and the specific social media platform.[42] One South African study of comments made on online news stories about a movement to end rape culture on college campuses found that many comments perpetuated victim blaming and demeaned the protesters.[43]

Beyond negative comments made by individuals, social networks provide a platform for like-minded users to form communities, which may create toxic echo chambers where the same harmful opinions are posted over and over with no rebuttal, which would seemingly validate and reinforce these beliefs. One example is the online "incel" movement. The term incel comes from "involuntary celibate," and the movement is composed of heterosexual men who have difficulty forming intimate relationships with women. A thematic analysis of 8000 posts made to online incel groups indicated that posts portrayed women as evil, men as being oppressed, and violence against women as legitimate.[44] A similar analysis of incel and men's rights groups indicated rhetoric suggesting that women use sex to manipulate men and gain power. That same rhetoric promoted other messages grouping men based on concepts rooted in toxic masculinity (eg, an "alpha male" is more dominant and of higher status, whereas "beta males" who "give in to women" are lesser men).[45] These groups have the capacity to encourage both small-scale and large-scale acts of GBV. For instance, an analysis of posts to a popular incel forum during the week following the 2018 attack in Toronto, in which Alek Minassian, a self-identified incel, drove a van into a group of pedestrians, resulting in numerous fatalities and injuries, found that less than 5% of the 3698 comments analyzed discouraged violence–on the grounds that violence would be ineffective at causing change for incels–and many of those posts were promptly ridiculed. Furthermore, 600 posts explicitly endorsed violence, with Minassian and Elliot Roger (another self-identified incel who murdered 6 people in a stabbing and shooting spree in 2014 as part of his planned "war on women") being portrayed largely as martyrs.[46] The posts in support of violence gave several reasons, including providing publicity for the incel movement, enacting revenge against the women who would not have sex with incels as well as men who were not supportive of incels, and promoting politic change.[46] For some users, Minassian's actions were described as a natural consequence of women "withholding" affection from men.

Social media can also be a vehicle for offenders to perpetrate further abuse against their victims, as was the case with teenager Rehtaeh Parsons, who died by suicide after a photo of her being sexually assaulted was disseminated on social media.[47] Despite the fact photographs of an assault can also be used against the perpetrator, it is possible that many who share these images do not see them as evidence of assault, but instead as an indictment of the victim's behavior, playing into various victim-blaming rape myths.[47] Similarly, another growing area of concern is "revenge pornography," in which a perpetrator maliciously releases sexually explicit material of another person (often an ex-lover) online, which is a form of psychological violence.[48] While there are legal protections against revenge pornography in some places,[49] legal consequences of revenge pornography may not assuage the psychological harm that has already been done. As with sharing images of sexual assault perpetration, victim blaming often occurs with revenge pornography (ie, blaming the victim for taking or sharing the photograph originally),[50] which may increase shame and distress.

Case Study

Case Study 6-1

A very highly publicized Netflix film that garnered significant media "hype" surrounded the infamous serial killer, Ted Bundy, and represents only 1 in a wave of works to focus on handsome men guilty of heinous acts. Bundy murdered at least 28 young women over a 4-year crime spree that also included kidnapping, burglary, and grand theft auto. While the title of the 2019 film is *Extremely Wicked, Shockingly Evil and Vile*, much of the discussion around the film focused not on the heinousness of Bundy's crimes, but rather on the attractiveness of the actor portraying Bundy, Zac Efron, as well as that of the serial killer himself.[51-54] While it could be argued that the film attempts to provide some commentary about how Bundy used his charisma and attractiveness to his advantage with both his victims and the public following his capture, it can likewise be argued that the filmmakers used a glamorized depiction of a "sexy serial killer" to draw in audiences. In 1 scene featured in the trailer that seems to break the fourth wall, Efron winks directly into the camera, a cheeky grin on his face. Such techniques are often employed in media to send a message to the audience.[55] In this case, that message seems to be a flirtatious one. In one person's online post, she opines[54]:

Ted Bundy was hot
John Wayne Gacy Jr was bae
Jeffery Dahmer looked like a snack
Jack the Ripper was a zaddy
Just bc they are serial killers doesn't mean they can't be attractive

Discussion

The "Bad Boy" media phenomenon, or even more troubling, the obsession with the "sexy psychopath," is becoming more evident in mass media online streaming releases or blockbuster movie premiers. In reference to the 2019 Bundy film, a disturbing feeling does not come from watching these things unfold. Rather, it stems from the fact that they seem almost irrelevant to the story. Are these exploring toxic masculinity or fetishizing it? An exploration of various journalistic media commentaries raises similar questions. *The Washington Post* asked if it portrayed "A Hot Ted Bundy?" and a "Romanticized Serial Killer?"[53] while, in another review of the movie, the headline read that the director "... cast a 'hot' Ted Bundy."

Typically, a good movie bad boy is an outcast within his society with a backstory he would rather forget, and who will eventually choose to do the right thing. A cool look paired with a nonchalant take on expectations and a judgmental, snide expression usually signals a bad boy who is loyal only to those he trusts.[53] "Basically, if you grab every single red flag in the history of mankind and stitch them together, you have him—and yet, the ladies adore him."[52] However, this is incredibly problematic, because it teaches men to equate romantic and sexual appeal with cruelty, or more comprehensively, toxic masculinity.

Although it is unlikely that clinicians will stop children or parents from entirely preventing television or media viewing, it is important to impart to them that learning gender roles from movies and TV shows has real consequences on self-esteem, relationships, and even their future life choices. Parents talking to their children about how boys and girls are portrayed in the media that they watch together, and making comments in the moment that address and counter stereotypes can have a significant impact and prevent role confusion. Clearly, mass media, in many forms, is having an ever-increasing influence in the lives of each subsequent generation of children; as such, parents must rise to the need to educate themselves to directly counteract potential detrimental developmental impacts.

Summary

As with all social tools and business platforms, the various forms of media bring both significant advantages and noteworthy limitations. Advantages for the global community have included the ability to expand awareness of social issues and happenings, including real-time updates, and the opportunity to give a voice to previously voiceless people or populations. On the other side of the scale, the disadvantages of media include the ability to spread and create damaging rumors and false information, and empowering people who choose to harm others. It is therefore important for clinicians to have a grasp of both problems and potential solutions, the impacts of, and potential resistance to, the intersections of gender violence, social media, and our complex lived environments across national boundaries. Throughout this volume, close attention is paid to the difficult issues highlighted when prior conceptions of basic foundations such as public space, individual rights, and professional responsibility are confronted by new examples that further trouble the boundaries of long-held frameworks of legal, social, professional understanding, and even the comprehension of the "real" versus the "portrayal" or "transmitted." Although continued debate exists regarding the impact of media violence exposure on viewers' thoughts and behaviors, clinicians should remain open to providing opportunities for clients to share and explore issues surrounding their own experiences as direct or vicarious victims related to social or mass media portrayals or interactions.

Resources

— National Domestic Violence Hotline. 24/7
Languages: English, Spanish and 200+ through interpretation service
800-799-7233
Live Chat: https://chat.thehotline.us/v2/index.html?dkey=783ea42e-3aa0-42f4-9899-ad886e4995b4&skill=g1b

— Department of Homeland Security (DHS) Resources on Gender-Based Violence: "The Department of Homeland Security (DHS) is committed to combatting gender-based violence and integrating protections for all individuals in our policies, programs, and activities across the Department. Gender-based violence (GBV) is defined as any harmful threat or act directed at an individual or group based on their actual or perceived: Biological sex; Gender identity; Gender expression; Sexual orientation; or Difference from social norms related to masculinity or femininity"
Free resources available from: https://www.dhs.gov/dhs-resources-gender-based-violence

— VAWnet (https://vawnet.org) – home to thousands of materials on gender-based violence and related issues.

References

1. Mapping the nexus between media reporting of violence against girls. UN Women. 2022. https://www.unwomen.org/sites/default/files/2022-08/Evidence-review-Mapping-the-nexus-between-media-reporting-of-violence-against-girls-en.pdf

2. Menon V, Pattnaik JI, Bascarane S, Padhy SK. Role of media in preventing gender-based violence and crimes during the COVID-19 pandemic. *Asian J Psychiatr.* 2020;54:102449. doi:10.1016/j.ajp.2020.102449

3. Gender stereotypes and stereotyping and women's rights. United Nations Human Rights Office of the High Commissioner. September 2014. https://www.ohchr.org/sites/default/files/Documents/Issues/Women/WRGS/OnePagers/Gender_stereotyping.pdf

4. Combating gender stereotyping and sexism in the media. Council of Europe. https://rm.coe.int/168064379b

5. Romero-Sánchez M, Megías JL, Carretero-Dios H. Sexist humor and sexual aggression against women: when sexist men act according to their own values or social pressures. *J Interpers Violence.* 2021;36(21-22):NP11322-NP11348. doi:10.1177/0886260519888518

6. Mallett RK, Ford TE, Woodzicka JA. What did he mean by that? Humor decreases attributions of sexism and confrontation of sexist jokes. *Sex Roles.* 2016;75(5-6):272-284. doi:10.1007/s11199-016-0605-2

7. O'Connor EC, Ford TE, Banos NC. Restoring threatened masculinity: the appeal of sexist and anti-gay humor. *Sex Roles.* 2017;77(2):567-580. doi:10.1007/s11199-017-0761-z

8. "Wifebeater." Merriam-Webster. Accessed October 2, 2022. https://www.merriam-webster.com/dictionary/wifebeater

9. "Wife beater." Urban Dictionary Online. Accessed October 2, 2022. https://www.urbandictionary.com/define.php?term=wife%20beater

10. Coyne SM, Ward LM, Kroff SL, et al. Contributions of mainstream sexual media exposure to sexual attitudes, perceived peer norms, and sexual behavior: a meta-analysis. *J Adolesc Health.* 2019;64(4):430-436. doi:10.1016/j.jadohealth.2018.11.016

11. Arbeit M. 5 ways sexual objectification in mainstream media can impact adolescent viewers. Society for Research on Adolescence. May 3, 2018. https://www.s-r-a.org/index.php?option=com_dailyplanetblog&view=entry&year=2018&month=05&day=02&id=62:5-ways-sexual-objectification-in-mainstream-media-can-impact-adolescent-viewers

12. Osborn M. US news coverage of transgender victims of fatal violence: an exploratory content analysis. *Violence Against Women.* 2022;28(9):2033-2056. doi:10.1177/10778012211025995

13. Hughto JMW, Pletta D, Gordon L, Cahill S, Mimiaga MJ, Reisner SL. Negative transgender-related media messages are associated with adverse mental health outcomes in a multistate study of transgender adults. *LGBT Health.* 2021;8(1):32-41. doi:10.1089/lgbt.2020.0279

14. United States strategy to prevent and response to gender-based violence globally 2022. US Department of State. 2022. https://www.state.gov/reports/united-states-strategy-to-prevent-and-respond-to-gender-based-violence-globally-2022/

15. Massey ZB, Wong NCH, Barbati JL. Meeting the (trans)parent: test of parasocial contact with transgender characters on reducing stigma toward transgender people. *Commun Stud.* 2021;72(2):232-250. doi:10.1080/10510974.2021.1876125

16. Schiappa E, Gregg PB, Hewes DE. Can one tv show make a difference? Will & Grace and the parasocial contact hypothesis. *J Homosex*. 2006;51(4):15-37. doi:10.1300/J082v51n04_02

17. Violence in the media and entertainment (position paper). American Academy of Family Physicians. 2022. https://www.aafp.org/about/policies/all/violence-media-entertainment.html

18. Ross T. Media and stereotypes. In: Ratuva S, ed. *The Palgrave Handbook of Ethnicity*. Palgrave Macmillan; 2019:1-17. doi:10.1007/978-981-13-0242-8_26-1

19. Violence in the media: psychologists study potential harmful effects. American Psychological Association. 2013. https://www.apa.org/topics/video-games/violence-harmful-effects

20. Turanovic JJ, Siennick SE. The causes and consequences of school violence: a review. National Institute of Justice. February 2022. https://www.ojp.gov/pdffiles1/nij/302346.pdf

21. Ridge RD, Hawk CE, McCombs LD, et al. 'It doesn't affect me!'—Do immunity beliefs prevent subsequent aggression after playing a violent video game? *J Media Psychol Theor Methods Appl*. 2023;35(4):234-240. doi:10.1027/1864-1105/a000369

22. Heng S, Zhou Z, Niu G, Liu Q. Priming effects of virtual avatars on aggression: influence of violence and player gender. *Acta Psychologica Sinica*. 2017;49(11):1460-1472. doi:10.3724/SP.J.1041.2017.01460

23. Martins N, Weaver A. The role of media exposure on relational aggression: a meta-analysis. *Aggress Viol Behav*. 2019;47:90-99. doi:10.1016/j.avb.2019.03.001

24. Contributing factors. Office for Violence Prevention and Victim Assistance, Rutgers University. 2022. https://vpva.rutgers.edu/info-resources/sexual-violence/contributing-factors

25. McInroy LB, Craig SL. Transgender representation in offline and online media: LGBTQ youth perspectives. *J Hum Behav Soc Environ*. 2015;25:606-617. doi:10.1080/10911359.2014.995392

26. Ekins R, King D. *The Transgender Phenomenon*. SAGE Publications; 2006.

27. Mocarski R, King R, Butler S, et al. The rise of transgender and gender diverse representation in the media: impacts on the population. *Commun Cult Crit*. 2019;12(3):416-433. doi:10.1093/ccc/tcz031

28. Transgender people over four times more likely than cisgender people to be victims of violent crime. UCLA School of Law. 2021. https://williamsinstitute.law.ucla.edu/press/ncvs-trans-press-release/

29. Billard TJ. Writing in the margins: mainstream news media representations of transgenderism. *Int J Commun*. 2016;10:4193-4218.

30. Reitz N. The representation of trans women in film and television. *Cinesthesia*. 2017;7(1):2. https://scholarworks.gvsu.edu/cine/vol7/iss1/2

31. Ford A. Whose club is it anyway?: The problematic of trans representation in mainstream films–"Rayon" and Dallas Buyers Club. *Screen Bodies*. 2016;1(2). doi:10.3167/screen.2016.010205

32. Feder S. *Disclosure: Trans Lives on Screen*. Streaming Video. United States: Disclosure Films, Bow and Arrow Entertainment, and Field of Vision; 2020.

33. Wood F, Carrillo A, Monk-Turner E. Visibly unknown: media depiction of murdered transgender women of color. *Race Justice*. 2019;12(2):368-386. doi:10. 1177/2153368719886343

34. Bagagli BP, Chaves TV, Zoppi Fontana MG. Trans women and public restrooms: the legal discourse and its violence. *Front Sociol*. 2021;6:652777. doi:10.3389/fsoc.2021.652777

35. Kaufman MR, Dey D, Crainiceanu C, Dredze M. #MeToo and Google inquiries into sexual violence: a hashtag campaign can sustain information seeking. *J Interpers Violence*. 2021;36(19-20):9857-9867. doi:10.1177/0886260519868197

36. Nutbeam M, Mereish EH. Negative attitudes and beliefs toward the #MeToo movement on Twitter. *J Interpers Violence*. 2022;37(15-16):NP13018-NP13044. doi:10.1177/08862605211001470

37. Kunst JR, Bailey A, Prendergast C, Gundersen A. Sexism, rape myths and feminist identification explain gender differences in attitudes toward the #metoo social media campaign in two countries. *Media Psychology*. 2019;22(5):818-843. doi:10.1080/15213269.2018.1532300

38. Nicolla S, Lazard AJ. Social media communication about sexual violence may backfire: online experiment with young men. *J Health Commun*. 2023;28(1):28-37. doi:10.1080/10810730.2023.2174214

39. PettyJohn ME, Muzzey FK, Maas MK, McCauley HL. #HowIWillChange: engaging men and boys in the #MeToo movement. *Psychol Men Masc*. 2019; 20(4):612-622. doi:10.1037/men0000186

40. Maes C, Schreurs L, van Oosten JMF, Vandenbosch L. #(Me)too much? The role of sexualizing online media in adolescents' resistance towards the metoo-movement and acceptance of rape myths. *J Adolesc*. 2019;77:59-69. doi:10.1016/j.adolescence.2019.10.005

41. Stubbs-Richardson M, Rader NE, Cosby AG. Tweeting rape culture: examining portrayals of victim blaming in discussions of sexual assault cases on Twitter. *Fem Psychol*. 2018;28(1):90-108. doi:10.1177/0959353517715874

42. Stevens H, Acic I, Taylor LD. Uncivil reactions to sexual assault online: linguistic features of news reports predict discourse incivility. *Cyberpsychol Behav Soc Netw*. 2021;24(12):815-821. doi:10.1089/cyber.2021.0075

43. Orth Z, Andipatin M, van Wyk B. "These women are making a statement against rape and yet the only thing y'all can focus on is 'Eww they're naked'": Exploring rape culture on Facebook in South Africa. *Gender Issues*. 2021;38(3):243-259. doi:10.1007/s12147-020-09268-x

44. O'Malley RL, Holt K, Holt TJ. An exploration of the involuntary celibate (incel) subculture online. *J Interpers Violence*. 2022;37(7-8):NP4981-NP5008. doi:10.1177/0886260520959625

45. Vallerga M, Zurbriggen EL. Hegemonic masculinities in the 'manosphere': A thematic analysis of beliefs about men and women on the red pill and incel. *Anal Soc Issues Public Policy*. 2022;22(2):602-625. doi:10.1111/asap.12308

46. O'Donnell C, Shor E. "This is a political movement, friend": Why "incels" support violence. *Br J Sociol*. 2022;73(2):336-351. doi:10.1111/1468-4446.12923

47. Dodge A. Digitizing rape culture: online sexual violence and the power of the digital photograph. *Crime Media Cult*. 2016;12(1):65-82. doi:10.1177/1741659015601173

48. Hearn J, Hall M. From physical violence to online violation: forms, structures and effects: a comparison of the cases of 'domestic violence' and 'revenge pornography.' *Aggress Violent Behav*. 2022;67:1-8. doi:10.1016/j.avb.2022.101779

49. Cole T, Policastro C, Crittenden C, McGuffee K. Freedom to post or invasion of privacy? Analysis of US revenge porn state statutes. *Vict Offender*. 2020; 15(4):483-498. doi:10.1080/15564886.2020.1712567

50. Mckinlay T, Lavis T. Why did she send it in the first place? Victim blame in the context of 'revenge porn.' *Psychiatr Psychol Law*. 2020;27(3):386-396. doi:10.1080/13218719.2020.1734977

51. Teske A. 10 movies that make the best use of the "Bad Boy" trope. Collider. February 25, 2023. https://collider.com/movies-bad-boy-trope/

52. Why the bad boy is bad for you. The Phillipian. May 27, 2022. https://phillipian.net/2022/05/27/why-the-bad-boy-is-bad-for-you/

53. Flynn M. Zac Efron as 'Hot Ted Bundy': A 'romanticized' serial killer? Or a convincing one? The Washington Post. January 28, 2019. https://www.washingtonpost.com/nation/2019/01/28/zac-efron-hot-ted-bundy-romanticized-serial-killer-or-convincing-one/

54. Wedemeyer A. For many online, Ted Bundy is "hot." The Ringer. January 31, 2019. Accessed May 20, 2024. https://www.theringer.com/tv/2019/1/31/18205088/why-do-people-think-ted-bundy-is-hot

55. Lauzen MM, Deiss Jr DM. Breaking the fourth wall and sex role stereotypes: an examination of the 2006-2007 prime-time season. *Sex Roles*. 2009;60(5-6):379-386. doi:10.1007/s11199-008-9553-9

Chapter 7

The Effects of Violence, Trauma, and Protective Factors on Individuals and Communities

Kaleigh Mancha, MS, LMFT, Certified Full Spectrum Doula
Natasha T. Stewart, MPA

Key Points

1. *In 2019, Child Protective Services (CPS) agencies received an estimated 4.4 million referrals involving the possible maltreatment of approximately 7 900 000 children, with an estimated 656 000 children identified as victims of abuse or neglect nationwide.*[1]
2. *50% of medical providers and 23% of behavioral health providers do not screen for intimate partner violence (IPV) at all.*[2]
3. *Regardless of type of the violence experienced, longitudinal research has identified 4 significant protective factors that enhance resilience: self-regulation, family support, school support, and peer support.*[3]

Background and Significance

To understand the purpose and value of identifying and assessing for risk and resilience factors, it is important to delineate the differences between stressors, toxic stress, violence, and trauma. While all individuals have unique inner worlds, strengths, and adaptabilities, each person, no matter how isolated, is part of multiple systems continuously engaged in constant exchanges and feedback loops. Humankind is permeable to influence, thus, responses and interactions ripple outward throughout each related system. What happens within and to an individual has a lasting impact on the individual and everyone in the systems they are connected to.

Toxic Stress

Stressors are external and internal stimuli that generate a stress response cycle. Some stressors are negative in their impact, while others are positive. An example of a negative stressor would be sitting in traffic while running late (external) or catching the flu (internal), while examples of positive stressors would be competing in a sports competition (external) or consuming caffeine (internal). Whether the stress benefits or harms the individual depends greatly on how the individual recovers from the experience, how often the individual is exposed to stressors and chronic stress response cycles, and what resources exist within and outside of the individual that facilitate a return to homeostasis or prohibit maintenance of a healthful internal homeostatic environment. The ***stress response cycle*** is a biologically adaptive response to stress, designed to equip an individual in navigating brief encounters of stress, completing the cycle when the individual returns to a state of balance or "normalcy." Note that homeostasis will shift and evolve over time, either due to increased resilience or as an adaptation to survival. This process is controlled by the central nervous system, which sends signals throughout the body about what is needed to meet the demands of an encounter when presented with a stressful situation. A cascade of hormones is released to activate the respiratory and cardiovascular systems; with increased oxygen flow to the brain, breathing becomes hastened, sharpening the senses and reflexes, allowing for the individual to be alert and responsive. With increased blood flow to the body, one's heart rate and blood pressure increases so blood and oxygen can saturate vital organs and limbs to prepare the body to react (ie, fight, flight, freeze, fawn). When an individual experiences this stress response cycle chronically, they are likely to notice a worsening of conditions such as panic attacks, asthma, emphysema, or bronchitis. The stress response cycle becoming a chronic physiological process due to toxic stress can also result in increased risk for developing high blood pressure, heart attacks, and strokes. One study states that "the chronic stress of living in impoverished and unhealthy conditions can overwhelm a child's stress response systems, causing what has been referred to as 'toxic stress.'"[4]

Violence is a toxic stress and can be part of environmental stressors an individual experiences via perpetuation, observation, or victimization. The American Psychological Association (APA) *Dictionary of Psychology* defines violence as "the expression of hostility and rage with the intent to injure or damage people or property through physical force."[5] In alignment with a systemic approach to trauma- and violence-informed care, this chapter will define and elaborate further on the impact of bilateral/bidirectional violence, unilateral perpetration and victimization, and systemic and structural violence.

Adverse Childhood Experiences

Adverse Childhood Experiences (ACEs) can have a lasting effect on children and adolescents well into adulthood. The Centers for Disease Control and Prevention (CDC) defines ACEs as potentially traumatic events that occur in childhood. ACEs can include violence, abuse, and growing up in a family system with mental health or substance use problems.[6] ACEs were identified and originally studied by the CDC in collaboration with Kaiser Permanente Insurance from 1995 to 1997, with over 17 000 participants.[7] The study was conducted to understand the effects on trauma exposure in children ages 0 to 17 years and observe associated health outcomes in adulthood, aiming to prove correlation and causation between early childhood experiences and the onset of preventable illnesses and ailments, disability, premature death, and diminished quality of life. While Kaiser's data collection process is ongoing, many states currently conduct their own data collection using the Behavioral Risk Factor Surveillance System (BRFSS). The results of the CDC-Kaiser Permanente study produced major insight into the understanding of ACEs' effects on specific populations and demographics. Of those findings, the data revealed that ACEs are common among all populations, with 1 in 5 of the original participants reporting exposure to 3 or more ACEs.[7] As the number of exposures to ACEs increases, so does the risk for negative outcomes if there are no or few protective or compensatory experiences to offset their impact. Among those participating in the CDC-Kaiser study, 54% were female and 46% were male, with 74% of participants identifying as White, non-Latinx, 11.2% Latinx, and the remaining population being other members of the Black, Indigenous, and people of color (BIPOC) community.[7] For the first time, a study of this size surveying affluent, middle class, White Americans, highlighted how common trauma exposure is in the United States regardless of privilege, sex, or socioeconomic status. This data also encouraged researchers, providers, and policy makers to think about the ways research around trauma has historically and erroneously focused on the pathologizing of BIPOC and marginalized individuals/communities, individuals identified as lower income earners, and those who live(d) in underresourced communities. A deeper data analysis of the ACEs study showed that some populations are more susceptible to ACEs due to a lack of resources available to or within their communities, poor economic conditions,[7] and the legacy of systemic and institutionalized racism, sexism, discrimination, and oppression.

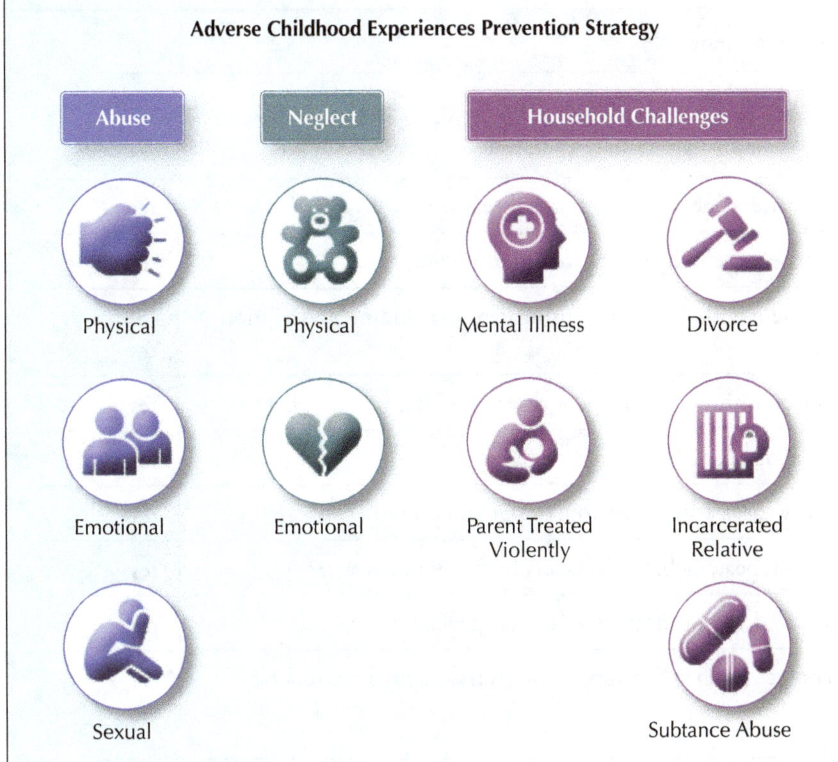

Figure 7-1

Figure 7-1. *National Center for Injury Prevention and Control: Adverse Childhood Experiences Prevention Strategy FY2021-FY2024.*[8]

The list of preventable traumatic events that contribute to ACEs is extensive and can be addressed in various ways with interventions implemented at the government, community, and familial level. The ACEs assessment surveys the following categories: abuse, neglect, and household challenges.

These categories reflect the most impactful forms of trauma on young children and adolescents. It is believed, for example, that 1 900 000 cases of heart disease and 21 000 000 cases of depression in the United States could be potentially avoided each year by preventing ACEs from occurring in the first place.[6] Additionally, 7 out of 10 leading adult causes of death (including heart disease, stroke, cancer, chronic obstructive pulmonary disease, diabetes, Alzheimer's, and suicide) are highly associated with exposure to ACEs.[6] In the United States, a survey conducted across 25 states noted that 61% of adults reported that they had experienced at least 1 type of ACE by the age of 18, and nearly 1 in 6 reported they had experienced 4 or more types of ACEs during childhood.[6]

The ACEs assessment (**Table 7-1**) is designed to serve as a measurement tool for adults to assess childhood violence and trauma exposure. If an adult scores 4 or more on this assessment and does not have compensatory experiences that neutralize the impact of these exposures, then existing research suggests that they are at extremely high risk of negative health outcomes later in life. These examples highlight just a few of the propensities for expected health outcomes with 4 or more ACEs[6]:

— 3 times the risk for heart disease or lung cancer

— 240% increased risk of hepatitis

— 390% increased risk of chronic pulmonary lung disease

— 460% increased risk of depression

— 1220% increased risk for attempted suicide

Table 7-1. Adverse Childhood Experiences Assessment

1. Did you ever feel that you did not have enough to eat, had to wear dirty clothes, or had no one to protect or take care of you?	Yes_____
2. Did you lose a parent through divorce, abandonment, death, or other reason?	Yes_____
3. Did you live with anyone who was depressed, mentally ill, or attempted suicide?	Yes_____
4. Did you live with anyone who had a problem with drinking or using drugs, including prescription drugs?	Yes_____
5. Did your parents or adults in your home ever hit, punch, beat, or threaten to harm each other?	Yes_____
6. Did you live with anyone who went to jail or prison?	Yes_____
7. Did a parent or adult in your home ever swear at you, insult you, or put you down?	Yes_____
8. Did a parent or adult in your home ever hit, beat, kick, or physically hurt you in any way?	Yes_____
9. Did you feel that no one in your family loved you or thought you were special?	Yes_____
10. Did you experience unwanted sexual contact (such as fondling or oral/anal/vaginal intercourse/penetration)?	Yes_____

Pediatric ACEs And Related Life-events Screener

In 2018, The **PE**diatric **A**CEs and **R**elated **L**ife-events **S**creener (PEARLS) was developed by the Bay Area Research Consortium on Toxic Stress and Health.[9] Much like the ACEs assessment, the PEARLS assessment measures the level of exposure one has had to adverse events during childhood; however, it expanded on the original ACEs assessment to include hardships and significant life events related to systemic and structural inequities and challenges. The ACEs assessment is for individuals over the age of 18 years, while the PEARLS assessment is designed for children 0 to 19 years of age. It is a tool rooted in the responsive nature of early intervention and treatment, designed to allow caregivers, clients, patients, and providers an opportunity to work in collaboration to identify a child's (or children's) current exposure to adversity or traumatic life events. There are 2 sections to the assessment: the first section includes the original questions from the ACEs assessment; the second section lists questions to assess toxic stress exposure. Research has supported the findings that the experiences listed in the second section of the assessment are "linked with poor physical, developmental, and behavioral health outcomes in childhood and throughout life."[4] There are 3 versions of the PEARLS assessment:

— ***Child P/C:*** Parent/caregiver reports on a child's (aged 0-11 years) experience; includes 17 questions.

— ***Teen P/C:*** Parent/caregiver reports on a teen's (aged 12-19 years) experience; includes 19 questions.

— ***Teen SR:*** Teen (aged 12-19 years) self-reports on his or her own experiences; includes 19 questions (**Table 7-2**).

Table 7-2. Part II of PEARLS Teen Self-Report Assessment[9]

1.	Have you ever seen, heard, or been a victim of violence in your neighborhood, community, or school? *(eg, targeted bullying, assault or other violent actions, war or terrorism)*	Yes_____
2.	Have you experienced discrimination? *(eg, being hassled or made to feel inferior or excluded because of your race, ethnicity, gender identity, sexual orientation, religion, learning differences, or disabilities)*	Yes_____
3.	Have you ever had problems with housing? *(eg, being homeless, not having a stable place to live, moved more than 2 times in a 6-month period, faced eviction or foreclosure, or had to live with multiple families or family members)*	Yes_____
4.	Have you ever worried that you did not have enough food to eat or that food would run out before you or your parent/caregiver could buy more?	Yes_____
5.	Have you ever been separated from your parent or caregiver due to foster care or immigration?	Yes_____
6	Have you ever lived with a parent/caregiver who had a serious physical illness or disability?	Yes_____
7.	Have you ever lived with a parent or caregiver who died?	Yes_____
8.	Have you ever been detained, arrested, or incarcerated?	Yes_____
9.	Have you ever experienced verbal or physical abuse or threats from a romantic partner?	Yes_____

Further, there are 2 formats for the PEARLS assessment: deidentified and identified. Deidentified allows respondents to indicate *how many* adverse life experiences have been experienced by the child or by themselves but does not require the person to indicate *which* life experiences. The deidentified assessment is for practices or providers wishing to identify vulnerable populations, namely those exposed to toxic stress or violence, in order to refer them out for further assessment and follow-up care. Scenarios wherein the deidentified version would be most appropriate include pediatrician offices during routine screening at well child visits. The provider could then refer a family to a counseling center if they screened as high risk. Another setting could include at a community-based organization during the intake process, such as an early head start program, who could refer the family to a social worker after completion of the assessment. The identified version requires respondents to specify, via a yes or no response, which experience(s) they have had or their child(ren) has had. It is best used by trained providers who have the skill and resources to address specific disclosure(s), can create a safety plan as needed, and can provide ongoing support for the child(ren) and family/caregivers.

Systemic and Community-Based Violence

The harm individuals suffer due to social structures and the institutions sustaining them is referred to as systemic violence. This violence prevents its victims from satisfying basic needs for survival and is ultimately avoidable.[10] Causes of systemic violence are rooted in social, economic, and political arrangements that limit or prevent individuals from actualizing wellness and wellbeing for themselves and their communities, echoing through politics, culture, law, and other arenas of power. These variables create an environment of injustice and oppression, reducing the quality of life and killing vulnerable populations prematurely. Examples of community adversity would be a lack of accessible or quality housing options, community violence, and community disruption, as seen in **Figure 7-2**.

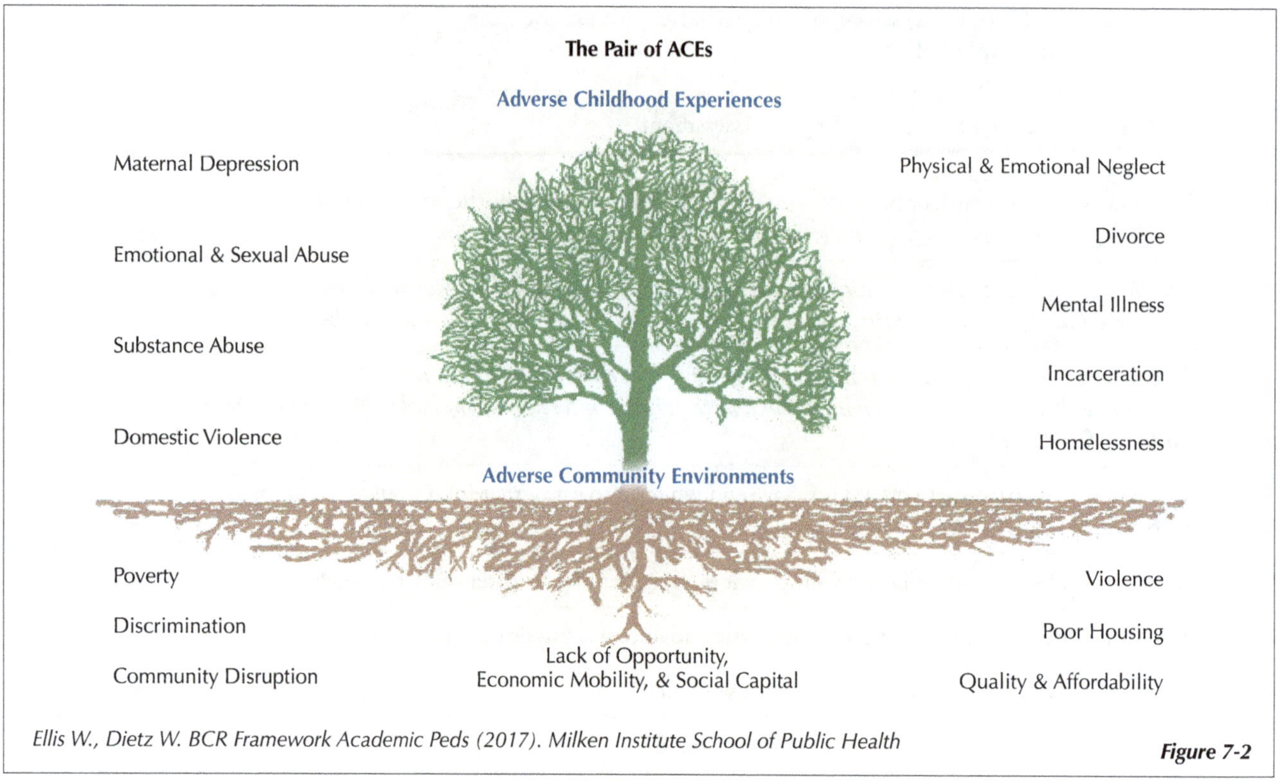

Figure 7-2. *The Pair of ACEs: In The Soil and in The Air.*[11]

More than 30 000 000 American children experience ACEs every year.[12] Parental perinatal mood and anxiety disorders (PMADs) are the number one complication of pregnancy and childbirth, affecting around 20% of birthing people, upwards of up to 60% of caregivers in specific populations.[13] PMADs is the term used to describe mood disorders that onset during pregnancy through the first year postpartum which include:

— Perinatal or postpartum mood disorder (depression)

— Perinatal or postpartum anxiety disorder

— Perinatal or postpartum psychosis

— Perinatal or postpartum obsessive-compulsive disorder (OCD)

All caregivers, birthing people, and support persons alike can be affected by PMADs. Research shows that parents navigating a PMAD have higher rates in the utilization of corporal punishment on their infants. Infants aged 0 to 12 months make up the highest rates of victimization for maltreatment and abuse, with 1/4 of all maltreatment and abuse happening before the age of 2 years.[14] The issue of PMADs is not an individual problem, it is a systemic failure; it is the manifestation of a lack of support at the personal and community level as well as the legal and political level. Research shows that parents who live in underresourced communities and households, identify as Black or Latinx, are recently migrated, or those who have become parents as adolescents have been associated with experiencing greater postpartum depressive symptoms.[15] However, studies have shown that racism and living in structurally marginalized communities, rather than parents' individual identities, are the factors that explain these increased occurrences of PMADs and the heightened severity of symptoms experienced.[15] When considering a solution to structural and socioeconomic inequities that increase the risk of ACEs, it is relevant to consider paid parental leave policies as 1 example of a systemic-level intervention. The United States has no national parental leave policy, though 178 other countries around the world do. As of 2021, only 9 states had paid leave programs with specific restrictions, and only 3 more states (Connecticut, Oregon, and Colorado) are expected to add similar policies by 2024. It is estimated that there could be in excess of 600 fewer infant deaths per year if the United States mandated national maternal leave, which calculates to a 2% to 3% decline in infant deaths for every guaranteed week of paid maternal leave.[16]

Limited economic upward mobility and opportunities are additional influences that contribute to adverse community environments. What this looks like in the real world goes against stereotypes and false narratives (eg, higher education is the antidote to poverty). College graduates without a college-educated parent have lower incomes and accumulate less wealth, on average, than those with a parent who has a bachelor's degree or higher.[16] "Cultural capital" is the privilege of generational knowledge that comes from having family members who have lived experiences of navigating often complicated or difficult to access processes, such as applying for and completing college successfully.

Figure 7-3. Pew Research Center.[17]

Adults with parents who are college-graduated are more likely to attain a bachelor's degree

% of adults who have completed at least a bachelor's degree, among those with...

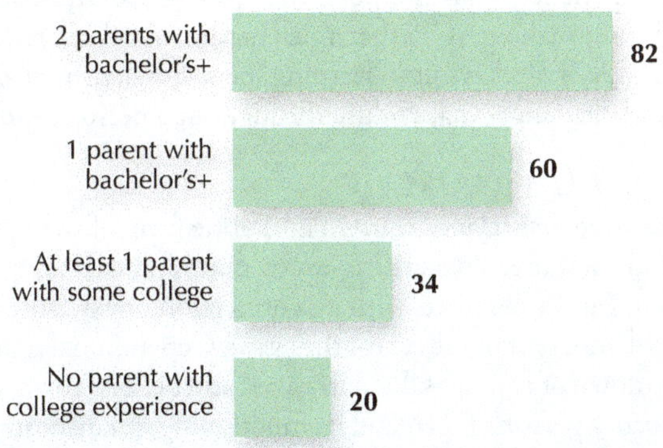

Note: Based on adults ages 22 to 59 with known parental education. "Some college" includes those with an associate degree, certificate, and those who attended college but did not obtain a degree

Source: Pew Research Center analysis of 2019 Survey of Household Economics and Decisionmaking

"First-Generation College Graduates Lag Behind Their Peers on Key Economic Outcomes"

Figure 7-3

Historically, the United States government and institutions therein have implemented systems with the purpose of intentionally excluding marginalized individuals from accessing resources equitably, such as purchasing a home or living in well-resourced and environmentally safe neighborhoods. In the 1940s and 1950s, "redlining" was a common practice meant to keep Black Americans out of suburban neighborhoods through racially restrictive covenants in home deeds and denials of loans to qualified applicants based on race, gender, religion, and ethnicity. While redlining became illegal when the Housing Act of 1968 was put into effect, the long-term impact of redlining is still prevalent in communities that are densely populated by BIPOC individuals even today. Neighborhoods in the United States, according to research conducted by the National Equity Project, are more racially segregated today than during the 1960s.[18] Concentrated levels of community-based violence occur in racially segregated and high poverty communities. In addition to a lack of adequate housing, BIPOC communities tend to experience fewer adequately funded and resourced schools within the community, minimal employment opportunities that foster economic stability, and an overall lack of opportunities for personal self-sufficiency. A report conducted by the 2018 Year Up Implementation and Early Impact Report noted that a lack of opportunities has a direct connection to increased substance misuse, increased health challenges, higher rates of crime and victimization, higher economic dependency, and higher rates of single parent, single income households.[19] On the opposite end of the spectrum, individuals who embody privileged identities and who live in communities primarily reflecting homogeneity in identity and socioeconomic status tend to experience little interaction with individuals that are a part of the BIPOC community. This lack of proximity forms implicit and explicit biases based on the portrayal of BIPOC individuals in the media.[18] This lack of exposure facilitates the perpetuation of harmful negative stereotypes in interpersonal interactions, retraumatization through culturally biased policy creation and service implementation, and continued institutionalized and systemic discrimination. Community disruption is the alteration, dysfunction, or breakdown of community-based social structures that serve to unify and strengthen a community.

If individuals are to be seen as intersectional beings in multitiered systems and structures, it must also be recognized how this pair of ACEs (ie, adverse childhood and community experiences) has the potential to foster dysfunction, disruption, disease, and death, only making ACEs that much harder to prevent, reduce, or address. The culmination of ACEs can result in learning, behavioral, mental, emotional, and physical delays and challenges that endure throughout a person's lifetime.[12]

Generational Trauma

Generational or ***intergenerational trauma*** is a subtle form of trauma that is passed down through families after a traumatic event occurs and healing has not been allowed to happen. Family members with no connection or exposure to the original traumatic event will inherent the effects of the event. Generational trauma is not only about the passing down of coping skills, narratives, and beliefs. Toxic stress caused by ACEs can transform a person's DNA and its functioning, predisposing and priming babies in utero for a world that is dangerous, thus requiring an altered expression of genetic material. This concept is referred to as epigenetic consequences.

Some individuals will go on to develop maladaptive, yet effective, coping strategies, such as negative or harmful behaviors that oppose social norms or engage in actions that lead to increased risk for harm to self or others. Generational inheritance of trauma can manifest as a learned fear or distrust of medical systems to access preventative medicine or treat new or chronic medical challenges and complications. This distrust in many communities is due to a long history of oppressive, racist, and discriminatory care practices in medical and mental health care systems. The challenge in addressing generational trauma is not necessarily rooted in a lack of desire or skill for healing; rather, there is a real barrier to move beyond assessment to treatment by connecting families with trauma-informed services designed to provide supportive interventions.[20] Building trust between providers and individuals is a crucial element in optimizing health outcomes for all. Trusting relationships between clients/patients and care providers can increase research around standardizing health treatments to become more equitable and inclusive, eliminating health care disparities and moving collectively towards health equity.[21]

Impact of Violence Exposure on IPV

During COVID-19, there was a significant increase in mental health challenges, barriers to seeking out and receiving health care, and heightened rates of violence and IPV. Research continues to support the undeniable correlational and causational nature of violence exposure on mental and physical health outcomes. Violence impacts both the micro and the macro, from an individual's worldview, beliefs, and actions to parenting philosophies, strategies, and skills, familial and community transmission of coping, and beliefs surrounding violence, resilience, and healing. This impact trickles out to shape society's overall profile of health and safety. It would then make sense that violence exposure has an impact on whether an individual will experience IPV or commit violence against another. There are 2 types of IPV: bilateral and unilateral. Within these types, violence is expressed through physical or sexual violence, stalking, and psychological (ie, mental and emotional) aggression.

Bilateral/Bidirectional Violence

Bidirectional violence is the engagement in violent behaviors by both people in a relationship. It can appear as both individuals being equally aggressive towards each other or one partner being more aggressive than the other, though the other partner is violent as well, often for the purpose of self-defense or to retaliate. A person who is experiencing violence and victimization that reacts with violence to resist or defend themselves is not likely to be violent in other relationships, though it is not unlikely for the primary aggressor to feel victimized as well. This is where the philosophy of trauma- and violence-informed language meets practical application. People have the capacity to both experience and perpetuate violence, which means a clearly defined "victim"/"perpetrator" binary can be harder to discern and inadequately meet the treatment needs of all individuals involved. According to Denise Hines, a leading IPV expert and researcher, "most studies, including recent national IPV studies (eg, National Intimate Partner and Sexual Violence Survey, National Crime Victimization Survey), ask about only victimization and do not assess perpetration of IPV, so we do not have strong current nationally representative data on bidirectionality. The National Family Violence Surveys in 1975 and 1985 did ask about victimization and perpetration, and they found high rates of both partners using violence. Unfortunately, that national study has not been conducted in more than 39 years."[22] In a review exploring 48 studies that had occurred over 20+ years, researchers found the following significant and illuminating data[23]:

- In 57.9% of violent relationships, both partners behaved violently.
- Regardless of the sample population studied, bidirectional violence was more common than unilateral violence.
- There are no gender differences when it comes to bidirectional violence.
- Men and women are equally likely to be the primary aggressor (if there is one).
- Women, much more often than men, report violence against them and seek help.
- There was no difference studied in directionality for gay, lesbian, or bisexual individuals.
- There appears to be higher rates of bidirectional violence among Black couples.

Unilateral/Unidirectional Violence

Unidirectional violence, or violence that is perpetrated by one person towards another, without reciprocal violence, occurs far less often than bidirectional violence. While unilateral violence is less common, female-perpetrated violence was seen as occurring in higher rates (than male to female perpetration) in 4 out of 5 sample types.[24] Unilateral violence perpetrated by a female partner against a male partner occurs in up to 37% of reported IPV cases, which is twice as prevalent as unidirectional violence committed by male partners towards female partners.[25]

The exception to this was "found only in criminal justice/legal studies that relied on police reports of IPV perpetration and/or in samples drawn from the United States' military."[25]

IPV, Family Violence, and Suicide: Childhood Exposure and Outcomes

"Violence becomes traumatic when the victim does not have the ability to consent or dissent, which, in turn, is linked with the universal experience of helplessness and hopelessness engendered by victimization."[24] Children are inherently dependent upon their caregivers, and therefore are unable to assert their will to avoid or engage in violence that may be happening around or to them. This dynamic of powerlessness creates an increased likelihood that violence experienced by children will be perceived and integrated as traumatic.

It is important to note the ways in which bilateral/bidirectional violence translates into loss of life, including its impact on families and children. Data from The National Family Violence Surveys further compel the necessity for deeper discussions and more consistently utilized screening tools to assess for IPV suicidality and homicidal tendencies in pediatric and adult clients receiving social services, medical care, and mental health care.

According to the CDC, women who are exposed to IPV are almost 5 times more likely to attempt suicide than women who have not been exposed, with more than 25% of female-completed suicides citing "intimate partner problems" when the precipitating factor was known.[26] Conversely, a study that collected data statewide found males who commit violence against their partners represented most IPV-related suicides and often disclosed suicidal ideations prior to attempting suicide.[27]

While IPV witnessed by a child is focused on adult violence that occurs to a caregiver, it is often not mutually exclusive from childhood maltreatment, which is violence directed specifically at the child. Understanding the rates of occurrence and compounding variables between violence, childhood maltreatment, IPV, suicide, and homicide, there is enough evidence to declare identifying those at risk for victimization as a high priority for providers in all fields, across all disciplines. The common co-occurrence of these violent experiences makes it difficult to separate one's impact from the other on childhood development, physically and psychologically. In addition to witnessing IPV, children are further impacted by their caregiver's response and recovery from violent experiences, which many times results in insufficient resources for sensitive and consistent caregiving.[28] For children to grow into healthy adults, they need attuned and responsive caregivers with whom they can form consistent and safe attachments. Safety and consistency, when modeled frequently in coping strategies reliant upon coregulation, is at the core of developing healthy emotional regulation and resilience. Investing in coordinated strategies to help young adults cope with childhood adversity could reduce IPV rates for individuals in their early 20s. Research shows young adults with scores of 1 to 3 and greater than 4 ACEs experience higher rates of verbal and physical victimization and perpetration, as well as a greater risk for escalation in IPV behaviors, as compared to individuals with 0 ACEs.[29]

Protective and Compensatory Experiences

Individuals are not static in their growth or capacity for learning. Specific positive experiences can reduce or cancel out the long-term impact and potential for adversity to manifest and enhance resilience within a person. A core belief care providers may consider adopting is the understanding that all people want to be well and live healthy, happy lives, free of violence. Bodies are in a constant cycle of repair and healing, doing everything in their power to keep themselves alive and functioning, even when dysfunction is present.

The protective and compensatory experiences (PACEs) questionnaire for adults is designed to assess one's propensity towards resilience and calculate an individual's potential to offset ACEs. A PACEs score subtracted from an ACEs score predicts a person's likelihood for reducing chronic physical ailments, increasing mental and emotional wellbeing, and decreasing the potential for suicidality, domestic violence, homicide, and substance misuse. The experiences listed in **Table 7-3** involve the consistent engagement of a child with systems outside of their family unit, as well as conditions in the home that require stability, predictability, and basic needs being met. Positive parenting practices, for example, have been studied to provide robust amounts of psychological protection, regardless of ACEs. This evidence suggests that positive parenting (ie, gentle parenting) is significant in mediating the impact of abuse and violence, especially for children who are chronically exposed to high levels of adversity or toxic stress.[30] While generational patterns of parenting can be learned and familial, social and cultural beliefs shape parenting choices and behaviors equally, if not more impactfully. The resources available to a caregiver influence whether they can be a responsive provider. Resources include system-wide screenings for mental health, suicide, and IPV; access to mental health services that are free of shame, punishment, or threat; investment in early childhood education and accessible childcare options; increased parenting education; and universal parental leave. When caregivers experience PACEs, they tend to have greater access to stable income and education as adults. Additionally, there is a positive correlation to nurturing parenting attitudes,[31] which decrease the likelihood for violence, abuse, and maltreatment and increase exposure to PACEs in children, fostering an environment of safety and a foundation for wellbeing.

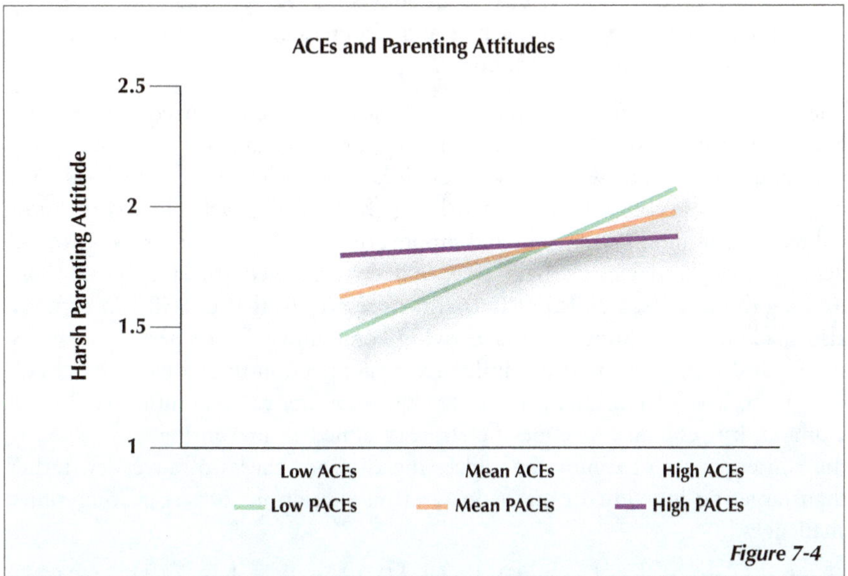

Figure 7-4. *ACEs and Parenting Attitudes: the role of cumulative protection in understanding resilience.*[31]

Table 7-3. PACEs Assessment[30]

1. Did you have someone who loved you unconditionally (you did not doubt that they cared about you)?	Yes_____
2. Did you have at least 1 best friend (someone you could trust and had fun with)?	Yes_____
3. Did you do anything regularly to help others (eg, volunteer at a hospital, nursing home, church) or do special projects in the community to help others (food drives, Habitat for Humanity)?	Yes_____
4. Were you regularly involved in organized sports groups (eg, soccer, basketball, track) or other physical activity (eg, competitive cheer, gymnastics, dance, marching band)?	Yes_____

(continued)

Table 7-3. PACEs Assessment[30] *(continued)*	
5. Were you an active member of at least 1 civic group or a non-sport social group such as scouts, church, or youth group?	Yes_____
6. Did you have an engaging hobby—an artistic or intellectual pastime either alone or in a group (eg, chess club, debate team, musical instrument or vocal group, theater, spelling bee, reading a lot)?	Yes_____
7. Was there an adult (not a parent) you could trust and could count on when you needed help or advice (eg, coach, teacher, minister, neighbor, relative)?	Yes_____
8. Was your home typically clean AND safe with enough food to eat?	Yes_____
9. Overall, did your school provide the resources and academic experiences that you needed to learn?	Yes_____
10. In your home, were rules clear and fairly administered?	Yes_____

Building Community Resilience

Community resilience is defined as[32]:

> "the ability of households, communities, and nations to absorb and recover from shocks, whilst positively adapting and transforming their structures and means for living in the face of long-term stresses, change and uncertainty. Resilience is about addressing the root causes of crises while strengthening the capacities and resources of a system in order to cope with risks, stresses, and shocks."

There is a complexity to the interconnected risks (eg, violence and conflict, natural hazards, economic shocks) and stressors (eg, urbanization, ageing populations) a community may face, which means health care and social service providers must intentionally and compassionately work together to collectively identify the most vulnerable community members and support them at all levels of care. **Figure 7-2** depicts a tree planted in soil that is steeped in systemic inequities and dysfunction, robbing the tree (ie, a child) of nutrients necessary to thrive, which in turn are also inadequate for supporting a thriving community. Every person, in every system and institution that has influence or connection to any part of a child's life or the lives of families, can positively contribute to community resilience. Community resilience is a specific strategy aimed at preventing and reducing the consequences of trauma by addressing the root causes of adversity, rather than targeting individual expressions and manifestations of larger community challenges.[12]

The goal of this targeted approach is to bridge the science behind ACEs/PACEs and the social determinants of health to begin actualizing trauma- and violence-informed care in real world health care settings, which also necessitates implementing comprehensive public policies designed with community stakeholders' integral feedback. PACEs paired with systemic changes towards a more just and equitable society create buffers or resilience characteristics with individuals. Community resilience aims to strengthen these characteristics at each level in the system by coordinating care across sectors and disciplines (**Table 7-4**).

Risk and Resilience Screening

Who Gets Screened?

There is a 20-year difference in life expectancy for children left untreated who have experienced 4 or more ACEs as compared to children who have experienced less than 3 ACEs.[3] Not to screen all patients and clients for chronic stress, violence, and trauma exposure would be a grossly irresponsible and blatantly problematic misstep for educational, social, medical, and mental health professionals and a disregard for medical professionals' ethical commitment to do no harm. The American Academy of Pediatrics and the American Academy of Nursing recommend primary care providers screen children for behavioral and emotional challenges during routine care visits, including the use of mental health screening tools for their caregivers.[4] There are gender differences present in individual willingness to disclose when trauma is separated out by childhood sexual abuse (CSA) and other forms of abuse. One study found victims of CSA were less likely to disclose their experiences, particularly when it was more severe (ie, involving physical contact) as compared to victims who experienced other forms of abuse, with young males being least likely to disclose CSA whether it involved physical contact or not.[33] All people, regardless of insurance status, in all social service and health care settings, need to be considered for IPV, trauma, and suicide screenings.

Table 7-4. Resilience Factors[12]

Individual-Level Buffers	Family-Level Buffers	Community-Level Buffers
Personal characteristics	Resources	Peer relationships
Personal traits	Supportive relationships	Nonfamily relationships
Intellect	Family coherence	Nonfamily social support
Self-efficacy	Parental relationship	Religion
Coping skills	Stable caregiving	Community cohesion
Appraisal of adversity or maltreatment	Spousal support	Civic engagement
Life satisfaction	Stable employment	Economic development

How Often?

As of 2020, the California Department of Health Care Services (DHCS) is working with the California Office of the Surgeon General to reduce ACEs exposure by 50% within 1 generation.[33] Currently, Medicaid will only allow providers to screen children when it is deemed medically necessary, once per year, per provider, per facility, and adults are allowed once in their adult lifetime up to age 65, per provider, per facility.[34] While these recommendations are a step in the right direction, most professionals are not routinely screening for violence exposure or suicidal ideations consistently, if at all, or in the case of Medicaid eligible reimbursable services, providers are limited in how often they can screen a patient and be reimbursed. When screening individuals for IPV, the American Psychiatric Association also recommends screening for suicide risk at the same time. 50% of medical providers and 23% of behavioral health providers did not screen for IPV at all in 2020.[2] Medical providers cited a lack of preparation to assess and respond to IPV disclosures as their biggest barrier to screening. Community organizations, educational institutions, and other social services can help bridge this gap in screening by coordinating with local agencies and organizations to identify sustainable networks of support to refer clients to once they have been screened. Deidentified screening tools and self-assessments can flag violence-impacted clients/patients for further assessment or referral without the necessity of additional expertise on the care provider's part.

When and Where Do Providers Screen?

How caregivers, community members, and providers handle disclosures can directly enhance or validate the traumatic experience(s) being shared, resulting in the potential for retraumatization or movement towards healing. If providers are to approach screening as a multidisciplinary effort, one needs only to look at data surrounding the power of screening in all care service environments, such as employment service programs. One study found a strong correlation with high trauma exposure and challenges with securing stable employment and employability.[35] When a trauma-informed protocol was put into place at an employment services program aimed at serving low-income urban residents, which included a trauma exposure screening paired with short-term interventions and referrals to treatment, they found that 90% of clients had experienced 2 or more traumatic life events, 49% of clients met the criteria for PTSD, 35% met the criteria for depression, and 48% met the criteria for generalized anxiety. Screening was received positively by 83% of clients and all clients completed all components of the protocol, which led to 57% of clients accepting a referral specifically to mental health care services and more than 75% accepting referrals to an outside service including primary or mental health care.[34] In 1 study where social workers provided universal trauma screenings (HITS: Hurt, Insult, Threaten, Scream and SAVE: sexual violence screening surveys) at Level I Trauma Centers in the United States over the course of a year, they found that 1 in 9 patients were at risk for IPV and sexual violence, regardless of sex or gender.[36] The Sumner M. Redstone Global Center for Prevention and Wellness suggests the strategies listed in **Table 7-5** for engaging across sectors, professions, and audiences in preventing ACEs (or increasing PACEs).[12]

Table 7-5. BCR Tools for Coalition Building, Communication, and Strategy Development[12]

Sector	Decision-maker	Where does their work/values align with prevention of the Pair of ACEs? Examples below	What is your ask? Examples below
Faith-based organizations	Local pastor, imam, youth minister, or faith-based homeless shelter director	— Serving their congregation to support health and wellbeing — Connecting with a variety of services and resources to provide the congregation and the community — Connecting with a larger network of trauma-informed support for congregation members in need	— Join the coalition — Become a trauma-informed organization or have staff trained to identify the Pair of ACEs in the congregation
Education	Elementary school principal, middle school counselor, day care director, or a school board member	— Building the foundation for lifelong success and learning — Developing school-based social supports so that children come to school fed, safe, healthy, and ready to learn — Supporting early detection of behavioral issues and healthy child development — Implementing alternatives to suspension	— Join the coalition — Become a trauma-informed organization or have staff trained to identify children exposed to the Pair of ACEs — Advocate for school board policy changes or additional resources to address issues in the classroom

(continued)

Table 7-5. BCR Tools for Coalition Building, Communication, and Strategy Development[12] *(continued)*

Sector	Decision-maker	Where does their work/values align with prevention of the Pair of ACEs? Examples below	What is your ask? Examples below
Parents and caregivers	Also consider caregivers of young children: mothers, fathers, grandparents	— Providing optimal environments and supports for their children (caregivers may experience barriers, such as working several jobs or long hours, an absent or abusive spouse, or lack of dependable transportation or safe spaces for their children to play)	— Join the coalition — Take a positive parenting class — Lead a parenting group in the neighborhood — Talk to the local leaders, neighborhood council, or school board for support, policy changes, or additional resources
Health care systems	CEO, community affairs director, head of pediatrics, or a physician-advocate	— Providing trauma-sensitive care — Bridging medical care with community resources to improve health outcomes	— Join the coalition — Introduce trauma-informed care within the health care system — Meet with local funders and policymakers to discuss Pair of ACEs in the community

Summary

The acknowledgment of the harm that is pervasive in our society cannot overshadow the unique abilities and strengths that individuals and communities have cultivated to rebound from trauma and grow forward. Likewise, no matter how many interventions or assessments are practiced or perfected, none of them replace the ongoing need for system-wide reform towards equitable and culturally responsive care. Providers are agents of social change and their work requires them to advocate and amplify the voices of those served. Violence prevention and the promotion of resiliency starts at the systemic and organizational levels. Through a commitment to advocacy, the inclusion of community stakeholders' voices, and collaboration across disciplines, providers can ensure that policy becomes practice.

Resources

Table 7-6. Resources

Organization	Description	Website
211	Most comprehensive source of information about local resources and services in the United States	https://www.211.org
Behavioral Risk Factor Surveillance System (BRFSS)	Largest continuously conducted health survey system in the world, with annual data about health behaviors and conditions from all 50 states and 3 territories	https://www.cdc.gov/brfss/index.html

(continued)

Table 7-6. Resources *(continued)*

Organization	Description	Website
PACES Connection	Connects those who are implementing trauma-informed and resilience-building practices based on ACEs science	https://www.acesconnectioninfo.com

References

1. US Department of Health and Human Services, Administration for Children and Families, Administration on Children, Youth and Families, Children's Bureau. *Child Maltreatment 2019.* US Department of Health and Human Services. 2021. https://www.acf.hhs.gov/sites/default/files/documents/cb/cm2019.pdf
2. Jackson EC, Renner LM, Flowers NI, Logeais ME, Clark CJ. Process evaluation of a systemic intervention to identify and support partner violence survivors in a multi-specialty health system. *BMC Health Serv Res.* 2020;20(1):996. doi: 10.1186/s12913-020-05809-y
3. Yule K, Houston J, Grych J. Resilience in children exposed to violence: a meta-analysis of protective factors across ecological contexts. *Clin Child Fam Psychol Rev.* 2019;22(3):406-431. doi:10.1007/s10567-019-00293-1
4. Francis L, DePriest K, Wilson M, Gross D. Child poverty, toxic stress, and social determinants of health: screening and care coordination. *Online J Issues Nurs.* 2018;23(3):2. doi:10.3912/OJIN.Vol23No03Man02
5. Violence. APA Dictionary of Psychology. https://dictionary.apa.org/violence
6. Adverse childhood experiences: preventing early trauma to improve adult health. Centers for Disease Control and Prevention. 2021. https://www.cdc.gov/vital-signs/ aces/index.html
7. About the CDC-Kaiser ACE study. Centers for Disease Control and Prevention. 2021. https://www.cdc.gov/violenceprevention/aces/about.html
8. National Center for Injury Prevention and Control. Adverse childhood experiences prevention strategy. Centers for Disease Control and Prevention. 2021. https://www.cdc.gov/injury/pdfs/priority/ACEs-Strategic-Plan_Final_508.pdf
9. PEARLS PEdiatric ACEs and Related Life Events Screener. ACEs Aware. 2019. https://www.acesaware.org/pdf_wrapper/pearls-tool-child-parent-care-giver-report-identified-english-rev-7-26-22/
10. Ruggiero V. *Visions of Political Violence.* Routledge; 2019.
11. Ellis WR, Dietz WH. A new framework for addressing adverse childhood and community experiences: the building community resilience model. *Acad Pediatr.* 2017;17(7S):S86-S93. doi:10.1016/j.acap.2016.12.011
12. Building community resilience: coalition building and communications guide. Ascend Aspen Institute. 2017. https://ascend.aspeninstitute.org/wp-content/uploads/2017/10/BCR20Coalition20Building20and20Communications-20Guide.pdf
13. Hodgkinson S, Godoy L, Beers LS, Lewin A. Improving mental health access for low-income children and families in the primary care setting. *Pediatrics.* 2017;139(1):e20151175. doi:10.1542/peds.2015-1175

14. US Department of Health and Human Services, Administration for Children and Families, Administration on Children, Youth and Families, Children's Bureau. *Child Maltreatment 2020.* US Department of Health and Human Services. January 19, 2022. https://www.acf.hhs.gov/cb/data-research/child-maltreatment

15. Feinberg E, Declercq E, Lee A, Belanoff C. The relationship between social support and postnatal anxiety and depression: results from the listening to mothers in California survey. *Women's Health Issues.* 2022;32(3):251-260. doi:10.1016/j.whi.2022.01.005

16. Byatt N, Levin LL, Ziedonis D, Moore Simas TA, Allison J. Enhancing participation in depression care in outpatient perinatal care settings: a systematic review. *Obstet Gynecol.* 2015;126(5):1048-1058. doi:10.1097/AOG.0000000000001067

17. Fry R. First-generation college graduates lag behind their peers on key economic outcomes. Pew Research Center. 2021. https://www.pewresearch.org/social-trends/2021/05/18/first-generation-college-graduates-lag-behind-their-peers-on-key-economic-outcomes/#:~:text=They%20tend%20to%20earn%20more,who%20have%20college%2Deducated%20parents.

18. Osta K, Vasquez H. Implicit bias and structural racialization. National Equity Project. https://www.nationalequityproject.org/frameworks/implicit-bias-structural-racialization

19. Fein D, Hamadyk J. *Bridging the Opportunity Divide for Low-Income Youth: Implementation and Early Impacts of the Year Up Program.* US Department of Health and Human Services; 2018.

20. Isobel S, McCloughen A, Goodyear M, Foster K. Intergenerational trauma and its relationship to mental health care: a qualitative inquiry. *Community Ment Health J.* 2021;57(4):631-643. doi:10.1007/s10597-020-00698-1

21. Griffith DM, Bergner EM, Fair AS, Wilkins CH. Using mistrust, distrust, and low trust precisely in medical care and medical research advances health equity. *Am J Prev Med.* 2021;60(3):442-445. doi:10.1016/j.amepre.2020.08.019

22. Cunningham M. Depp-Heard trial shines light on bidirectional intimate partner violence. George Mason University. 2022. https://www.gmu.edu/news/2022-06/depp-heard-trial-shines-light-bidirectional-intimate-partner-violence

23. Langhinrischsen-Roling J, Misra TA, Selwyn CN, Rohling ML. Rates of bidirectional versus unidirectional intimate partner violence across samples, sexual orientations, and race/ethnicities: a comprehensive review. *Partner Abuse.* 2012;3(2):1-2. doi:10.1891/1946-6560.3.2.e3

24. Hine B, Noku L, Bates EA, Jayes K. But, who is the victim here? exploring judgments toward hypothetical bidirectional domestic violence scenarios. *J Interpers Violence.* 2022;37(7-8):NP5495-NP5516. doi:10.1177/0886260520917508

25. Murphy EM. Predicting the likelihood of dating violence perpetration in a sample of women: unidirectional versus bidirectional violence. Old Dominion University. 2020. https://digitalcommons.odu.edu/psychology_etds/349

26. National Violent Death Reporting System (NVDRS). Centers for Disease Control and Prevention. 2019. https://www.cdc.gov/violenceprevention/datasources/nvdrs/index.html

27. Kafka JM, Moracco KBE, Taheri C, et al. Intimate partner violence victimization and perpetration as precursors to suicide. *SSM Popul Health*. 2022;18:101079. doi:10.1016/j.ssmph.2022.101079

28. Mueller I, Tronick E. Early life exposure to violence: developmental consequences on brain and behavior. *Front Behav Neurosci.* 2019;13:156. doi:10.3389/fnbeh.2019.00156

29. Forster M, Rogers CJ, Rainisch B, et al. Adverse childhood experiences and intimate partner violence; findings from a community sample of hispanic young adults. *J Interpers Violence.* 2022;37(19-20):NP18291-NP18316. doi:10.1177/08862605211035881

30. Yamaoka Y, Bard D. Positive parenting matters in the face of early adversity. *Am J Prev Med.* 2019;56(4):530-539. doi:10.1016/j.amepre.2018.11.018

31. Morris AS, Hays-Grudo J, Zapata MI, Treat A, Kerr KL. Adverse and protective childhood experiences and parenting attitudes: the role of cumulative protection in understanding resilience. *Advers Resil Sci.* 2021;2(3):181-192. doi:10.1007/s42844-021-00036-8

32. Risk and resilience. OECD. 2017. https://www.oecd.org/dac/conflict-fragility-resilience/risk-resilience/

33. Lev-Wiesel R, First M. Willingness to disclose child maltreatment: CSA vs other forms of child abuse in relation to gender. *Child Abuse Negl.* 2018;79:183-191. doi:10.1016/j.chiabu.2018.02.010

34. Trauma screenings and trauma-informed care provider trainings. Department of Health Care Services. 2019. https://www.dhcs.ca.gov/provgovpart/Pages/TraumaCare.aspx

35. Topitzes J, Mersky JP, Mueller DJ, Bacalso E, Williams C. Implementing trauma screening, brief intervention, and referral to treatment (T-SBIRT) within employment services: a feasibility trial. *Am J Community Psychol.* 2019;64(3-4):298-309. doi:10.1002/ajcp.12361

36. Zakrison TL, Ruiz X, Gelbard R, et al. Universal screening for intimate partner and sexual violence in trauma patients: an EAST multicenter trial. *J Trauma Acute Care Surg.* 2017;83(1):105-110. doi:10.1097/TA.0000000000001495

Chapter 8

Implications of Personality Structure on Violent Offenders

Deborah St. Germain, DNP, RN, AFN-C, SANE-A, SANE-P
Paul Thomas Clements, PhD, RN, AFN-C™, ANEF, DF-IAFN, DF-AFN

Key Points

1. *The strongest risk factors for interpersonal violence include maladaptive substance use, psychotic disorders, and externalizing personality traits.*
2. *Perpetrators with personality disorders show a higher prevalence of anxiety, drug dependence, and alcohol use, which facilitates violent behavior among this group and is a predictor for recidivism for sexually violent offenders.*

Background and Significance

Since the 1980s, interpersonal violence in the United States has become a major public health issue resulting in an immense amount of violence research, which has impacted the development and implementation of violence prevention programs. Yet, the number of victims of violence, survivors, and perpetrators has continuously risen.[1] This violence encompasses many behaviors, not only physical, but also verbal, sexual, emotional, economic, social, and psychological harming behaviors.[2] It can appear as intimate partner violence (IPV), child abuse, elder abuse, and other forms of familial violence.[1] Even a mother and her growing fetus in an unwanted pregnancy may be the target of violence. Others at risk for violence can include siblings, parents, neighbors, friends, acquaintances, or strangers.[3]

Perpetration of violence may take many forms to create fear by leveraging threats and taking actions through the use of technology, photography, digital platforms, and in-person.[4] Certain communities and their members are increasingly vulnerable and at higher risk for interpersonal violence. Globally, lifetime rates of interpersonal violence in females older than 15 years is approximately 30%.[2] Frequently, this violence results in life-altering changes, including physical and psychological injury, substance and alcohol misuse, post-traumatic stress symptomology, suicidal ideation, premature death from stress-induced diseases, and homicide.[5-8] According to the Centers for Disease Control and Prevention (CDC), more than 55% of homicides are related to IPV. Notably, Black, Indigenous, and Hispanic women are murdered at significantly higher rates than women of other races.[7]

For centuries, researchers have studied populations and identified risk factors that increase vulnerability to interpersonal violence *victimization*.[1] However, a growing body of literature focuses on risk factors for interpersonal violence *perpetration*.[5] And, even though men are identified as the main perpetrators of such violence, women are also known to perpetrate interpersonal violence and are not to be overlooked.[8,9] Interestingly, the results of multiple systematic reviews have revealed that those who engage in violent behavior engage in multiple forms of violence.[8,9] Worldwide, a—typically male—partner or spouse is the killer in 38% of women's homicides.[10] In the findings from one large-scale systematic review, many male perpetrators revealed they rationalized killing their intimate partner, deflected responsibility for their actions, and adhered to strict gender norms.[9]

Fazel et al[4] reviewed 22 meta-analyses that identified risk factors for interpersonal violence. The findings noted that neuropsychiatric disorders, specifically personality disorders (PD), were among the strongest risk factors, followed by substance use disorders, and witnessing or being a victim of violence in childhood. Two reviews focused on homicides only, which revealed 2 neuropsychiatric risk factors: schizophrenia and substance misuse. In a contemporary article appearing in *Clinical Psychology Review*, Collison & Lynam[10] took an in-depth look at IPV and the personality characteristics of both victims and perpetrators of violent IPV. Their research revealed that PDs were significantly and positively related to IPV perpetration. Results were more mixed for IPV victimization.

PDs are classified by one's way of thinking, feeling, and behaving that deviates from culture's expectations, causing distress or problems functioning, and lasts over time.[11] PDs affect at least 2 of the following areas: ways of thinking about oneself and others, responding emotionally, relating to other people, and controlling one's behavior.[11] It is believed to be caused by a combination of genetic and environmental factors.[12] Traits of PD may become less severe with age, but certain traits may persist to some degree after acute symptoms have prompted a diagnostic evaluation.[13] The *Diagnostic and Statistical Manual of Mental Disorders, Fifth Edition Text Revision* (DSM-5-TR)[14] groups the 10 types of personality disorders into 3 clusters (A, B, and C), based on similar characteristics. However, the clinical usefulness of these clusters has not been established. According to Zimmerman[13]:

Table 8-1. DSM-5 Personality Disorders

Cluster A	Cluster B	Cluster C
Characterized by appearing odd or eccentric	Characterized by appearing dramatic, emotional, or erratic	Characterized by appearing anxious or fearful
Paranoid: Mistrust and suspicion	*Antisocial:* Social irresponsibility, disregard for others, deceitfulness, and manipulation of others for personal gain	*Avoidant:* Avoidance of interpersonal contact due to rejection sensitivity
Schizoid: Disinterest in others	*Borderline:* Inner emptiness, unstable relationships, and emotional dysregulation	*Dependent:* Submissiveness and a need to be taken care of
Schizotypal: Eccentric ideas and behavior	*Histrionic:* Attention seeking and excessive emotionality	*Obsessive-compulsive:* Perfectionism, rigidity, and obstinacy
	Narcissistic: Self-grandiosity, need for admiration, and lack of empathy	

However, in 2013, the American Psychiatric Association included an alternative model of personality disorders (AMPD) in the *Diagnostic and Statistical Manual for Mental Disorders, Fifth Edition* (DSM-5), which focused heavily on the trait model. Following this reframing, a large number of publications focused on the AMPD's Criterion B, which consists of 25 trait facets arranged in 5 broad domains that are similar to the established five-factor model (FFM) of personality.[15] According to Krueger & Hobbs,[16] the AMPD's general criteria for PD consist of 7 individual criteria, A through G.

The first, Criterion A, refers to personality functioning. In the AMPD, the prerequisite of PD is evidence that the patient encounters difficulties with personality functioning, where functioning is understood as impairment in the sense of self and corresponding impairment in interpersonal functioning. Criterion B refers to pathological personality traits. These traits are organized around 5 broad domains: Negative Affectivity, Detachment, Antagonism, Disinhibition, and Psychoticism. These domains are generally well understood as maladaptive variants of the domains of the FFM of normative personality structure. In the AMPD, PD is defined as the combination of clinically significant problems in functioning along with 1 or more pathological traits. In addition to these 2 primary criteria, Criteria C and D refer to inflexibility and stability across time, respectively. Criteria E, F, and G refer to ensuring that the PD is not better explained by "another mental disorder" (E), the effects of a substance, or a medical condition (F), and is not normative for the person's developmental stage or sociocultural environment (G).

These personality domains frequently correlate with the personality characteristics of offenders who perpetrate IPV.[17-19] In addition to social and environmental factors, individual personality traits have become noted to be intricately linked with maladaptive behavior.[20,21] Thus, studies have included examining the link between individual personality traits and criminality.[20-22] Substantial empirical research suggests that psychopathy is a robust predictor of criminal behavior, mainly focusing on instrumental violence, which refers to violence that is employed as a means to an end to attain a subsidiary goal and can be contrasted with reactive violence, which involves a response to a perceived threat or provocation.[17,20] Furthermore, many scholars agree that instrumental violence among psychopathic offenders is significantly determined by the affective traits of psychopathy.[17,20,22] Factors that contribute to high recidivism include a lack of understanding of legal concepts, lack of control over their desires, high degree of impulsivity and aggression, lack of shame, distorted emotions, irresponsible and superficial emotions, inability to benefit from past experiences of punishment, and damage to conscience.[23-25]

When framed within the FFM[26] personality traits, in particular low agreeableness, low conscientiousness, and high neuroticism, have previously been associated with increased aggression, low stress tolerance, and antisocial behavior. Interestingly, the same personality characteristics have also been consistently linked to mental distress and increased risk of psychopathology. This is of relevance as both individual personality differences and mental distress (ie, subclinical symptoms of stress and depression) have been found to influence important factors in the treatment of violent offenders (eg, treatment motivation).

The Effect of Personality Disorders on Relationships

People who have untreated PDs may demonstrate the following traits[14,20]:

— Sensitivity to rejection or abandonment

— Poor social skills

— Hostility toward a gender

— High levels of dependence

— Controlling behaviors

— Heightened feelings of rage

— Acts of mental and/or physical abuse

— Extreme jealousy

— Unpredictability

— Extreme sensitivity

— Low self-esteem

— Morbid insecurity

Therefore, it is not surprising that a person with an abusive PD might commit spousal abuse or relational abuse, including abuse of a parent, child, or elder.[26,27] These behaviors can take a serious toll on a relationship and undermine the safety of those being victimized.[1,2,28] More significant is that these behaviors will often be repeated and at times be more intense than previous events.[22] The cycle repeats itself when the abusive partner shows remorse after an abusive incident, but while their condition remains untreated, and typically unmanageable, repeating violent events will eventually occur again.[1,4,21,22] This is why IPV is seldom a "one-and-done" event. It is invariably chronic and may even escalate to murder.[29] Therefore, a person who suffers from a PD and has a tendency toward aggression may be at higher risk of perpetrating IPV.[10,30,31] While the initial signs may not always be easily identifiable, listed[11,32-34] are some signs to carefully monitor for that can indicate personality traits of an abuser and behaviors associated with IPV:

— Routine criticizing

— Blames the victim for their outbursts/behaviors

— Makes unfounded accusations

— Displays controlling behaviors (eg, instructs partner what to wear)

— Throws objects

— Punches walls or kicks furniture

— Physically attacks their partner

— Prevents partner from getting medical care

— Shows aggression toward household pets

— Prevents partner from seeing friends/family

— Restricts partner's access to money

— Prevents partner from working

— Forces partner to engage in sex

— Refuses to wear a condom

The Power and Control Wheel in Interpersonal Relationships,[35] found in **Figure 8-1**, demonstrates the cyclical nature of the abuse and shows additional examples of behaviors the abuser may engage in to control the person in an interpersonal relationship with them.

Unfortunately, offenders with PD rarely recognize they need to seek out help because they are typically not motivated to engage in self-awareness and are resistant to reflecting on their behaviors.[36] Their egocentricity drives their desire to always maintain power and control over others. They manipulate others into trusting and believing in them. Their abusive, violent, or nonviolent actions may be focused on 1 person, such as their intimate or domestic partner, or on several people as they attempt to control others with whom they have a relationship, such as a parent or friend.[36] Adding to the lack of proper diagnosis and treatment, when they do seek help, it is often due to conditions such as anxiety, depression, substance use, or because of the problems created by their PD, such as divorce or unemployment,

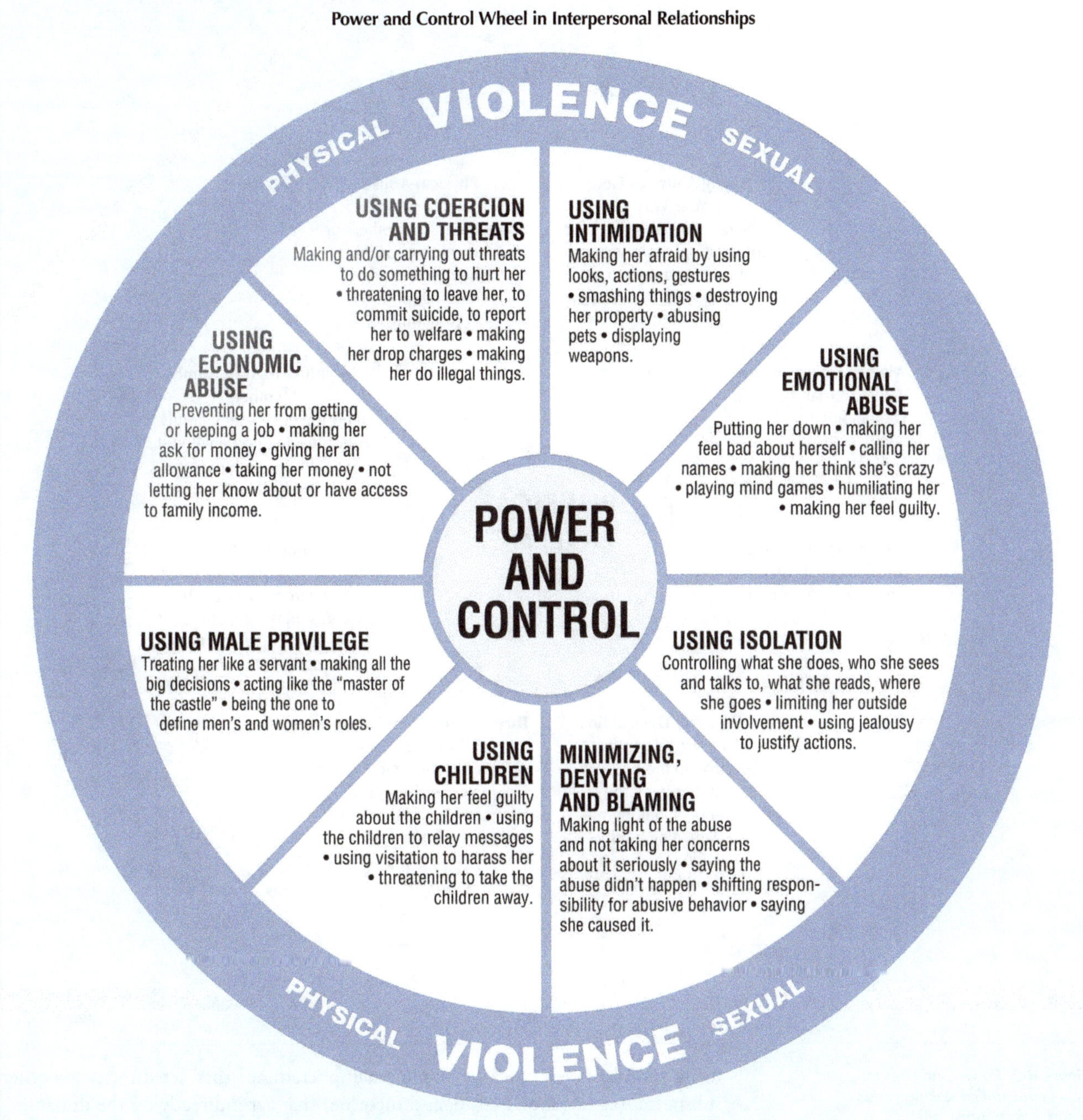
Power and Control Wheel in Interpersonal Relationships
PHYSICAL VIOLENCE SEXUAL
USING COERCION AND THREATS
Making and/or carrying out threats to do something to hurt her • threatening to leave her, to commit suicide, to report her to welfare • making her drop charges • making her do illegal things.
USING INTIMIDATION
Making her afraid by using looks, actions, gestures • smashing things • destroying her property • abusing pets • displaying weapons.
USING ECONOMIC ABUSE
Preventing her from getting or keeping a job • making her ask for money • giving her an allowance • taking her money • not letting her know about or have access to family income.
USING EMOTIONAL ABUSE
Putting her down • making her feel bad about herself • calling her names • making her think she's crazy • playing mind games • humiliating her • making her feel guilty.
POWER AND CONTROL
USING MALE PRIVILEGE
Treating her like a servant • making all the big decisions • acting like the "master of the castle" • being the one to define men's and women's roles.
USING ISOLATION
Controlling what she does, who she sees and talks to, what she reads, where she goes • limiting her outside involvement • using jealousy to justify actions.
USING CHILDREN
Making her feel guilty about the children • using the children to relay messages • using visitation to harass her • threatening to take the children away.
MINIMIZING, DENYING AND BLAMING
Making light of the abuse and not taking her concerns about it seriously • saying the abuse didn't happen • shifting responsibility for abusive behavior • saying she caused it.
PHYSICAL VIOLENCE SEXUAL

Figure 8-1

Figure 8-1. *Power and Control Wheel (used with permission).*

not the disorder itself.[37] The Power and Control Wheel in Familial Relationships[37] is found in **Figure 8-2** and demonstrates behaviors the abuser may engage in to control family members in an interpersonal relationship with them.

Alcohol and substance use are robust predictors of IPV perpetration and victimization.[38-41] Men with PD traits are at an increased risk for consuming alcohol and perpetrating IPV.[42] However, previous research has neglected malleable mechanisms potentially responsible for the link between PD traits, alcohol problems, and IPV perpetration.[42,43] Teva et al[17] found that perpetrators with PDs showed a higher prevalence for anxiety, drug dependence, and alcohol use, which facilitates violent behavior among this group. Further research[39-42] has linked drug use as a predictor for recidivism for sexually violent offenders with psychopathic traits. For example,

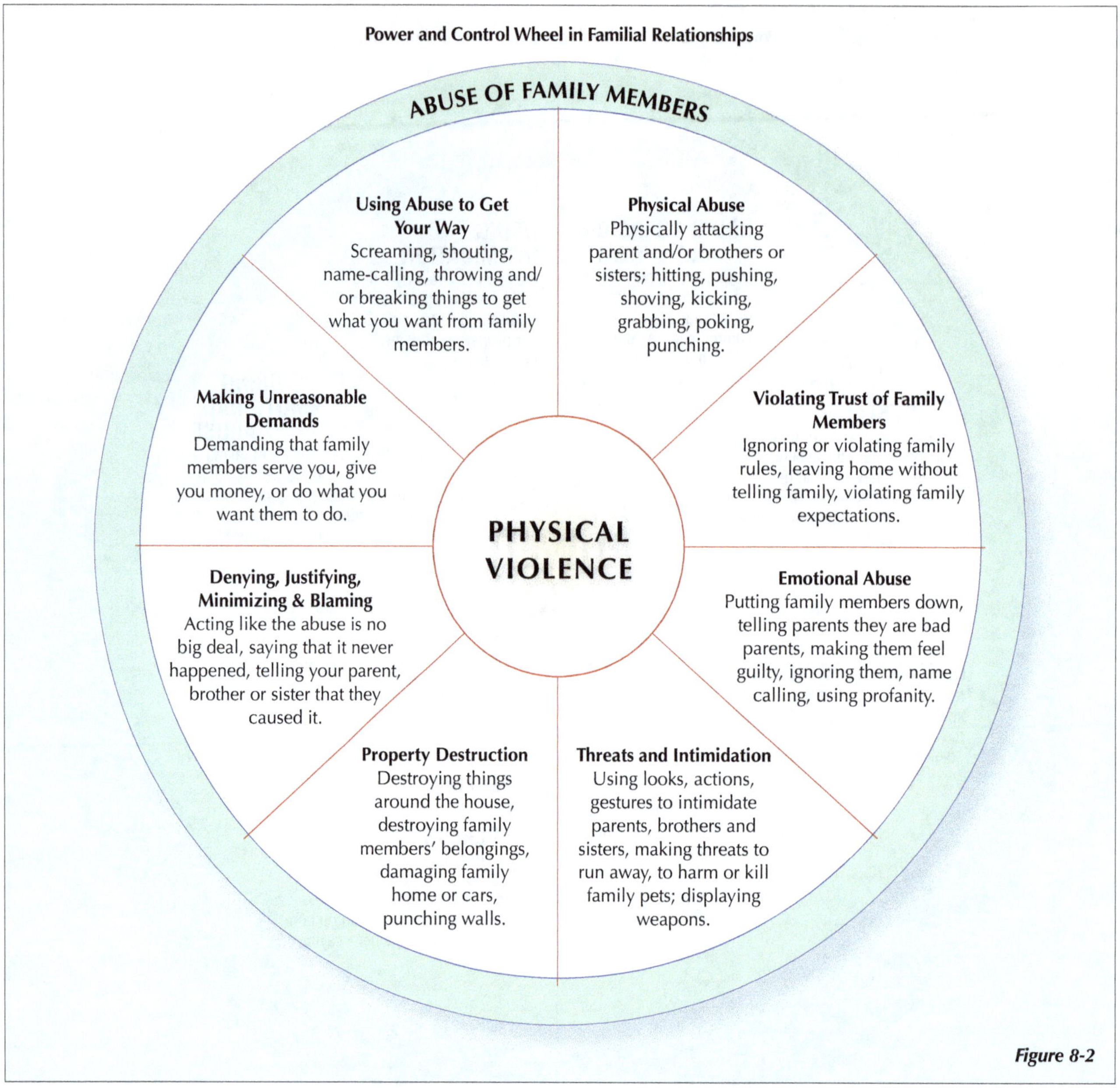

Figure 8-2. Power and Control Wheel in Familial Relationships (used with permission).

using stimulants (eg, cocaine and methamphetamine) that act directly, or other substances (eg, alcohol, heroin, and nicotine) that act indirectly on the dopamine system, affect the structures of the brain that control moral reasoning, executive functioning, and behavioral monitoring.[44,45] Additionally, using substances that increase pleasurable sensations and experiences can promote criminal behavior by creating disinhibition and reinforcing the biological reward pathway.[18]

Assessing for Violence Potential

One of the most widely used instruments in the psychiatric assessment of psychopaths is the Hare Psychopathy Checklist-Revised (PCL-R), which rates a person's psychopathic or antisocial tendencies.[46,47] In addition, it is a well-validated measurement tool with 2 correlated dimensions that underlie PCL-R scores, Factor 1 (F1), affective and interpersonal traits, and Factor 2 (F2), impulsive, antisocial lifestyle. These 2 factors can be further subdivided into correlated lower-order dimensions: F1 can be parsed into arrogant, deceitful interpersonal style (Interpersonal facet), and deficient affective experience (Affective facet); F2 can be parsed into impulsive, irresponsible lifestyle (Lifestyle facet) and prodigious antisocial behavior (Antisocial facet). Most evidence suggests relationships between psychopathy and violence are chiefly reliant on F2.[47]

The Psychopathic Personality Inventory (PPI-Revised) is a personality test for traits associated with psychopathy in adults.[48] The PPI was developed in the early 1990s by Scott Lilienfeld and Brian Andrews to assess personality traits associated with psychopathy in a nonclinical context, and addressing the need for a psychopathy measure suitable for the general population.[49] Although initially used to assess these traits in noncriminal (eg, university students) populations, it is still used in clinical (eg, incarcerated) populations as well.[48,49]

In contrast to other psychopathy measures, such as the PCL, the PPI is a self-report scale, rather than an interview-based assessment. It is intended to comprehensively index psychopathic personality traits without assuming particular links to antisocial or criminal behaviors.[50] The PPI-R is a robust and versatile tool for assessing psychopathic traits across a range of settings. Its development and refinement have ensured its reliability and validity, making it a valuable instrument for both clinical assessment and psychological research. Through its detailed measurement of various psychopathic dimensions, the PPI-R contributes to a deeper understanding of psychopathy and its implications for individual behavior and societal outcomes.[51,52]

The Personality Inventory for DSM-5 (PID-5) is a psychological assessment tool developed to measure maladaptive personality traits in alignment with the DSM-5-TR.[14,53] Its development and implementation represent significant steps toward refining the understanding and diagnosis of PDs. Over the years, there has been a growing recognition of the limitations of categorical models. Dimensional models, which view personality traits on a continuum rather than as discrete categories, have gained traction. These models better captured the complexity and variability of personality pathology. The DSM-5, published in 2013, included a hybrid model in Section III (for further study) that combined categorical and dimensional assessments of PDs.[54] This hybrid model proposed the use of specific personality trait domains and facets to describe personality pathology, leading to the development of the PID-5.[55,56] The PID-5 was designed based on the FFM of personality, which includes 5 broad domains: Negative Affectivity, Detachment, Antagonism, Disinhibition, and Psychoticism.[55-57]

Table 8-2. Five-factor Model of Personality

Negative Affectivity	Detachment	Antagonism	Disinhibition	Psychoticism
Traits include emotional lability, anxiousness, separation insecurity, and submissiveness	Traits include withdrawal, intimacy avoidance, anhedonia, and restricted affectivity	Traits include manipulativeness, deceitfulness, grandiosity, attention seeking, and callousness	Traits include irresponsibility, impulsivity, distractibility, risk-taking, and rigid perfectionism	Traits include unusual beliefs and experiences, eccentricity, and perceptual dysregulation

IPV and the LGBTQIA+ Community

Research[58] indicates that lesbian, gay, bisexual, transgender, queer/questioning, intersex, and asexual/aromantic/agender, etc (LGBTQIA+) individuals are at high risk of victimization by others. Only 1 study[58] was found that sought to examine PDs and their related clinical variables in a sample of gay, lesbian, bisexual, and transgender (GLBT) individuals. The study population was 145 GLBT patients who were admitted to a residential chemical dependency treatment program and diagnosed with mental health disorders. A total of 136 (93.8%) had at least 1 PD and 64 (44%) were diagnosed with antisocial personality disorder (ASPD). However, this study did not explore the relationship between interpersonal violence victimization and perpetration.

What is known is that rates of IPV are similar in heterosexual relationships and relationships in the LGBTQIA+ community.[59-61] Notably, there are some differences, as some of the tactics used by abusive partners can be unique to an LGBTQIA+ relationship. Some psychologically abusive examples are threats of outing, such as threats to expose the victim's sexual orientation, gender identity, or HIV status; controlling their partner's expressions of gender identity and connection to the larger LGBTQIA+ community; using children to control or manipulate the victim, which may happen particularly in cases where the children are related to the abusive partner but do not have an established legal relationship with the other parent; preventing their partner from spending time with friends, claiming that the friends are sexual partners; telling the victim they will not be believed because of their LGBTQIA+ identity; and making fun of their transgender partner's body or appearance.[57,58] The Power and Control Wheel in LGBTQIA+ Relationships,[60] found in **Figure 8-3**, demonstrates behaviors the abuser may engage in to control persons in an interpersonal relationship with them.

Figure 8-3. *Power and Control Wheel in LGBTQIA+ Relationships (used with permission).*

Power and Control Wheel in LGBTQIA+ Relationships

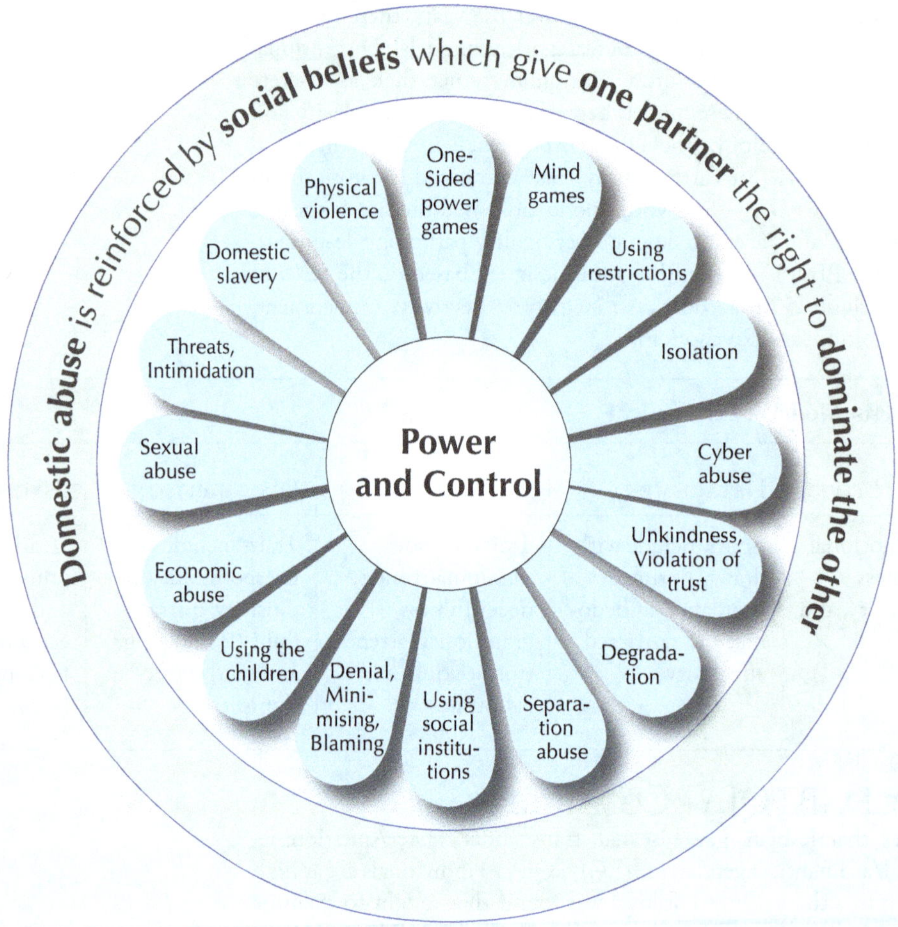

Figure 8-3

Culturally created beliefs regarding masculinity may discourage IPV victims from openly discussing their experiences, especially when gender-related stereotypes exist purporting that homosexual men are less masculine than heterosexual men. These men reported being raped, physically assaulted, or stalked by their male partners.[62,63]

The "Bad Boy" Phenomenon: Cultural Archetype Males and Toxic Masculinity Archetype

Male phenotypes that correlate with masculine power and testosterone are characterized by confidence and adventurousness. It has been described that "bad boys" display qualities of a psychological dark triad[64] of 1) Narcissism-entitlement and a grandiose view of themselves, 2) Machiavellian-callousness and prone to exploiting others, and 3) Psychopathy-antisocial and impulsive behaviors. However, emotionally unavailable, these men choose physical intimacy over emotional intimacy and thus remain "distant" in the relationship.[65]

One of the primary causes of toxic masculinity is societal expectations of male behavior.[39] With their inflated sense of self-importance, they often lack empathy for others. These beliefs and behaviors can lead to manipulative behavior and a desire for control over their partners. Toxic men exhibit harmful behaviors to those around them as their need to assert their dominance over others, leading to aggressive and abusive behavior, including emotional manipulation and abuse to physical violence and death.[64]

There are several reasons that women are attracted to toxic men[65]:

1. Attachment style developed in childhood; Insecure/Anxious (eg, emotionally unavailable parents, fear of abandonment, etc; tend to seek out familiar patterns in adult relationships)
2. Learned helplessness – "victim role"
3. Vulnerability – low self-esteem
4. Desire to "fix" the abuser

Needless to say, none of these reasons justify the stress these unstable relationships bring. As one survivor stated, "Bad boys aren't necessarily super-hot, but they usually have a bit of a sexy mystery: they've got a ruggedness, an edginess, a smoldering exterior that thinly veils an aggressive, rules-be-damned attitude."[40] Additionally, "they encourage a girl to release her wild side, but ...they won't stick by her when she needs support." Nice guys, meanwhile, are often portrayed as homely or uninteresting, and perhaps they only win the girl by exhibiting some bad-boy qualities.[64,65] They are soft and geeky, but their personality overcomes their looks (or lack thereof) in the end.[66] As often portrayed in mass media, their love interest finally falls for them upon learning how moral and courageous they are.

The bad boy phenomenon, however, is not new. An example can be found in a mainstream pop culture song released by country and western star, Skeeter Davis (with words and lyrics written by the well-known duo Carole King and Gerry Goffin in 1963), titled "I Can't Stay Mad at You."[67] The singer lists the various wrongs she catches her love interest doing to her, including lying and even seeing him with another girl, but clearly telling him that none of these will cause her to be the one "to find someone new," and that in the end she is so enmeshed with him that she will always "bounce right back into your arms."

In the meantime, it is worth noting that the lyrics of this song are still readily translatable to many current-day relationships, requiring clinicians to actively examine assumptions about people's love for bad boys/girls and how those attitudes permit victim-blaming.[68] No one—male, female, or otherwise—ever deserves abuse by an intimate partner. The key is to stop assuming that the reasons are superficial and to start empowering victims.

Case Study

Case Study 8-1

Jeremiah was born with significant illnesses requiring frequent hospitalizations in the first 5 years of his life. He was the first of 2 children born to his parents. His mother, the primary caretaker and disciplinarian of the family, had a permissive parenting style and rarely held him accountable for his actions. Growing up, he and his mother shared an unusually strong bond. In his teenage years, both parents worked 2 jobs to support the family. As he grew into childhood and adolescence, he had difficulty making friends with his peers, so he gravitated toward younger children and teachers for acceptance. His teachers would comment to his parents about his charming personality and how helpful he was around school. Early in his adolescence, Jeremiah began excessively lying about his homework, grades, and activities he was involved in at school. When his parents found out, he did not accept any responsibility for his actions. In high school, he decided that he was going to become an astronaut. He talked excessively about it, so much so that he cut out pictures to decorate his bedroom walls and put together models of spaceships. Yet, he was failing multiple classes, did nothing to improve his grades, and complained that the teachers were poor educators. Upon completing high school, he attended multiple colleges but frequently moved to different places when he was not performing well or failed to pay tuition. His lying continued throughout adulthood and he began engaging in criminal behavior including theft, coercion, extortion, and drug-related offenses. However, his charming personality convinced elders in the community that he was a kind and helpful person. Whenever he would accumulate excessive debt from overspending on his multiple credit cards, he would steal money from others, including family members, and would manipulate others to give him things he wanted. His mother would always come to his rescue by helping him file bankruptcy multiple times and pay off his debts as a result of multiple civil lawsuits, all to prevent him from going to jail. He took no responsibility for his actions and often blamed others when he was caught. He would befriend younger people and bring them to his parents' home to stay when his parents were out of town. There, he would provide alcohol to underaged persons and engage in sexual activity, even though he was much older. When he would go to work, these adolescents and young adults were left at his parents' home unattended, sometimes for days at a time. On multiple occasions, this resulted in extensive damage to the home, stolen jewelry, money, expensive personal items, guns, tools, and vehicles. Again, he blamed everything on the other people and was never held accountable by his parents. Several years later, he began engaging in relationships with imprisoned men who were incarcerated for felony convictions, including attempted murder, child abuse, and sexual assault. While in prison, he would send them letters with pictures and money, some of which was stolen from family members. He would promise them a supportive relationship and integration back into society, which would ensure their happiness and a productive life after prison. Once paroled, he used deception, manipulation, drugs, and alcohol to abuse them sexually, emotionally, physically, and financially. He had no empathy, guilt, or remorse for what he had done. He blamed the victims for choosing to engage in this relationship with him.

Discussion

Jeremiah demonstrates several traits of having a PD. From some of the examples provided, he demonstrated selective bonding with his mother and then vulnerable groups including teenagers, young adults, and those incarcerated or formerly incarcerated. Parental absence due to working multiple jobs left only the mother to tend to the children. As a result of his early childhood illnesses, he was overly protected by his mother who continued a permissive parenting style for decades into his adult life. He engaged increasingly in risk-taking behaviors, which impacted his ability to maintain employment, as a result of the theft of money, goods, property, and lying. He continues to show no remorse for the harm he has caused his parents, other family members, friends, or former employers.

Eventually, Jerimiah was arrested for crimes he committed. While incarcerated, he was referred for psychological and counseling services. The PCL-R[29,30] diagnostic for PD was administered. The average neurotypical person receives a score between 3 and 6, with 4 being the average estimate. The average non-psychopathic person receives a score between 16 and 22. Jerimiah scored 24, which is reflective of a person with a sociopathic or ASPD (range 22 to 26).

Sample Assessment

Assessing Jeremiah for psychopathology involves a comprehensive evaluation of his behavioral, cognitive, and emotional patterns over his lifespan. Here are the key steps and considerations in this assessment:

1. Clinical Interview and History Taking

   Developmental History: Documenting his early childhood illnesses, hospitalizations, and family dynamics, particularly his relationship with his permissive mother

   Educational and Social History: Evaluating his difficulties in making friends, his tendency to lie about school-related activities, and his unrealistic aspirations

   Criminal and Behavioral History: Analyzing his patterns of deceit, criminal activities, and manipulation

   Interpersonal Relationships: Investigating his relationships with younger individuals, his interactions with his family, and his manipulative behavior towards others

2. Behavioral Observation

   Interviews: Observing his behavior during interviews for signs of charm, deceit, or lack of remorse

   Interactions: Noting how he interacts with different individuals (eg, family members, professionals)

3. Psychological Testing

   Personality Assessments: Administering tools like the Minnesota Multiphasic Personality Inventory (MMPI-2) or the PCL-R to assess traits associated with psychopathy

   Cognitive Assessments: Evaluating his cognitive functioning, problem-solving abilities, and executive functioning

4. Collateral Information

   Family Interviews: Gathering information from family members about his behavior and history

   School and Employment Records: Reviewing records to confirm patterns of behavior, academic performance, and employment stability

   Legal Records: Examining his criminal record for patterns of offenses and legal issues

5. DSM-5 Criteria for Psychopathology

   ASPD: Jeremiah exhibits many traits consistent with ASPD, which include:

- Failure to Conform to Social Norms: Engaging in criminal behavior repeatedly
- Deceitfulness: Repeated lying, use of aliases, or conning others for personal profit or pleasure
- Impulsivity or Failure to Plan Ahead: Frequently changing colleges and jobs without a clear plan
- Irritability and Aggressiveness: Engaging in fights and assaults
- Reckless Disregard for Safety: Leaving younger individuals unattended, providing alcohol to minors
- Consistent Irresponsibility: Failing to sustain consistent work behavior or honor financial obligations
- Lack of Remorse: Indifference or rationalizing having hurt, mistreated, or stolen from others

Narcissistic Personality Disorder (NPD):

- Grandiosity: Unrealistic aspirations of becoming an astronaut without academic effort
- Need for Admiration: Seeking validation and admiration from younger individuals and teachers
- Lack of Empathy: Exploiting others without remorse or guilt

6. Risk Assessment
   - Violence and Criminal Behavior: Evaluating the risk of future criminal activities and potential harm to others
   - Self-Harm and Substance Abuse: Assessing risks related to his substance use and reckless behavior
7. Formulation and Diagnosis

   This involves combining all the collected data to form a comprehensive picture of Jeremiah's mental health. A likely diagnosis could include:
   - ASPD due to his pervasive pattern of disregard for the rights of others
   - NPD given his grandiosity and lack of empathy
   - Possible comorbid conditions such as Substance Use Disorder
8. Treatment and Management Recommendations
   - Psychotherapy: Focusing on cognitive-behavioral therapy (CBT) to address distorted thinking patterns and behaviors
   - Medication: Considering pharmacotherapy for any comorbid conditions, such as mood stabilizers for impulsivity
   - Social and Legal Interventions: Coordinating with legal and social services to manage his behavior and protect potential victims

By conducting a thorough and multifaceted assessment, clinicians can better understand Jeremiah's psychopathology and develop an effective treatment plan.

Summary

The relationship between PD and violence is well-established. However, the extent to which psychopathy is related to different types of violent behavior warrants further study. The ultimate goal of research into psychopathy and antisocial personality types relative to IPV is to explore the etiological factors that underlie violent behavior. This will facilitate the development of more effective treatment options.

References

1. Niolon PH, Treves-Kagan S, Dahlberg LL, Mercy JA. The evolution of interpersonal violence research and prevention across the lifespan in the United States: the past, present, and future. In: Geffner R, White JW, Hamberger LK, Rosenbaum A, Vaughan-Eden V, Vieth VI, eds. *Handbook of Interpersonal Violence Across the Lifespan*. Springer, Cham; 2020. doi:10.1007/978-3-319-62122-7_95-1

2. Violence against women. World Health Organization. March 25, 2024. https://www.who.int/news-room/fact-sheets/detail/violence-against-women

3. Sardinha L, Maheu-Giroux M, Stöckl H, Meyer S, García-Moreno C. Global, regional, and national prevalence estimates of physical or sexual, or both, intimate partner violence against women in 2018. *Lancet.* 2022;399(10327): 803-813. doi:10.1016/S0140-6736(21)02664-7

4. Fazel S, Smith E, Chang Z, Geddes J. Risk factors for interpersonal violence: an umbrella review of meta-analyses. *Br J Psychiatry.* 2018;213(4):609-614. doi:10.1192/bjp.2018.145

5. Mercy JA, Hillis SD, Butchart A, et al. Interpersonal violence: global impact and paths to prevention. In: Mock CN, Nugent R, Kobusingye O, Smith KR, eds. *Injury Prevention and Environmental Health*. 3rd ed. The International Bank for Reconstruction and Development / The World Bank; 2017. doi:10.1596/978-1-4648-0522-6_ch5

6. Trauma and violence. Substance Abuse and Mental Health Services Administration. Updated May 29, 2024. Accessed September 27, 2022. https://www.samhsa.gov/trauma-violence

7. Petrosky E, Blair J, Betz C, Fowler K, Jack S, Lyons B. Racial and ethnic differences in homicides of adult women and the role of intimate partner violence – United States, 2003-2014. *MMWR Morb Mortal Wkly Rep*. 2017;66 (28):741-746. doi:10.15585/mmwr.mm6628a

8. Evans DP, Di Marco MH, Narasimhan S, Vieytes MM, Curran A. Male perpetrators' accounts of intimate femicide: a global systematic review. Presented at: Global Meeting of Law and Society: Rage, Reckoning and Remedy. July 2022. https://www.researchgate.net/publication/362160171_Male_Perpetrators%27_Accounts_of_Intimate_Femicide_A_Global_Systematic_Review

9. Garcia-Vergara E, Almeda N, Martín Ríos B, Becerra-Alonso D, Fernández-Navarro F. A comprehensive analysis of factors associated with intimate partner femicide: a systematic review. *Int J Environ Res Public Health*. 2022;19 (12):7336. doi:10.3390/ijerph19127336

10. Collison KL, Lynam DR. Personality disorders as predictors of intimate partner violence: a meta-analysis. *Clin Psychol Rev*. 2021;88:102047. doi:10.1016/j.cpr.2021.102047

11. What are personality disorders? American Psychiatric Association. September 2022. https://www.psychiatry.org/patients-families/personality-disorders/what-are-personality-disorders

12. What causes personality disorders? American Psychological Association. 2010. https://www.apa.org/topics/personality-disorders/causes

13. Zimmerman M. Overview of personality disorders. MSD Manual Professional Version. Updated September 2023. https://www.msdmanuals.com/professional/psychiatric-disorders/personality-disorders/overview-of-personality-disorders

14. *Diagnostic and Statistical Manual of Mental Disorders*. 5th ed, text rev. American Psychiatric Association; 2022.

15. Clark LA, Watson D. The trait model of the DSM-5 alternative model of personality disorder (AMPD): a structural review. *Personal Disord.* 2022;13(4): 328-336. doi:10.1037/per0000568

16. Krueger RF, Hobbs KA. An overview of the DSM-5 alternative model of personality disorders. *Psychopathology*. 2020;53(3-4):126-132. doi:10.1159/000508538

17. Teva I, Marin-Morales A, Bueso-Izquierdo N, Perez-Garcia M, Hidalgo-Ruzzante N. Personality characteristics in specialist and generalist intimate partner violence perpetrators. *Clin Psychol Psychother*. 2023;30(1):86-96. doi: 10.1002/cpp.2778

18. DeMatteo D, Olver ME. Use of the Psychopathy Checklist-Revised in legal contexts: validity, reliability, admissibility, and evidentiary issues. *J Pers Assess.* 2023;104(2):234-251. doi:10.1080/00223891.2021.1955693

19. Tharshini NK, Ibrahim F, Kamaluddin MR, Rathakrishnan B, Che Mohd Nasir N. The link between individual personality traits and criminality: a systematic review. *Int J Environ Res Public Health*. 2021;18(16):8663. doi:10.3390/ijerph18168663

20. Antisocial personality disorder: often overlooked and untreated. American Psychiatric Association. December 29, 2022. https://www.psychiatry.org/news-room/apa-blogs/antisocial-personality-disorder-often-overlooked

21. Fisher KA, Torrico TJ, Hany M. *Antisocial Personality Disorder*. StatPearls Publishing; 2024. https://www.ncbi.nlm.nih.gov/books/NBK546673/

22. Schnittker J, Larimore SH, Lee H. Neither mad nor bad? The classification of antisocial personality disorder among formerly incarcerated adults. *Soc Sci Med.* 2020;264:113288. doi:10.1016/j.socscimed.2020.113288

23. Yukhnenko D, Blackwood N, Fazel S. Risk factors for recidivism in individuals receiving community sentences: a systematic review and meta-analysis. *CNS Spectr*. 2020;25(2):252-263. doi:10.1017/S1092852919001056

24. Alper M, Duros MR, Markman J. 2018 update on prisoner recidivism: a 9-year follow-up period (2005-2014). US Department of Justice, Office of Justice Programs, Bureau of Justice Statistics. May 2018. https://www.bjs.gov/content/pub/pdf/18upr9yfup0514.pdf

25. Recidivism. National Institute of Justice. Accessed March 8, 2022. https://nij.ojp.gov/topics/corrections/recidivism

26. Dam VH, Hjordt LV, da Cunha-Bang S, Sestoft D, Knudsen GM, Stenbaek DS. Trait aggression is associated with five-factor personality traits in males. *Brain Behav*. 2021;1(7):e02175. doi:10.1002/brb3.2175

27. Huecker MR, King KC, Jordan GA, et al. *Domestic Violence*. StatPearls Publishing; 2023. https://www.ncbi.nlm.nih.gov/books/NBK499891/

28. Spencer CM, Stith SM, Cafferky B. What puts individuals at risk for physical intimate partner violence perpetration? A meta-analysis examining risk

markers for men and women. *Trauma Violence Abuse.* 2022;23(1):36-51. doi:10.1177/1524838020925776

29. van Baak C, Eichelsheim V, Weenink D, Rosenkrantz Lindegaard M. Why do bystanders report intimate partner violence? Insights into real-life reasoning from those who actually intervened. *J Interpers Violence.* 2024;39(13-14):3207-3238. doi:10.1177/08862605241227156

30. Yu R, Nevado-Holgado AJ, Molero Y, et al. Mental disorders and intimate partner violence perpetrated by men towards women: a Swedish population-based longitudinal study. *PLoS Med.* 2019;16(12):e1002995. doi:10.1371/journal.pmed

31. Johnson SA. Understanding the violent personality: antisocial personality disorder, psychopathy, & sociopathy explored. *Forensic Res Criminol Int J.* 2019;7(2):76-88. doi:10.15406/frcij.2019.07.00267

32. Skodol AE. Personality traits play a major role in the alternative DSM-5 model for personality disorders. *Psychiatr News.* 2018;53(7):680-687. doi:10.1176/appi.pn. 2018.4a20

33. Young C, Habarth J, Bongar B, Packman W. Disorder in the court: cluster B personality disorders in United States case law. *Psychiatr Psychol Law.* 2018;25(5):706-723. doi:10.1080/13218719.2018.1474816

34. Freilich CD, Krueger RF, Hobbs KA, Hopwood CJ, Zimmermann J. The DSM-5 maladaptive trait model for personality disorders. In: Krueger RF, Blaney PH, eds. *Oxford Textbook of Psychopathology.* 4th ed. Oxford Academic; 2023:604-627. https://doi.org/10.1093/med-psych/9780197542521.003.0026

35. Gatner DT, Douglas KS, Hart SD. Examining the incremental and interactive effects of boldness with meanness and disinhibition within the triarchic model of psychopathy. *Personal Disord.* 2016;7(3):259-268. doi:10.1037/per0000182

36. Robb-Dover K. Domestic violence and personality disorders: the eye-opening link. FHE Health. Updated January 27, 2022. https://fherehab.com/learning/domestic-violence-personality-disorder

37. Focht J, Chu A. The cycle of domestic violence. National Center for Health Research. 2023. https://www.center4research.org/the-cycle-of-domestic-violence/

38. Eckhardt CI, Parrott DJ, Massa AA. Substance use and intimate partner violence perpetration. In: Geffner R, White JW, Hamberger LK, Rosenbaum A, Vaughan-Eden V, Vieth VI, eds. *Handbook of Interpersonal Violence and Abuse Across the Lifespan.* Springer, Cham; 2020:1-20. https://doi.org/10.1007/978-3-319-62122-7_156-1

39. Graham K, Bernards S, Laslett AM, et al. Children, parental alcohol consumption, and intimate partner violence: a multicountry analysis by perpetration versus victimization and sex. *J Interpers Violence.* 2021;36(11-12):5608-5634. doi:10.1177/0886260518804182

40. Cafferky BM, Mendex M, Anderson JR, Stith SM. Substance use and intimate partner violence: a meta-analytic review. *Psychol Violence.* 2018;8(1):110-131. doi:10.1037/vio0000074

41. Brem MJ, Florimbio AR, Elmquist J, Shorey RC, Stuart GL. Antisocial traits, distress tolerance, and alcohol problems as predictors of intimate partner violence in men arrested for domestic violence. *Psychol Violence.* 2018;8(1):132-139. doi:10.1037/vio0000088

42. Etherington NA, Baker LL. The link between boys' victimization and adult perpetration of intimate partner violence: opportunities for prevention across the life course. Western University Centre for Research & Education on Violence Against Women & Children. 2016. https://gbvlearningnetwork.ca/our-work/reports/report_2016_4.html

43. The neurobiology of substance use, misuse, and addiction. In: Substance Abuse and Mental Health Services Administration (US); Office of the Surgeon General (US), eds. *Facing Addiction in America: The Surgeon General's Report on Alcohol, Drugs, and Health.* US Department of Health and Human Services; 2016. https://www.ncbi.nlm.nih.gov/books/NBK424849/

44. How stimulants affect the brain and behavior. In: *Treatment Improvement Protocol (TIP) Series, No. 33, Treatment for Stimulant Use Disorders: Updated 2021.* Substance Abuse and Mental Health Services Administration (US); 1999. https://www.ncbi.nlm.nih.gov/books/NBK576548/

45. Volkow ND, Michaelides M, Baler R. The neuroscience of drug reward and addiction. *Physiol Rev.* 2019;99(4):2115-2140. doi:10.1152/physrev.00014.2018

46. Hare RD. The Hare PCL-R: some issues concerning its use and misuse. *Legal Criminol Psychol.* 1998;3(1):99-119. doi:10.1111/j.2044-8333.1998.tb00353.x

47. Benning SD. Psychopathic Personality Inventory (PPI). In: Zeigler-Hill V, Shackelford T, eds. *Encyclopedia of Personality and Individual Differences.* Springer, Cham; 2016. doi:10.1007/978-3-319-28099-8_1098-1

48. Lilienfeld SO, Andrews BP. Development and preliminary validation of a self-report measure of psychopathic personality traits in noncriminal populations. *J Pers Assess.* 1996;66(3):488-524. doi:10.1207/s15327752jpa6603_3

49. Dutton K. *The Wisdom of Psychopaths: Lessons in Life from Saints, Spies and Serial Killers.* William Heinemann; 2012.

50. Malterer MB, Lilienfeld SO, Neumann CS, Newman JP. Concurrent validity of the psychopathic personality inventory with offender and community samples. *Assessment.* 2010;17(1):3-15. doi:10.1177/1073191109349743

51. Neumann CS, Malterer MB, Newman JP. Factor structure of the Psychopathic Personality Inventory (PPI): findings from a large incarcerated sample. *Psychol Assess.* 2008;20(2):169-174. doi:10.1037/1040-3590.20.2.169

52. Sörman K, Nilsonne G, Howner K, et al. Reliability and construct validity of the psychopathic personality inventory-revised in a Swedish non-criminal sample - a multimethod approach including psychophysiological correlates of empathy for pain. *PLoS One.* 2016;11(6):e0156570. doi:10.1371/journal.pone.0156570

53. Krueger RF, Derringer J, Markon KE, Watson D, Skodol AE. Initial construction of a maladaptive personality trait model and inventory for DSM-5. *Psychol Med.* 2012;42(9):1879-1890. doi:10.1017/S0033291711002674

54. Few LR, Miller JD, Rothbaum AO, et al. Examination of the Section III DSM-5 diagnostic system for personality disorders in an outpatient clinical sample. *J Abnorm Psychol.* 2013;122(4):1057-1069. doi:10.1037/a0034878

55. Miller JD, Bagby RM, Hopwood CJ, Simms LJ, Lynam DR. Normative data for PID-5 domains, facets, and personality disorder composites from a representative sample and comparison to community and clinical samples. *Personal Disord.* 2022;13(5):536-541. doi:10.1037/per0000548

56. Thimm JC, Jordan S, Bach B. The Personality Inventory for DSM-5 Short Form (PID-5-SF): psychometric properties and association with big five traits and pathological beliefs in a Norwegian population. *BMC Psychol.* 2016;4(1):61. doi:10.1186/s40359-016-0169-5

57. Maples JL, Carter NT, Few LR, et al. Testing whether the DSM-5 personality disorder trait model can be measured with a reduced set of items: an item response theory investigation of the Personality Inventory for DSM-5. *Psychol Assess.* 2015;27(4):1195-1210. doi:10.1037/pas0000120

58. Grant JE, Flynn M, Odlaug BL, Schreiber LR. Personality disorders in gay, lesbian, bisexual, and transgender chemically dependent patients. *Am J Addict.* 2011;20(5):405-411. doi:10.1111/j.1521-0391.2011.00155.x

59. Health considerations for LGBTQ youth. Centers for Disease Control and Prevention. Updated December 20, 2019. https://www.cdc.gov/healthyyouth/disparities/health-considerations-lgbtq-youth.htm

60. Murphy C. The dynamics of intimate partner abuse has some unique perspectives in LGBTIQ relationships. Speak Out Loud. 2017. https://speakoutloud.net/lgbtiq/lgbtiq-intimate-partner-abuse

61. APA guidelines for psychological practice with sexual minority persons. American Psychological Association. 2021. https://www.apa.org/about/policy/psychological-sexual-minority-persons.pdf

62. Rhodes LR. Addressing intimate partner violence with LGBTQ+ clients. American Counseling Association. June 2023. https://www.counseling.org/publications/counseling-today-magazine/article-archive/article/legacy/addressing-intimate-partner-violence-with-lgbtq-clients#

63. Understanding intimate partner violence in the LGBTQ+ community. Human Rights Campaign. Updated November 4, 2022. https://www.hrc.org/resources/understanding-intimate-partner-violence-in-the-lgbtq-community

64. Bloxsom C, Firth J, Kibowski F, Egan V, Sumich AL, Heym N. Dark shadow of the self: how the dark triad and empathy impact parental and intimate adult attachment relationships in women. *Forensic Sci Int Mind Law.* 2021;2(2):100045. doi:10.1016/j.fsiml.2021.100045

65. Wayne R. Bad boys: why women love them. Medium. May 19, 2019. https://rachelwayne.medium.com/bad-boys-why-women-love-them-b4ff43cd8967

66. Pace R. 17 telling signs of the nice guy syndrome & ways to handle it. Marriage.com. Updated February 28, 2024. https://www.marriage.com/advice/relationship/nice-guy-syndrome/

67. Goffin G, King C. *I Can't Stay Mad at You.* Nashville: RCA Victor; 1963.

68. Friman PC. There is no such thing as a bad boy: the circumstances view of problem behavior. *J Appl Behav Anal.* 2021;54(2):636-653. doi:10.1002/jaba.816

Section II

Assessment

Chapter 9

Intimate Partner Violence: *Assessment, Medical Issues, and Collaborative Intervention*

Nilesh N. Gokal, MD, FAAFP
Gaurav Zirath, MD, MBA, DABOM, FAAFP
Justine Suba-Cohen, DO, MHS, DABOM, FAAFP
Gerica Alvarado, MD, FAAFP

Key Points

1. *Improved understanding for screening and intervention for intimate partner violence (IPV) is necessary to increase awareness and accurately assess vulnerable populations with more up-to-date data.*
2. *The impacts of IPV on an individual's physical and emotional health are multifactorial and many times severe and long-lasting.*
3. *Certain marginalized groups are impacted differently by IPV due to lifestyle, cultural expectations, socioeconomic status, or religious beliefs.*

Background and Significance

IPV is known to be underreported in the United States, making it essential for health care providers to implement screening in their practices. With the expanded use of virtual visits as a result of COVID-19, it is crucial for clinicians to be vigilant of atypical behaviors and physical examination findings in their patients that may indicate physical or nonphysical forms of IPV. Patients who screen positive for IPV may not always be ready for direct intervention or even for safety mitigation, and they may require frequent office visits to develop a long-term plan. In the interim, health care providers should address the many negative health outcomes that can be associated with IPV, including a range of acute and chronic conditions involving various organ systems, mental health problems, and engagement in high-risk behaviors. Patients should also be informed of the many local and national resources available at the time of IPV identification.

Effects of IPV on Health

The data confirming the relationship between IPV and poor mental and physical health outcomes of victims are overwhelming. While there are a number of confounding variables that can combine with IPV to have an effect on an individual, research associates IPV with several chronic conditions, including depression, post-traumatic stress disorder (PTSD), anxiety, sleep disorders, self-harm, and suicide, with depression and PTSD being the most prevalent.[1,2] As with many statistics surrounding IPV, there are no consistent data regarding the strength of the association, the amount of exposure required for these conditions to develop, or which forms of IPV lead to physical or psychological consequences.

The complicated interactions between IPV, childhood trauma, substance use, and PTSD make it difficult to assess causality and timing. However, consistently, victims of IPV have a higher incidence of mental health diagnoses when compared to the rest of the population. Depending on the population studied, women who have experienced IPV are 4 to 7 times more likely to exhibit suicidal ideation than women who have not experienced IPV.[3,4] This increase in suicidal ideation extends to several cultural contexts beyond the United States.[5]

While physical violence can cause chronic injuries such as fractures or traumatic or anoxic brain injuries that increase the risk of seizures or cognitive disorders, it can also have long-term consequences not directly attributable to the primary injuries. All forms of IPV increase the prevalence of poor functional health, somatic disorders, chronic disorders, chronic pain, gynecological symptoms, unwanted pregnancies, and increased risk of sexually transmitted infections, including HIV. Women who have experienced IPV are 3 times more likely to have gynecological problems, even if the abuse they experienced was not sexual in nature.[6] The severity and effects of IPV are multiplied in pregnancy, when violence becomes more severe and pregnancies higher risk.[7] Examples of chronic disorders seen in victims of IPV include higher incidences of debilitating headaches, asthma, irritable bowel syndrome, and substance use. There are many hypotheses but no concrete data to explain what mechanisms lead to these chronic diseases. An estimated 40% to 60% of murders of women in North America are done by intimate partners, which does not include data on suicide associated with IPV.[5] Not only are effects of IPV seen clinically, but they are also manifested socially, with missed days at school or work while simultaneously experiencing increased financial pressures and demands secondary to the need for medical visits or legal, housing, and counseling services.

Current evidence suggests that the only psychological consequences of IPV that abate after removal from the abusive situation are depression and suicidality. According to 1 study, a woman who has experienced IPV and has left her abuser will not have better psychological health outcomes 5 years later than a woman who has remained in an abusive relationship for that time.[8] Similarly, a Norwegian study looked at physical health functions of women after leaving an abusive partner. They found that victims of IPV had significantly lower functional health scores than the national average 12 months after leaving their partners.[9] Finally, a study using data from the World Health Organization across 11 countries found no difference in health outcomes between those who had experienced recent abuse (within the last 12 months) and historical abuse (more than 1 year ago), except for suicidal thoughts.[2] This indicates that even a transient IPV experience can have long-lasting effects on the physical and mental health of victims, and survivors of historical IPV require similar support from the health care system as those currently experiencing IPV.

Disproportionate Effects on Marginalized Groups

IPV disproportionally affects minority populations. Studies consistently cite higher rates of IPV in Black and Native American/Alaska Native women (43%–46%) when compared to White women (30%–35%). The same is true for foreign-born women, who also reported that violence tends to escalate after immigrating to the United States.[10] The related disparities of income, immigrant status, racism, and other sources of victimization and social determinants of health that often coexist within these populations can exacerbate or confound the health effects of IPV. For example, ethnic minority women tend to have lower levels of education, lower income, and lower access to health care,[11] and immigrant women often have language difficulties and a lack of knowledge regarding their rights.[12,13] A review by Stockman et al[14] looked at 36 studies within the United States focusing on women from ethnic minority groups, including Black/African Americans, Hispanic/Latinx,

Native American/Alaska Natives, and Asian Americans, including immigrants. This was the first published review focusing on the effects of IPV on ethnic minority women in the United States. For physical effects of IPV, studies looking at African American women and African Caribbean women found higher rates of disordered eating, which was more likely after physical abuse than psychological abuse. Studies looking at Latina and South Asian women found a correlation between IPV and generalized pain as well as sleeping difficulties.

The effects of IPV on minority populations also extend to mental health outcomes, adding to the well-studied psychological health of marginalized populations. Stockman et al[14] found 1 study that looked specifically at Black women. This study found an association between IPV, PTSD, and depression. Among Latina women, studies indicate prevalence of depression among IPV-exposed women to be 2 times that of nonexposed women and overall worse functioning when compared with nonexposed women. When looking at sexual health outcomes, 1 study found that Puerto Rican women born in the United States were at greater risk of IPV and risky sexual practices than those born in the Commonwealth of Puerto Rico. There is limited data from Native American/Alaska Native women as well as Asian American women, but the available data suggest an association between IPV and mood disorders similar to that of the general population. There are no studies specifically looking at substance use and IPV among ethnic minorities. More research, appropriately powered, should be directed toward these populations to best serve them, finding appropriate prevention strategies, interventions, and treatments that are specific to their unique social, cultural, and often political barriers.

While the majority of studies focus on the effects of IPV on the health and lives of women, there has been an increasing call for data surrounding the effects on other populations. A review by Randle[15] looking specifically at the effects of IPV on men suggested that while IPV perpetrated toward men by women is more likely to be psychological than physical, the rates of PTSD and depression in some data sets did not differ between the genders. Conflicting data exists, as Ehrensaft et al[16] measured psychiatric disorders in men and women before and after experiencing IPV and did not find increased risk of depression or PTSD in men who had experienced IPV. Again, societal, cultural, and gender expectations play a role in underreporting or recognition of IPV and depression or PTSD in men. Overall, men who are victims of IPV seem to be at higher risk for PTSD and depression, but more data are required to ascertain to what degree.

Even fewer data exist when looking specifically at men within same-sex couples. Research so far suggests higher rates of mental health problems among gay men than heterosexual men, even when excluding the effects of IPV. The research reviewed by Randle et al in 2011 seems to suggest IPV in male same-sex couples leads to similar psychological consequences as in heterosexual couples, with increased rates of depression, anxiety, low self-esteem, and PTSD.[15] This finding was confirmed in a study by Buller et al.[17] IPV is associated with higher rates of HIV within the lesbian, gay, bisexual, transgender, queer, intersex, asexual+ (LGBTQIA+) community and within ethnic minority women. This may be due to forced sex, limited negotiation of safe sex, and abuse-related immunocompromisation.

There are also few data in the medical literature regarding effects of IPV on the health of the transgender population. This scarcity of data is startling, especially given the high rates of violence they experience outside of intimate partner relationships. The 2015 Transgender Survey Report found that 54% of transgender people have experienced IPV.[18] However, a review conducted by Peitzmeier et al,[19] which included data from 85 articles, found the median lifetime prevalence of physical IPV within the transgender population to be 37.5%, while reporting of any

IPV by victims within the transgender population ranged from 6.3% to 83.3%. This discrepancy in the findings suggests there is not yet reliable data to help quantify the burden on this population. When compared to cisgender reports, transgender patients are 1.66 times more likely to experience any IPV and 2 times more likely to experience physical and sexual IPV. Among the existing data, there is no difference between rates of IPV experienced by individuals assigned male at birth or assigned female at birth. Although, outside of the scope of IPV, transgender women of color have exceedingly high rates of death by homicide when compared to the rest of the population. Limited data seem to suggest an association between IPV and worse mental health outcomes as well as higher rates of substance use. One study[20] focusing on health outcomes of those aged 50 years and older found 57% of respondents to the United States Transgender Survey reported IPV in their lifetimes with 41% of respondents reporting transgender-specific IPV, which was the most commonly reported form of abuse. Transgender victims of IPV were more likely to report abuse of illicit or prescription drugs, psychological distress, or to carry a diagnosis of disability. Additionally, 1 in 4 reported suicide attempts.[20] Notably, the study population above was composed of mostly White, non-Latinx, college-educated, legally partnered (eg, married, in a domestic partnership, or common law marriage) adults.

Spectrum of Violence and Cultural Considerations

IPV is a global phenomenon, existing in various forms in most societies throughout the world; however, there may be many cultural differences and experiences that lead to normalization or acceptance of what is known to be abusive behavior.[21,22] The signs and symptoms of IPV can be and often are subtle. This is especially so when the violence is nonphysical or the victim does not see themselves as a victim. The effects of IPV on a victim's health are comparable regardless of the type of violence they experience. When looking at data from the National Intimate Partner and Sexual Violence Survey (NISVS), 47% of men and women in the United States reported having experienced psychological aggression, such as humiliating or controlling behaviors.[10] These statistics are likely an underestimation, as the Centers for Disease Control and Prevention (CDC) and Bureau of Justice Statistics estimate less than 1/2 of IPV victims actually report the incident or pattern of behavior to the police or medical professionals, and less than 1/4 report to domestic violence centers. Accurate statistics are even more difficult to obtain when looking at underrepresented groups, as quoted rates are greatly influenced by how data are gathered and which victims are willing to disclose their abuse. Therefore, there is no clear consensus on the current rates of IPV within many underrepresented groups.

While it may not be possible to exhaustively cover all the cultural intricacies that influence a victim's decision to recognize or disclose IPV, it is important to acknowledge and explore some of them. It is also important to note that the following examples are based on research but are not intended to be nor should they be taken as a generalization of any one group. Within groups, there are regional and generational differences as well as intersectional influences. One example of the effects of culture on normalization is how it can be deeply influenced by gender roles. For instance, the concept of "machismo" within many Hispanic cultures sets the expectation that men are to be sexually aggressive, dominant, and maintain control of the household and their partners while emphasizing subservience of women to their husbands.[7] Within the context of marriage, it can prove difficult to identify abuse if the societal expectation is to submit to the will of one's husband. By contrast, men in these and many other cultures who are victims of IPV will also face challenges in recognizing, disclosing, and receiving aid for their abuse.

Another important concept, common to many cultures, is the idea of "familism," which prioritizes the good of the family over that of the individual. This not only prevents victims from seeking help but also from perceiving their treatment as abusive. When comparing Gender Inequality Indexes to IPV acceptance or normalization, countries with greater gender equality have societies more supportive of IPV being a public matter and vice versa. In a report by Daniela Barba[21] at Vanderbilt University, she analyzed normalization of IPV in 7 countries in the Americas (Dominican Republic, Ecuador, Guyana, Jamaica, Mexico, El Salvador, and Peru). When responding to her question of "Physical violence between members of a couple is a private matter and should be handled by the couple or close family," between 42% and 62% of study participants agreed with that statement. When asked about IPV under circumstances of infidelity or household neglect, normalization of IPV was even higher. Victims may not disclose their abuse due to fear of bringing shame or distress to their families.

The LGBTQIA+ community has also had a history of underreporting violence, despite same-sex couples having rates of IPV similar to those of heterosexual couples. This is partially due to the fact that campaigns to raise awareness of IPV have mostly focused on heterosexual relationships. Research, although limited, shows that victims may also be less likely to report abuse due to fear of being "outed" or fear of stigmatizing the community itself and leading to further oppression and marginalization, similar to the concept of familism above. A study by Toro-Alfonso et al[23] looked at Puerto Rican gay men and found 48% reported nonphysical violence, but very few perceived this to be IPV. Theories suggest this discrepency may be due to expectations of masculinity, especially within a community that experiences the stigma of being gay while also belonging to a culture heavily influenced by machismo. By contrast, lesbian couples report a fear that a disclosure of lesbian IPV could lead to minimization of male violence. Rolle et al[24] report that relationships with at least 1 bisexual partner may experience even further stress due to stigmatization from the heterosexual community as well as biphobia from the homosexual community. Importantly, there is evidence that the LGBTQIA+ community has been subjected to significant violence by police departments and medical institutions,[24,25] making trust a notable obstacle for clinicians to overcome when attempting to identify IPV as a member of these institutions or while holding affiliation or collaboration with them.

Repeated exposure to a particular experience causes changes in a person's cognitive, behavioral, and emotional processes of that experience. In this way, not only can cultural differences and generational trauma affect personal and societal perceptions of IPV, but media and social media exposures can also influence these views. In the public eye, depictions of weakness or jokes directed toward men who are the victims of violence trivialize such violence while upholding and strengthening the gendered stigma of IPV. These depictions make it difficult for male victims or those close to them to seek help.[26]

Nonphysical violence, specifically, has been relegated to the private realm even within the legal code. Across the United States, legal definitions of IPV vary, and only 38 states include it within their criminal code, which, even then, often limit the definition to mean physical violence. Those that do include nonphysical violence limit it to acts of harassment, stalking, or intimidation.[27] Additionally, most states do not explicitly include same-sex or queer couples in their legal code. This makes it especially difficult to prosecute these cases and decreases the likelihood that victims will come forward if they fear they have no legal recourse or protection. Gender biases also permeate the United States legal system, with only 2% of suspected female perpetrators being arrested after a report of violence.[15] While it may be difficult to identify, intervene, and prosecute nonphysical violence, its effects on the lives of victims should not be underestimated. Per Dillon et al,[28] only 0.6% of the burden of disease was attributed to physical injuries as a result of

IPV. Several studies have found psychological IPV to be as detrimental as physical IPV, especially for depressive symptoms. Because IPV disproportionately affects multiracial, Indigenous, Black, and Hispanic men and women, sexual minorities, and those with disabilities—the same groups who are often marginalized within society and the health care system—it is imperative that a conscientious effort is made to create a safe space that allows these groups in particular to disclose their abuse.

Impacts of COVID-19 on IPV

The impact of COVID-19 on behavioral health is enormous. Numerous publications have reported a significant increase in mental health illnesses among both adults and children. Despite the release of COVID-19-related lockdowns, prevalence of mental health illness remains a large concern around the world.[29] It has become imperative that clinicians ensure all patients, regardless of age, sexual orientation, or ethnicity, are screened for mental health-related changes. It has become more important than ever to recognize and treat mental health-related illnesses, including but not limited to developing new-onset or worsening of depression, anxiety, attention deficit hyperactivity disorder (ADHD), PTSD, panic attacks, and suicidal thoughts and attempts. Furthermore, similar trends of significant increases in substance abuse and domestic violence have also been reported around the world resulting from the effects of COVID-19.[30] During the course of COVID-19, many people were able to remain connected through the use of technology and experienced how much of an asset it is to daily life. Technology continues to advance the public's lives in many ways and positively impacted day-to-day activities, but it has also added another consideration within the realm of IPV. Technology that is designed to protect and safeguard families is being used for abuse (see **Case Study 9-3**).

Screening

The United States Preventive Services Task Force's (USPSTF) recommendations regarding screening for IPV have dramatically changed throughout the years. In the 1990s, the USPSTF found "insufficient evidence to recommend for or against the use of specific instruments to detect domestic violence" because there was "limited evidence that directly addressed the harms of screening and whether interventions actually reduce harm to women."[31] By 2013, the USPSTF updated screening recommendations and recommended that "clinicians screen women of childbearing age [approximately 14-46 years old[31]] for intimate partner violence (IPV) and provide or refer women who screen positive to intervention services," including emergency services, behavioral health specialists, community resources, home visits, and mentoring support.[32] Age is not the only consideration when deciding to screen for IPV. Those with low income, mental health disorders, current state of pregnancy, or history of adverse childhood events should also be screened carefully.[33] Even though there is no current evidence on appropriate intervals for screening, it is important to screen for IPV more than once due to varying comfort levels of patients and because IPV tends to be repetitive, with an escalation in frequency and severity over time.[34]

Despite patients and clinicians agreeing that IPV screenings should take place regularly, only a small percentage of clinicians follow through on this, largely because of time constraints, perceived inability to change the situation, and unfamiliarity with how to approach a delicate topic.[34-36] Providing validated resources, education, and training to instill a certain comfort level may be impactful in empowering clinicians to approach screening. In addition to clinicians, the medical staff should be appropriately trained on IPV screening, as they are usually the first to use screening tools during the initial intake process at every clinical visit. It is important to note that patients may answer untruthfully during these short encounters, especially when asked by a staff member with whom they are unfamiliar. Regardless, IPV screening should be incorporated into every possible health care services encounter.

There are several instruments (**Table 9-1**) that have shown the most sensitivity and specificity in identifying IPV. These tools can be self-administered or used in a clinical interview format. It is important to note that screening tools are limited by the patient's readiness to disclose the abuse. Patients may respond in different ways, including not feeling ready to admit that they are in an abusive situation or fearing retaliation from their partner despite promises of confidentiality by the clinician.[35,37,38]

Table 9-1. Recommended IPV Screening Tools

Screening Tool	Description
Humiliation, Afraid, Rape, Kick (HARK)	4-question tool that represents different components of IPV including emotional, sexual, and physical abuse[32]
Hurt, Insult, Threaten, Scream (HITS)	4-question tool that assesses the frequency of certain components of IPV using a 5-point Likert scale from 1=Never to 5=Frequently[32]
Ongoing Violence Assessment Tool (OVAT)	4-question tool created to detect IPV in emergency settings[39]
Slapped, Threatened, and Throw (STaT)	3-question tool that asks about being slapped, threatened with violence, or having objects thrown at/around the victim[40]
Women Abuse Screening Tool (WAST)	Includes 8 items that assess physical and emotional IPV[32]

Case Studies

Case Study 9-1

Julia was a 27-year-old, Black-Hispanic female noted to have had several no-shows at her primary care clinician's office over the last few months despite reminder texts and phone calls from the office staff. Her clinician was concerned about potential social barriers that may have been impacting her ability to make it to her appointments and called her directly to inquire about transportation, copays, job schedule, childcare, and other factors that may have been impacting Julia's attendance of scheduled appointments. During the discussion, Julia disclosed that her husband liked to be present for all of her appointments, and he was unable to leave his work until after 5:00 PM, at which time the clinic closed for the day. To accommodate his schedule, the clinic offered Julia a 4:45 PM visit and reassured her that it was okay if she and her husband were late; the team would wait for her.

Julia and her husband, Paul, presented for her wellness visit. They appeared to have good rapport, as Julia was relaxed and laughing. Paul was pleasant and engaging. Julia responded to all questions relating to her health without the input of her husband. In preparation for the physical exam, the clinician asked Paul to step outside, which he did without hesitation. During the physical exam, with Paul outside of the room, Julia's clinician asked if she felt safe at home. Julia assured her clinician that she did.

Her clinician then asked, "Is there anything we could do to make you more comfortable with coming to your appointments alone?"

Appearing to be confused, Julia replied that she felt extremely comfortable being in the office, "It's just that my husband doesn't like me to leave the house without him. He's very jealous that way."

This led to several follow-up questions from her clinician regarding what else Julia was not permitted to do on her own. The clinician learned that Julia was not allowed to work, go grocery shopping, or be with her friends without Paul. She was allowed to visit her mother, who lived nearby. Paul also checked her phone regularly and kept it with him when he was home, including when they were sleeping. Throughout the conversation, Julia was calm, direct, and matter-of-fact. She did not see a problem with this behavior, as it meant Paul cared for her and her safety, as this is what her family taught her about roles within a marriage in a community that strongly valued machismo ideologies.

Her clinician received permission from the patient to discuss further and inquired about whether there had ever been a problem with infidelity in the relationship, which Julia denied, and then proceeded to explain her concerns over these behaviors to Julia.

"In my experience, when a partner prevents you from leaving your home without supervision or having your own private phone, this may be an early sign of abusive behavior. Has Paul ever hit you or threatened to hit you? Has he ever threatened to kick you out of the home?"

Julia denied both statements and the clinician expressed her relief. As the conversation progressed, Julia disclosed that she missed seeing her friends and became tearful, but she maintained that this is just how their relationship was. The clinician gave Julia resources to call if she ever felt unsafe, or if the behavior progressed and she would like to talk to someone about it. She reassured Julia that the conversation would remain confidential and that she would always be able to speak privately with her clinician during her visits.

Discussion

Julia's case exemplifies the importance of maintaining an open and curious line of questioning during an assessment to create a safe space and elicit a history of IPV without using alienating or judgmental language. Julia's pattern of no-shows to her medical appointments and inability to come to her appointments without her husband present were indicators that there may be some concerning behaviors her clinician should explore further. It may be that this is Julia's choice due to past experiences with the medical system or due to anxiety, depression, fear, lack of transportation or childcare, cultural expectations, or a myriad of reasons that clinicians may not initially consider. It is worth noting how her clinician's question regarding certain behaviors places the responsibility on the clinic and medical system, "what can we do to make it easier for you…to make this more comfortable for you," rather than an accusatory or judgment-filled statement, such as "Why is your husband so controlling?" or "Why can't you come to the clinic by yourself?" The former statements divert responsibility and burden from Julia, creating a safe space and allowing her to candidly explain her situation in her own words. The latter statements are more likely to elicit a defensive response, especially from a patient like Julia, who has coded Paul's behavior as protective rather than abusive. Due to the value placed on machismo, Julia has been socialized to accept her abuse as a show of love.

Open, curious, nonjudgmental questions about home life and safety lead to quicker rapport and reduce the risk of alienating potential victims. The same is true when providing information regarding abuse and resources for victims. Using terms such as "in my experience" or "this can be a sign of" again gives a general, indirect idea of concern without any unintended accusation. Once IPV has been disclosed, it is not a clinician's job to "fix" the situation or "rescue" the victim. It is, however, imperative to educate, empower, and reduce feelings of guilt. A statement of "you do not deserve to be hurt, no matter what" can be incredibly powerful. Empowering victims by allowing them to decide when and how they are ready to intervene or accept help for their situation is integral.

Case Study 9-2

Aged 35 years, Peter has had multiple health issues, including obesity, sleep apnea, diabetes, heart failure, asthma, and bipolar disorder. He presented to the clinic for an Emergency Department (ED) follow-up, where he was recently evaluated for sharp chest pain which radiated from his neck down to his left arm and fingertips. Review of his hospital visit showed an unremarkable chest X-ray and normal cardiac workup including blood tests that ruled out heart failure exacerbation and heart attack. He was discharged home the same day.

During his follow-up with his primary care clinician, Peter denied persistence of chest pain, though still complained of constant pain and numbness from his neck down to his left hand. When given a physical examination, he had chest wall tenderness as well as stiffness around his neck and left upper back muscles. Most notably, he had a positive Spurling's examination, which indicated nerve impingement in his neck. His physician gently questioned him about potential causes of his neck pain including any history of trauma to the neck. Peter broke down and admitted that 2 weeks prior to his presentation to the ED, his husband had struck him on the left side of his head and placed him in a chokehold. His primary care clinician comforted him and discussed options and resources moving forward. Peter confided that he had been contemplating leaving his husband over the last few months; however, he did not wish for the clinician to report this incident. After assessing that Peter was in no immediate danger at home, his clinician agreed not to report the abuse, ordered an MRI of the cervical spine for diagnostic evaluation, and scheduled Peter for a close follow-up visit.

At the next appointment, Peter was very excited to share that he had moved in with his mother. He said that this was very difficult to do because his husband had hidden his underwear in a safe. He was able to slowly pack his car with essentials and waited for the ideal opportunity to sneak out. Peter was also able to complete the MRI of the cervical spine, which showed minimal disc bulging. His left arm numbness continued to worsen, so his clinician ordered a nerve conduction test of the left upper extremity and referred him to pain management. In addition, his clinician completed paperwork for Peter so that he could take medically indicated time off from his job as he completed his evaluation for his left arm and was able to speak with a therapist.

Peter continued to follow up with his primary care clinician every 2 to 4 weeks for the next 6 months with successively longer intervals. He agreed to starting an anti-depressant medication as he completed an intensive outpatient therapy program (IOP) and established care with a therapist who specialized in PTSD.

Discussion

Obtaining candid details surrounding instances of IPV is not always an easy task in a primary care clinic. A well-established, trusting, longitudinal relationship with the same clinician promotes patient openness to safely discuss vulnerable topics such as IPV.

Clinicians can provide a secure environment and ensure that they maintain their patient's integrity by keeping the patient fully clothed and undressing only when required for physical examination. Ideally, patients should not be accompanied by other guests so that they will not feel inhibited in disclosing their honest experiences.[34,35,41] There should also be detailed documentation of all observed injuries as well as direct quotes from the patient, which are extremely helpful should the patient pursue legal action.[34]

Clinicians are not obligated to report IPV to state agencies unless there are children or seniors involved. Patients usually prefer to keep their story confidential within the walls of the examination room. This is why it is critical to assess the risk of immediate harm at the time of IPV disclosure and during all follow-ups.[34,35,41] Snider et al[42] developed a 5-question prediction instrument that can help predict which patients are at increased risk for severe harm or lethal assault. If the patient answers "yes" to at least 3 of those questions, they are at high risk of harm, with a sensitivity of 83% and a specificity of 56%:

1. Has physical violence increased over the past 6 months?
2. Has your partner used a weapon or threatened you with a weapon?
3. Do you believe your partner is capable of killing you?
4. Have you been beaten while pregnant?
5. Is your partner violently and constantly jealous of you?

Case Study 9-3

Amelia, a 61-year-old female immigrant from the Philippines, married to her husband for 41 years, was an established patient of a clinic for over 2 years. As a result of COVID-19, Amelia and her husband, a veteran, retired early. During a routine appointment, screening for IPV led to the patient sharing nearly 1 year of emotional, mental, and physical trauma. During COVID-19, Amelia's husband started using marijuana daily, purchased by selling valuable mutual assets. Marijuana use also led to enormous credit card debt. She used the entirety of her 401k retirement savings to pay off the credit card debt accumulated from marijuana purchases. The husband sold most of the valuables from the co-owned lock box without the permission of the patient. Both received their social security funds into their joint checking account. The husband not only changed the passwords, but also set up notifications for all banking transactions taking place. He also installed cameras inside and outside of the home to track the patient. She was unsure if her phone calls and location were also being tracked, resulting in her apprehension with pursuing therapy and receiving external support.

Amelia also endured mental trauma from an incident involving a firearm, which led to 911 being called. Her recollection of the event is numerous police cars, sirens, firetrucks, ambulances, and a helicopter at the scene as both Amelia and her husband walked out of the house with their hands in the air, and firearms pointed at both by the officers.

The physical and emotional extremities of the situation were openly abated by the police, and all firearms were removed from the home. The husband was subsequently taken to a local mental health institution for concerns of severe depression. Amelia continued to receive follow-up care with her primary care clinician and received telephone support from a local organization.

Amelia was relieved with the firearms being removed from the home; however, this incident added to her trauma, as many neighbors witnessed the entire scene, leading to embarrassment and guilt. She continued to care about her husband, who was "very good" to her for all the years of their marriage, except the last few years since COVID-19. She felt guilty that she ruined her husband's reputation in the neighborhood, further limiting his already grim social life with the neighbors. With no firearms, the form of abuse shifted to verbal and emotional intimidation. She avoided leaving the house when he was also home to avoid being questioned by him. She considered moving out of the house, but due to the finances being primarily managed by her husband, she was unable to obtain independent housing. She was also afraid that her husband would not be able to afford the bills without her contribution and did not want him to lose the home they purchased together.

Discussion

Amelia's IPV and abuse was discovered by screening during a routine follow-up. The importance of routine screening for IPV cannot be emphasized enough, especially in the setting of increasing prevalence of mental illness resulting from COVID-19. The United States Department of Health and Human Services recommends IPV screening and counseling for all women during their preventative health visit.[30] Screening should be conducted routinely and not only when abuse is suspected. Amelia's finances, as described in the case, are controlled by her husband, limiting her access to essential funds. Her case is also complicated by the use of technology as a means of further intimidation, control, and abuse.

She was afraid to use funds due to concerns about her husband being notified. She was also afraid of leaving the house and needing to provide her husband with an explanation. The husband was able to track her location easily with her mobile phone, which also placed her in a dangerous situation if she was found at a shelter or other supportive place without her husband's knowledge. Cameras inside the house limited Amelia's ability to call for therapy or help without her conversations being recorded. She was unable to find secure housing with her social security income or pay for day-to-day expenses. She did not have any family support in town, and her only social support was a few close friends from her previous employment.

There is a wide array of resources available for those who are victims of IPV and abuse aided by the use of technology. Actions to consider for patients such as Amelia include:

- Establishing a personal bank account (there are online accounts that can be opened without going into the branch)
- Not using personal savings to depletion
- Keeping bank account login information private
- Keeping mobile phone passwords protected

— Setting up alerts for all banking transactions for joint accounts

— Obtaining professional legal advice

Summary

The CDC reviews data from United States crime reports, which suggest that about 1 in 5 homicide victims are killed by an intimate partner. This fails to corroborate with reporting or documenting of IPV within outpatient medical settings, further highlighting the integral need for improved methods of screening and detection as well as resources for continued care. Current gaps lead to loss of patient safety and poor health outcomes. While marginalized groups are at increased risk, data clearly demonstrates the need for improved screening methods and intervention for all populations. The USPSTF currently recommends that clinicians screen women of childbearing age for IPV, and it is important to recognize that IPV can be present at any age in any gender. Though there is no current consensus on what methods are best to employ, several tools exist for self-administration or for use during clinical interviews. Empowering both patients and clinicians with a focus on enhanced screening, paired with an understanding of local and national resources, is vital to addressing IPV and improving outcomes.

All forms of IPV are associated with adverse health outcomes and chronic, sometimes irreversible conditions in all victims. Victims of IPV have higher use of the medical system, with some estimates suggesting women who are victims of IPV generating 92% more costs per year than the rest of women,[5] and Stockman et al estimated in 2015 that $5.8 billion is spent annually for medical and mental health costs and loss of productivity from IPV.[14] Overall, data suggest that women present to health care settings before they present to law enforcement or social services. It is important for clinicians to be aware of these relationships as attempts at addressing mental health, chronic disease, or substance use will be unsuccessful without addressing IPV. The paucity of data when it concerns minority populations and men is telling, but current research that strives to close this gap will allow clinicians to better care for these patients in the long run.

Resources

Community Resources:

— It is imperative to have resources readily available. Most of the resources are now available electronically and can be accessed quickly.

— A brief list of important national resources is provided in **Table 9-2**. It is important to highlight that the organizations such as The National Domestic Violence Hotline are accessible 24 hours a day, with advocates available via telephone, text messages, and online chat.

— Veterans and their families have access to additional support with The Intimate Partner Violence Assistance Program (IPVAP), which is a program led by the US Department of Veterans Affairs. The link provided in the table can be used to locate state coordinators for support.

— In addition to the national resources, clinicians are recommended to have local resources available, including shelters and counseling, legal, and financial advice.

— Building strong relationships with local community centers and resources will be most advantageous for quick response.

— A comprehensive list of local and national resources is available on the Centers for Disease Control and Prevention website: https://www.cdc.gov/violenceprevention/intimatepartnerviolence/index.html

Table 9-2. National IPV Resources

National Domestic Violence Hotline	800-799-SAFE (7233) 800-787-3224 (TTY) thehotline.org	— 24/7 — Free — Confidential
National Sexual Assault Hotline	800-656-HOPE (4673)	— 24/7 — Free — Confidential
Intimate Partner Violence Assistance Program (IPVAP) US Department of Veterans Affairs	855-VA-WOMEN womenshealth.va.gov https://www.socialwork.va.gov/IPV/Index.asp Locating state coordinator: https://www.socialwork.va.gov/IPV/Coordinators.asp	— Community-based support, advocacy, and legal services — Domestic shelters — Access to IPV coordinators
Safe House	(205) 669-7233 (SAFE) – collect calls accepted safehouse@safehouse.org	— 24-hours — Counseling — Legal assistance
WomensLaw	womenslaw.org info@hotline.womenslaw.org	— Email-based legal advice

References

1. Gilbert LK, Zhang X, Basile KC, Breiding M, Kresnow M. Intimate partner violence and health conditions among US adults—national intimate partner violence survey, 2010–2012. *J Interpers Violence.* 2023;38(1-2):NP237-NP261. doi:10.1177/08862605221080147

2. Potter L, Morris R, Hegarty K, García-Moreno C, Feder G. Categories and health impacts of intimate partner violence in the World Health Organization multi-country study on women's health and domestic violence. *Int J Epidemiol.* 2021;50(2):652-662. doi:10.1093/ije/dyaa220

3. Hurwitz EJ, Gupta J, Liu R, Silverman JG, Raj A. Intimate partner violence associated with poor health outcomes in US South Asian women. *J Immigr Minor Health.* 2006;8(3):251-261. doi:10.1007/s10903-006-9330-1

4. Ellsberg M, Jansen HA, Heise L, Watts CH, Garcia-Moreno C; WHO Multi-country Study on Women's Health and Domestic Violence against Women Study Team. Intimate partner violence and women's physical and mental health in the WHO multi-country study on women's health and domestic violence: an observational study. *Lancet.* 2008;371(9619):1165-1172. doi:10.1016/S0140-6736(08)60522-X

5. Campbell JC. Health consequences of intimate partner violence. *Lancet.* 2002;359(9314):1331-1336. doi:10.1016/S0140-6736(02)08336-8

6. Campbell J, Jones AS, Dienemann J, et al. Intimate partner violence and physical health consequences. *Arch Intern Med.* 2002;162(10):1157-1163. doi:10.1001/archinte.162.10.1157

7. Ahrens CE, Rios-Mandel LC, Isas L, Del Carmen Lopez M. Talking about interpersonal violence: cultural influences on Latinas' identification and disclosure of sexual assault and intimate partner violence. *Psychol Trauma.* 2010;2(4):284-295. doi:10.1037/a0018605
8. Zlotnick C, Johnson DM, Kohn R. Intimate partner violence and long-term psychosocial functioning in a national sample of American women. *J Interpers Violence.* 2006;21(2):262-275. doi:10.1177/0886260505282564
9. Alsaker K, Moen BE, Kristoffersen K. Health-related quality of life among abused women one year after leaving a violent partner. *Soc Indic Res.* 2008;86(3): 497-509. doi:10.1007/s11205-007-9182-7
10. Smith SG, Chen J, Basile KC, et al. *The National Intimate Partner and Sexual Violence Survey (NISVS): 2010-2012 State Report.* National Center for Injury Prevention and Control, Centers for Disease Control and Prevention; 2017. https://www.cdc.gov/violenceprevention/pdf/nisvs-statereportbook.pdf
11. Williams DR, Rucker TD. Understanding and addressing racial disparities in health care. *Health Care Financ Rev.* 2000;21(4):75-90.
12. Erez E, Hartley CC. Battered immigrant women and the legal system: a therapeutic jurisprudence perspective. *West Criminol Rev.* 2003;4(2):155-169.
13. Bauer HM, Rodriguez MA, Quiroga SS, Flores-Ortiz YG. Barriers to health care for abused Latina and Asian immigrant women. *J Health Care Poor Underserved.* 2000;11(1):33-44. doi:10.1353/hpu.2010.0590
14. Stockman J, Hayashi H, Campbell J. Intimate partner violence and its health impact on ethnic minority women. *J Women's Health.* 2015;24(1):62-79. doi:10.1089/jwh.2014.4879
15. Randle AA, Graham CAA. A review of the evidence on the effects of intimate partner violence on men. *Psychol Men Masculinity.* 2011;12(2):97-111. doi:10.1037/a0021944
16. Ehrensaft MK, Moffitt TE, Caspi A. Clinically abusive relationships in an unselected birth cohort: men's and women's participation and developmental antecedents. *J Abnorm Psychol.* 2004;113(2):258-270. doi:10.1037/0021-843X.113.2.258
17. Buller AM, Devries KM, Howard LM, Bacchus LJ. Associations between intimate partner violence and health among men who have sex with men: a systematic review and meta-analysis. *PLOS Med.* 2014;11(3):e1001609. doi:10.1371/journal.pmed.1001609
18. James SE, Herman JL, Rankin S, Keisling M, Mottet L, Anafi M. The report of the 2015 US transgender survey. National Center for Transgender Equality. 2016. https://transequality.org/sites/default/files/docs/usts/USTS-Full-Report-Dec17.pdf
19. Peitzmeier S, Malik M, Kattari S, et al. Intimate partner violence in transgender populations: systematic review and meta-analysis of prevalence and correlates. *Am J Pub Health.* 2020;110(9):e1-e14. doi:10.2105/AJPH.2020.305774
20. Hillman J. Lifetime prevalence of intimate partner violence and health-related outcomes among transgender adults aged 50 and older. *Gerontol.* 2022;62(2): 212-222. doi:10.1093/geront/gnab067
21. Barba D. Insights series #150: socialization matters more than circumstance in predicting the normalization of intimate partner violence in the Americas. LAPOP Lab. May 3, 2022. https://www.vanderbilt.edu/lapop/insights/IO950en-1.pdf

22. Kohlman S, Baig A, Balice G, et al. Contribution of media to the normalization and perpetuation of domestic violence. *Austin J Psychiatry Behav Sci.* 2014; 1(4):1018.

23. Toro-Alfonso J, Rodríguez-Madera S. Domestic violence in Puerto Rican gay male couples: perceived prevalence, intergenerational violence, addictive behaviors, and conflict resolution skills. *J Interpers Violence.* 2004;19(6):639-654. doi:10.1177/0886260504263873

24. Rolle L, Giardina G, Caldarera AM, Gerino E, Brustia P. When intimate partner violence meets same sex couples: a review of same sex intimate partner violence. *Front Psychol.* 2018;9(1506):1-10. doi:10.3389/fpsyg.2018.01506

25. Brown TNT, Herman JL. Intimate partner violence and sexual abuse among LGBT people: a review of existing research. The Williams Institute UCLA School of Law. November 2015. https://williamsinstitute.law.ucla.edu/wp-content/uploads/IPV-Sexual-Abuse-Among-LGBT-Nov-2015.pdf

26. Taylor JC, Bates EA, Colosi A, Creer AJ. Barriers to men's help seeking for intimate partner violence. *J Interpers Violence.* 2022;37(19-20):NP18417-NP18444. doi:10.1177/08862605211035870

27. McCann M. Domestic violence/domestic abuse definitions and relationships. National Conference of State Legislatures. Updated June 13, 2019. Accessed September 12, 2022. https://www.ncsl.org/research/human-services/domestic-violence-domestic-abuse-definitions-and-relationships.aspx#:~:text=(7)%20%22Intimate%20partner%20violence,in%20a%20domestic%20partnership%3B%20or

28. Dillon G, Hussain R, Loxton D, Rahman S. Mental and physical health and intimate partner violence against women: a review of the literature. *Int J Family Med.* 2013;2013:313909. doi:10.1155/2013/313909

29. Patel K, Robertson E, Kwong ASF, et al. Psychological distress before and during the COVID-19 pandemic among adults in the United Kingdom based on coordinated analyses of 11 longitudinal studies. *JAMA Netw Open.* 2022;5(4):e227629. doi:10.1001/jamanetworkopen.2022.7629

30. Galea S, Merchant RM, Lurie N. The mental health consequences of COVID-19 and physical distancing: the need for prevention and early intervention. *JAMA Intern Med.* 2020;180(6):817-818. doi:10.1001/jamainternmed.2020.1562

31. US Preventive Services Task Force. Screening for family and intimate partner violence: recommendation statement. *Ann Intern Med.* 2004;140(5):382-386. doi:10.7326/0003-4819-140-5-200403020-00014

32. Moyer VA. Screening for intimate partner violence and abuse of elderly and vulnerable adults: US Preventive Services Task Force recommendation statement. *Ann Intern Med.* 2013;158(6):478-486. doi:10.7326/0003-4819-158-6-201303190-00588

33. ACOG Committee Opinion No. 518: Intimate partner violence. *Obstet Gynecol.* 2012;119(2 Pt 1):412-417. doi:10.1097/AOG.0b013e318249ff74

34. US Preventive Services Task Force. Screening for intimate partner violence, elder abuse, and abuse of vulnerable adults: recommendation statement. *Am Fam Physician.* 2019;99(10).

35. Dicola D, Spaar E. Intimate partner violence. *Am Fam Physician.* 2016; 94(8): 646-651.

36. O'Doherty LJ, Taft A, Hegarty K, Ramsay J, Davidson LL, Feder G. Screening women for intimate partner violence in healthcare settings: abridged Cochrane systematic review and meta-analysis. *BMJ*. 2014;348(g2913):1-14. doi:10.1136/bmj.g2913

37. Chang JC. Intimate partner violence: how you can help female survivors. *Cleve Clin J Med*. 2014;81(7):439-446. doi:10.3949/ccjm.81a.13069

38. Modi MN, Palmer S, Armstrong A. The role of Violence Against Women Act in addressing intimate partner violence: a public health issue. *J Womens Health (Larchmt)*. 2014;23(3):253-259. doi:10.1089/jwh.2013.4387

39. Weiss SJ. Ongoing violence assessment tool (OVAT). MDCalc.com. Accessed September 30, 2022. https://www.mdcalc.com/calc/10418/ongoing-violence-assessment-tool-ovat#evidence

40. Paranjape A, Liebschutz J. STaT: a three-question screen for intimate partner violence. *J Womens Health*. 2004;12(3):233-239. doi:10.1089/154099903321667573

41. MacMillan HL, Wathen CN, Jamieson E, et al. Approaches to screening for intimate partner violence in health care settings: a randomized trial. *JAMA*. 2006;296(5):530-536. doi:10.1001/jama.296.5.530

42. Snider C, Webster D, O'Sullivan CS, Campbell J. Intimate partner violence: development of a brief risk assessment for the emergency department. *Acad Emerg Med*. 2009;16(11):1208-1216. doi:10.1177/08862605221080147

Chapter 10

Sexual Assault Assessment

Christine Foote-Lucero, MSN, RN, CEN, SANE-A, SANE-P, AFN-C, DF-AFN
Erin M. Aschman, BSN, RN, SANE-A, GFN-C

Key Points

1. *Sexual assault (SA) is any sexual contact or act performed upon a person by 1 or more persons without consent.*
2. *The medical, emotional, and forensic needs of a patient affected by sexual violence should be met through a comprehensive medical forensic examination (MFE) and should include examination, treatment, testing, documentation, follow-up, and reporting options.*
3. *Having the ability to provide trauma- and violence-informed care (TVIC) is an essential skill when caring for patients affected by sexual violence, and clinicians should seek to mitigate retraumatization and minimize negative outcomes.*

Background and Significance

SA is a complex form of violence with medical, psychological, and legal components and can have profound and lasting effects on patients. SA is defined as any sexual act performed by 1 or more persons on another without explicit consent and can include force or threat of force.[1] SA encompasses many types of sexual behaviors or contact and can include penetration or attempted penetration of body orifices, unwanted sexual touching, forced sexual activities, exposure to pornography, viewing or recording private grooming or dressing, exhibitionism, verbal and emotional sexual harassment, and attempts to force someone into sexual activity with others. All genders are affected by SA and should be screened and treated without bias. The Joint Commission (TJC) requires hospitals to assist patients affected by SA by either providing appropriate examinations or referring them to a private or public community agency that can provide the service.[2] All members of the health care team who respond to patients affected by SA must provide compassionate, coordinated, and competent TVIC. This approach should include realizing how trauma can affect individuals and communities, recognizing signs of trauma, responding with TVIC language and behaviors, and ensuring that revictimization is prevented.[3] In addition, health care providers (HCP) should always use the term "patient," a health care term, rather than "victim," a legal term. Similar to any area of health care, the complex and multidimensional approach needed to properly care for a patient experiencing SA necessitates the HCP to have undergone specialized training. The HCP must be knowledgeable in the medical, psychological, social, and safety needs of these patients, in addition to the legal implications and processes of the state and jurisdiction of their practice. Many institutions have established sexual assault nurse examiner (SANE) or forensic nurse examiner (FNE) programs to address the specific and unique needs of patients affected by sexual violence.

Prevalence and Epidemiology

Providing for the post-SA needs of a patient requires the HCP to deliver care with dignity, recognizing SA as a human rights issue. SA does not discriminate between ability, wealth, or social status, and all ages, genders, and races may be vulnerable. In the United States, approximately 1 in 4 women and 1 in 5 men experience some form of sexual violence in their lifetime.[4] These numbers are likely understated due to the substantial underreporting of sexual violence. A variety of factors contribute to underreporting of SA, such as embarrassment and stigma, ambiguity about what constitutes SA, perceptions by victims that they will not be believed or that the criminal justice system will be ineffective, and perception that some incidents are not serious enough.[5] Other factors may include prior encounters with law enforcement or negative experiences with HCPs who were not compassionate and understanding in the implementation of TVIC. These factors can be seen especially in transgender patients who experience health care disparities at a higher rate than their cisgender counterparts.[6] Research repeatedly concludes that lesbian, gay, bisexual, transgender, queer or questioning, intersex, and asexual/aromantic/agender, among other sexual and gender minority (LGBTQIA+) populations are at an elevated risk of sexual violence victimization, as seen in **Figures 10-1-a** and **10-1-b** below.[7]

Figure 10-1-a. *Prevalence of sexual assault by female gender identity.*[7]

Figure 10-1-b. *Prevalence of sexual assault by male gender identity.*[7]

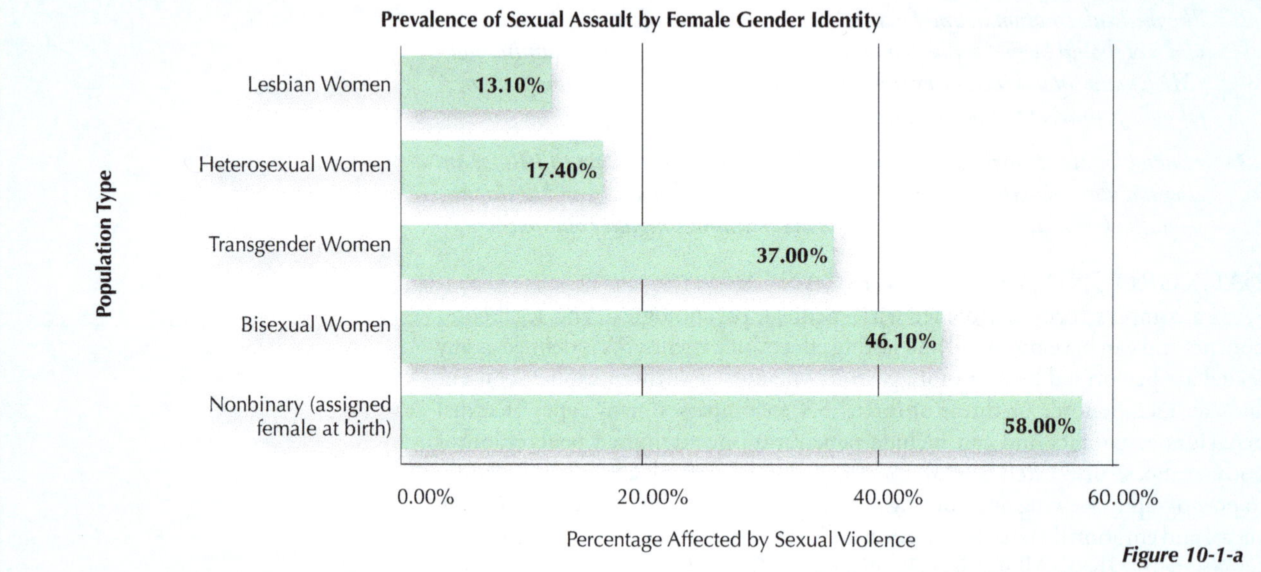

Figure 10-1-a

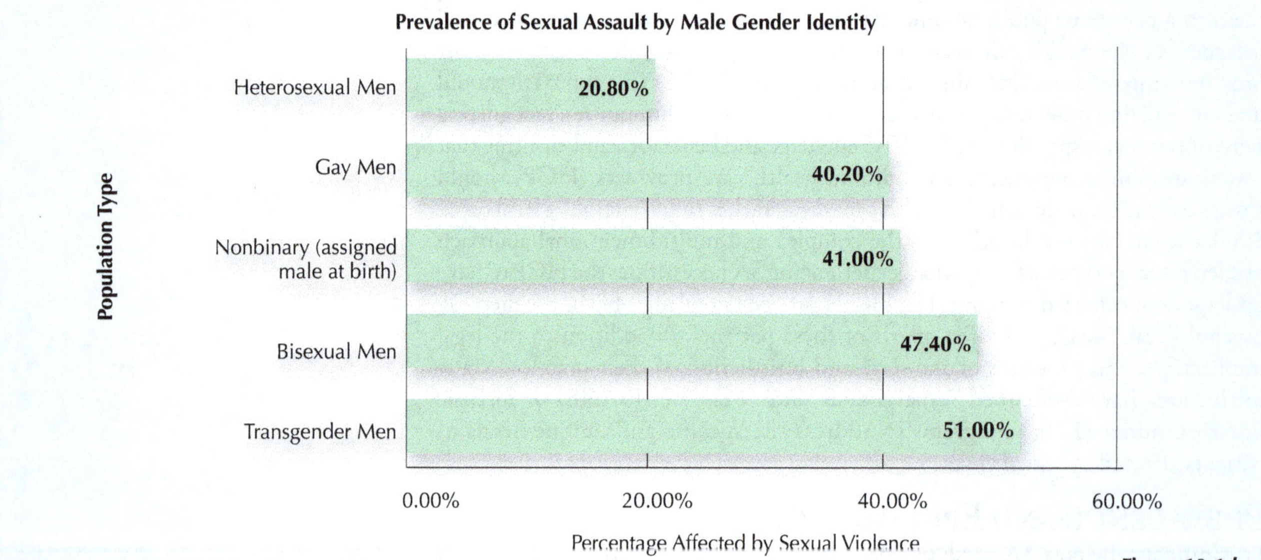

Figure 10-1-b

Health Consequences

In addition to medical issues, SA can also affect social functioning, health perceptions, and quality of life.[8] Clinicians responding to SA patients are uniquely positioned to help mitigate physical, sexual, and psychological consequences and sequelae.[8,9] Physical sequelae include but are not limited to migraines, concussion, postconcussive syndrome, chronic pain, sleep disturbances, sexually transmitted infections (STIs), unplanned pregnancy, and miscarriage. Sexual sequelae include but are not limited to fear of sexual coercion, increased casual sex, and increased sexual risk-taking behaviors, such as multiple sexual partners, sexual activities at a young age, unprotected sexual activities, and exchanging sexual activities for money.[8] Psychological sequelae include but are not limited to acute or post-traumatic stress disorder, suicide, self-harm, depression, and substance abuse.[8] The knowledge and attitude of the HCP toward sexually assaulted patients are important aspects that influence the patient's perception of care, as well as their physical and psychological wellbeing.[9] The experience of the initial medical visit post-SA can mitigate many of the poor health outcomes that these patients may develop.

Medico-Legal Examination

There are many health care and legal challenges that are specific to patients affected by SA. These include negligence in follow-up or disregard for those that do not demonstrate physical injuries; underestimation of patients' complaints; long waiting hours; inability to eat or drink while waiting for the medico-legal examination; unqualified HCPs conducting the exam, which may lead to unintentional revictimization; contamination of viable evidence that could be used in a court of law; and noncompliance with jurisdictional legal requirements.[9] Because of this, many health care facilities have implemented SANE or FNE programs. These HCPs receive specialized education and preparation to perform a medico-legal examination, often referred to as an MFE. This examination can validate a patient's concerns, allow for increased sense of control, mitigate trauma, provide safety, and promote healing. Accommodations must be provided for patients that have hearing or visual impairments, as well as patients in need of translation services. Certified medical interpreters fluent in both the patient's language as well as cultural customs should be used for any translation needs, and the HCP must recognize the risks of using a family member or friend to interpret, such as inaccuracies in interpretation, misunderstanding of medical terminology, or preconceived bias surrounding the event or person involved.

The role of the SANE is to conduct a high-quality MFE while providing patient-centered care. Some SANEs are also trained in the collection of evidence in suspect examinations. Studies have shown that patients feel humanized and better cared for during their hospital encounters with SANEs than during prior experiences with non-SANE providers.[3] In addition, studies have also shown that Emergency Departments (EDs) with SANE programs are more likely to provide STI prophylaxis, emergency contraception (EC), comprehensive medical services, and proper completion of forensic exams.[3] Many nursing organizations have recommended the use of a SANE, and the American College of Emergency Physicians (ACEP) has endorsed a policy that recommends selective triage to specialized SANE treatment centers as well as providing SANE resources for these patients.[10]

The HCP should be prepared to address the needs—forensic as well as medical and emotional—of the SA patient. There are many components to a thorough MFE, and the HCP performing these exams should include the following:

- Discuss the MFE, including risks, benefits, and alternatives required for informed consent.
- Assess and treat physical injuries.

- Obtain a current medication list, allergies, and past medical, surgical, and gynecologic history, including the patient's current mode of contraception and last menstrual period.
- Document a history of the assault for medical diagnosis and treatment.
- Perform a physical examination, including a head-to-toe assessment with detailed anogenital and pelvic examinations.
- Document body and genital findings with diagrams and photographs.
- Obtain appropriate evidence specimens while maintaining chain of custody.
- Consider and collect applicable STI testing.
- Provide infectious disease prophylaxis as indicated.
- Evaluate for exposure to Human Immunodeficiency Virus (HIV) and discuss the risks and benefits of postexposure prophylaxis.
- Provide or arrange for the provision of EC if indicated.
- Provide acute crisis intervention and referral for advocacy.
- Counsel the patient regarding their findings, recommendations, and prognosis.
- Complete a psychosocial assessment.
- Arrange referrals for medical and psychological follow-up.
- Report to authorities as required by local jurisdictional statutes.
- Ensure chain of evidence.
- Present findings and opinions in court.

The HCP should also ensure that the medical forensic chart, which includes the history and images, is kept separate from the general hospital records in compliance with the Violence Against Women Act (VAWA).[10]

Therapeutic communication, trust, rapport, and support are the cornerstones of an MFE. TVIC techniques that the clinician should implement may include maintaining eye contact and engaging in active listening with the patient; minimizing distractions like ringing phones; environment modification such as private MFE rooms that provide safety and are segregated from general wards; clear, unrushed, transparent communication with explanations that are tailored to the patient's educational, developmental, and cognitive level; collaboration with the patient regarding the plan of care; and establishing the patient's empowerment to accept or decline any component of the MFE. Crucial to TVIC is also the consideration of any structural barriers to accessing services, such as a lack of money for prescriptions or transportation. These should be addressed prior to making treatment recommendations. Thoughtful use of language that is not construed as offensive or implies that the assault occurred due to the patient's actions, known as victim blaming, is imperative.[9] The HCP should also use gender-neutral language; be sensitive to cultural, historical and gender issues; and explain to patients what to expect both before and during the examination.

Consent

All patients affected by SA should be offered an MFE. This discussion should include risks and benefits of the MFE, including topics such as reporting options, mandatory reporting obligations, legal implications, and evidentiary value of specimens based upon time that has lapsed since the assault. It is necessary for the

HCP to obtain verbal and written informed consent from patients who are older than 18 years. Children and developmentally delayed adults who do not make their own medical decisions will typically require the consent of a parent, guardian, health care proxy, or Medical Durable Power of Attorney (MDPOA) in order to perform an MFE with evidence collection, although this may vary based upon whether that person is the suspected offender or based upon local jurisdictional statutes. Even when the patient is not the party providing legal consent, the HCP is still required to acquire the patient's assent, or agreement, before proceeding with any part of the MFE. Both the informed consent process and the assent process are meant to be an ongoing conversation throughout the duration of the MFE. The patient has the right to cooperate with or decline any or all of the MFE, and a patient must never be held down or forced to cooperate with any part of the examination. The HCP should consider these questions when initiating consent for the MFE: (a) Can the patient give legal informed consent? (b) Can a patient younger than 18 years give assent with a parent, guardian, health care proxy or MDPOA providing legal consent, per jurisdictional statutes? (c) Can the patient understand the role of the HCP and any other care provider assisting in the MFE? (d) Does the patient understand the long-term implications of the consent given? Patients under the influence of any substance may be able to give consent if they appear to be clinically sober, such as providing correct information for orientation questions and demonstrating alertness with linear, organized speech. If SA is suspected but the patient is unable to provide consent, it is controversial as to whether or not to perform this examination. However, in the absence of a surrogate decision-maker, portions of the examination might be done if routine examination already requires examination of those areas, if examination would not induce additional discomfort, or if a medical procedure is to be done that would destroy evidence.[9] It is imperative that the HCP follows their institutional policy and local jurisdictional mandates in these situations.

History

After written consent is acquired, a history of the assault should be obtained. It is imperative to include the patient's exact statements, word for word, in quotations, to ensure accuracy and avoid misinterpretation. This is a medical history for the purposes of diagnosis and treatment, and not a statement or inquisition for investigatory purposes. It is therefore not appropriate for law enforcement to be in the room during the history obtained by the HCP. This may even negate the provider's medical exception to hearsay, Rule 803(4), which would allow the HCP to discuss the statements that the patient made in a court of law.

The history should focus on specific details of the assault for the purposes of medical diagnosis and treatment, with those details including but not limited to: considerations for bodily and anogenital injury, assessment for risk of pregnancy and STIs, identification of applicable specimens, determination of a possibility of loss of consciousness or memory, and to ascertain if there was use of weapons, force, restraint, or threats. The history should be obtained in a sensitive and supportive manner, starting with least invasive questions before moving onto more invasive questions. Any support persons at the bedside should refrain from interrupting or asking questions in a leading or suggestive manner.[1] The HCP should be careful to note in the history what body parts could have been touched, kissed, licked, or are otherwise a potential source of DNA transfer so that these areas can be swabbed per the evidence collection kit protocol. If a slang term or nickname is used to describe a body part or a sexual act, that term should be used in quotations as the patient said it, but then the examiner should clarify its meaning. Once a disclosure of the assault has been made, the HCP should validate the patient's experience. Responses can include "Thank you for sharing that with me," "Thank you for trusting me," "I know that must have been very hard," "There is nothing you did to cause this," and "I am so sorry that has happened to you." Legal terms, such as alleged, should not be used in a medical chart for an SA patient, just as a provider would not use the terms "alleged headache" or "alleged abdominal pain."

Trauma is defined as an event that combines fear, horror, or terror with an actual or perceived lack of control and overwhelms a person's coping mechanisms.[11] The individual hard-wiring of a person's brain, combined with a lifetime of learning and their lived experiences, results in trauma being subjective from one person to another. The experience of a traumatic event has physiologic implications to the body. The release of specific chemicals within the body, most notably catecholamines, trigger the body's survival reflexes and can have implications to the brain's ability to chronologically store, form, and categorize memories. Higher functioning systems within the prefrontal cortex which allow logical and rational thinking can also be impacted.[11] During trauma, this chemical flood is activated to aid the body in survival, effectively directing the body to shunt resources to bodily systems that allow the body to react with a survival response such as fight, flight, freeze, or fawn. Bursts of adrenaline also activate the amygdala, an area of the brain involved with the processing of emotions, which may lead to isolated sensory fragments being recorded into memory.[11] Specific sensory details such as visual images, smells, sounds, or felt experiences can be strongly imprinted and recalled. Simultaneously, the body directs resources to vital functions and directs resources away from nonvital bodily functions.[11]

It is important to note that the body's initial and immediate reaction to a traumatic event is automatic and therefore cannot be consciously controlled. This can be very distressing to patients who have experienced trauma. These effects can be observed in a myriad of emotional responses from the patient. While providing the history, the patient may have fragmented or poor memory recall, which can cause increased stress and retraumatization.[11] It is important that the HCP creates a safe environment with uninterrupted time for the patient to provide the history. A trained HCP can use prompts, like sensory questions such as "Do you remember hearing anything during the assault?" to aid in the patient's memory recall. A clear understanding of the physiological implications of trauma can aid in decreasing distress in the SA patient and promote an understanding and acceptance of the individual's traumatic experience. Therefore, the HCP taking a history should understand TVIC and key elements of how patients are affected by trauma to mitigate retraumatization. The way in which a history is taken can also have long-term impacts on the patient's recovery (see **Volume 2, Chapter 12: Consent and Alcohol-Enabled and Drug-Facilitated Sexual Assault**).

Physical and Anogenital Exam with Evidence Collection

A thorough head-to-toe examination with a detailed anogenital examination should be performed on all patients who experience SA. The HCP should refer to institutional policy regarding timeframes for collecting physical DNA evidence, although facilities will generally collect if patients present within 7 days of their assault. It is imperative to include subjective symptoms such as complaints of pain, lightheadedness, and nausea, as well as objective findings. During the examination, the patient's body should be covered, only exposing necessary areas for the shortest possible time. Each injury should be carefully recorded to include size (using metric measurements), shape, color, type of injury, and anatomical location. It is also good practice to include if the patient recalls how the injury was sustained. Supplemental photo documentation is recommended to support written documentation. The HCP should be able to identify if these injuries are consistent with the history provided by the patient. While many patients may not have any body surface trauma, extragenital findings are typically more common than genital findings and can include bruises, abrasions, or erythema to the thigh, upper arm, face, or neck.[12] Based upon the information provided in the history, the HCP should also swab any bodily areas throughout the head-to-toe assessment that could have possible evidentiary value per their local jurisdictional guidelines. If the HCP determines that there may be evidentiary value in oral swabs, in cases of oral penetration, the mouth should be swabbed early in the MFE so that the patient can eat and drink if desired.

After the head-to-toe assessment is complete, the HCP should proceed to the detailed anogenital exam (see **Figures 10-2** through **10-8** and **Table 10-1**). The patient's comfort should influence their positioning for this portion of the examination. Possible positions include lithotomy, supine knee chest, supine frog leg, or side lying. For females, the HCP should begin with a gross visual inspection of the mons pubis and outer labia majora. Then gentle labial traction is performed to visualize the vestibule. This is the mucosal area within the labia majora, and includes the labia minora, clitoris and clitoral hood, urethra and periurethral tissue, hymen, posterior fourchette, and fossa navicularis. Traction may be performed toward the examiner, laterally, and to some degree anteriorly and posteriorly depending upon the structure within the vestibule that is being visualized. Each structure should be assessed and photographed with a colposcope (binocular microscope), or an equivalent substitute, that allows for magnification and lighting. Once genital evidence collection of this area is complete, the HCP should proceed with inspection of the buttocks, perineum, anus, and anal folds. Collection of evidence from this area should occur before placement of a vaginal speculum or vaginal instrumentation, as consideration must be given to the natural gravitational flow of secretions from the vaginal vault to the anal folds upon speculum removal.[13] Then, in patients who have reached a Tanner Stage 3 sexual maturity rating and are noted to have an estrogenized hymen, the clinician may proceed with speculum insertion to assess and perform evidence collection from the vagina and cervix.[14] The HCP should also consider the collection of STI swabs. If the patient is not appropriate for a speculum insertion, such as a patient who has not started menses or is postmenopausal and does not have an estrogenized hymen, a blind vaginal swab may be considered. After all evidence has been collected, the final step will be for the HCP to perform a detailed assessment of the estrogenized hymen, using either a large cotton-tipped swab or a foley catheter if required due to the redundancy of the tissue.[15] The foley catheter technique is far superior in allowing for circumferential visualization and utilizes an inflated foley balloon in the distal vaginal vault to expand the estrogenized hymen to its full capacity so that the hymenal edge may be readily visualized for signs of trauma. The swab or foley should always be done after evidence collection to ensure that any DNA that was present was preserved and collected prior to the procedure.

On male patients, the detailed anogenital examination should begin with a thorough inspection of the penis, including the shaft, glans, and the scrotum.[15] If the patient is not circumcised, the foreskin should be retracted gently and thoroughly to perform a comprehensive examination. As with female patients, each structure should be assessed, photographed, and evidence collected per protocol. Once external genital assessment and evidence are completed, the clinician should inspect the buttocks, perineum, anus, and anal folds, followed by evidence ccollection of this area.[15] In both male and female patients, the HCP should consider anoscopy in cases of reported anal penetration, reported anal pain, or concerns for anal or rectal injury.

The HCP performing the anogenital exam should be proficient in identifying acute and healed injury, normal variants that are commonly mistaken for injury, iatrogenic findings, and sexual maturity rating such as Tanner Staging. Normal variants could include hymenal notches (or clefts), cervical ectropion, Nabothian cysts, and nevi. Generally, genital injury findings are uncommon after SA.[14,16] However, when injury findings are present, prevalence nearly triples in women that were examined in the first 72 hours compared with those presenting later, likely due to the rapid and remarkable healing capacity of the mucosal tissue within the female genitalia. The most common location for injury in women is the posterior fourchette, but other anatomical locations include the labia minora, hymen, fossa navicularis, vulva, vagina, perineum, and cervix.[16] Anal injuries are also more likely to be found when examining patients affected by intimate partner violence (IPV).[16] Anal lacerations, swelling, and bruising are also markers for nonconsensual sexual intercourse and should increase the index of suspicion for lack of consent.[16] However, failure to find these markers should not waive suspicion, as lack of injury does not indicate absence of SA. It is crucial for the HCP to understand that many patients will have minor or no extragenital or genital injuries. While studies have noted both the presence of anogenital injuries in cases of consensual sexual intercourse, as well as the absence of anogenital injuries in cases of nonconsensual sexual intercourse, the presence of external genital lacerations is more than 2 times as likely to be a finding in nonconsensual sexual intercourse.[16]

In cases where the HCP is unsure of whether findings are acute injury versus normal variant, or in cases where there is injury that requires re-evaluation for healing, the HCP should have the patient return for a follow-up visit in 1 to 2 weeks.[1] At the follow-up visit, additional photographs of injuries can be taken to assess and document healing or any changes from initial findings. Further treatment in order to complete vaccinations, repeat testing for STIs, and consult with specialists may be necessary as indicated by the Centers for Disease Control and Prevention (CDC).[1] A follow-up phone call may also be considered to

Figure 10-2-a and *10-2-b*. Structures of the female genitalia.

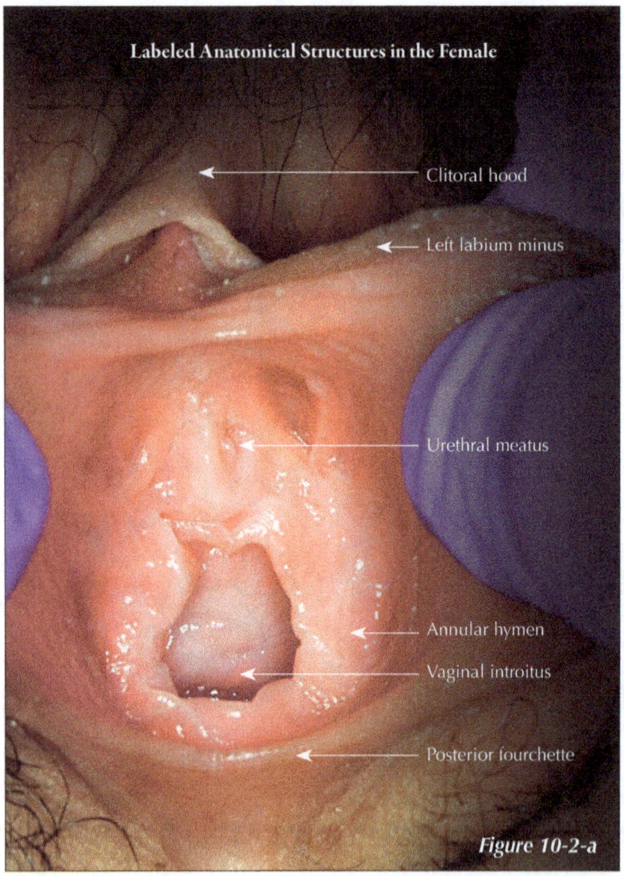

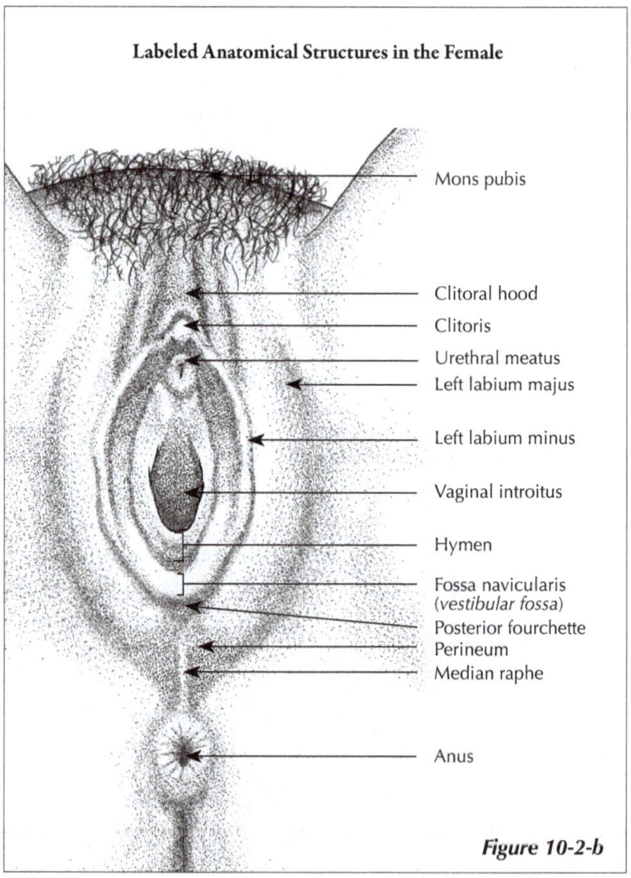

address further questions, communicate medical results, or evaluate further medical or safety needs. A discussion with the patient regarding follow-up phone calls should occur at the initial visit and should be completed within 48 hours after discharge.

The HCP performing an MFE must also be competent and proficient at providing trans-affirming care to the transgender patient who has experienced SA. Transgender patients are individuals whose gender identity does not correspond with their assigned sex at birth, and these patients have differing needs from other patients affected by SA.[17] The HCP should perform an anatomical inventory so that appropriate and applicable assessments and interventions are performed. The HCP should also understand the unique concerns relevant to transgender patients, such as added psychological and bodily trauma, hormone replacement therapy, transition-related surgeries, and body dysmorphia. Consideration may also be given to allow the patient to self-collect STI samples or self-insert instruments such as a speculum.

Table 10-1. Structures of the female genitalia
— ***Cervical os:*** The opening in the cervix that leads to the endometrial cavity of the uterus. This area consists of unstratified columnar epithelium cells.
— ***Cervix:*** The portion of the uterus between the isthmus and the vagina.
— ***Clitoral hood:*** A fold of skin covering the clitoris.
— ***Clitoris:*** A small, cylindrical erectile body at the anterior portion of the vulva, covered by the clitoral hood.
— ***Fossa navicularis:*** The concavity of the lower part of the vestibule, posterior and inferior to the hymen corona.
— ***Hymen:*** A collar or semicollar of tissue surrounding the vaginal orifice.
— ***Labia majora:*** Two folds of skin on either side of the labia minora. This area usually is covered with hair that appears during puberty.
— ***Labia minora:*** The longitudinal thin folds of nonkeratinized skin medial to the labia majora. The labia minora are hairless but have many sensory nerve endings that engorge when stimulated.
— ***Median raphe:*** A visible line of tissue extending from the anus to the perineum. It is located between the vestibule and the anus in the female and the scrotum and the anus in the male.
— ***Mons pubis:*** The rounded fleshy prominence created by adipose tissue overlying the pubic symphysis bone.
— ***Perineum:*** The external surface or base of the perineal body, lying between the vulva and anus. This network of muscles, located between and around the vagina and anus, supports the pelvic cavity and maintains the structure of the pelvic floor by keeping the organs in place.
— ***Periurethral bands*** (also called vestibular bands or urethral ligaments): Structures that support the urethra and the pelvic floor and are often confused with adhesive scarring. When seen, these bands are usually symmetrical, found in pairs, and attached to the pubic symphysis area.
— ***Posterior fourchette*** (also called Hart's line or the posterior commissure): An area where the 2 labia meet posteriorly.

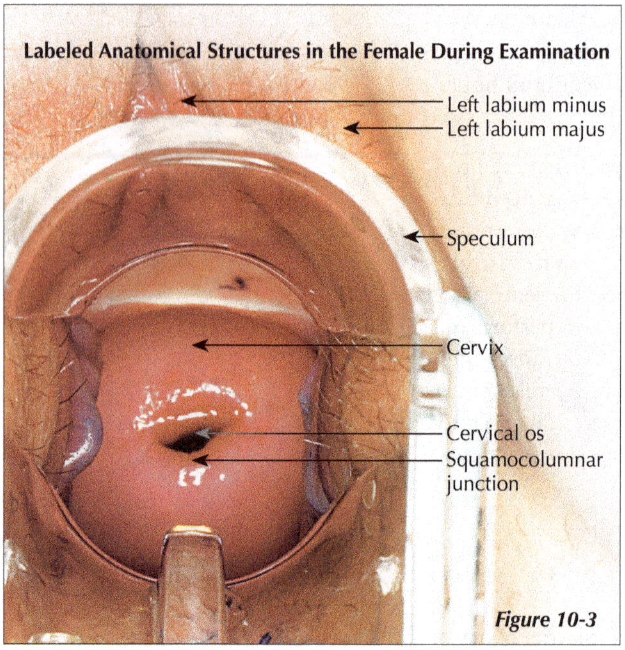

Figure 10-3

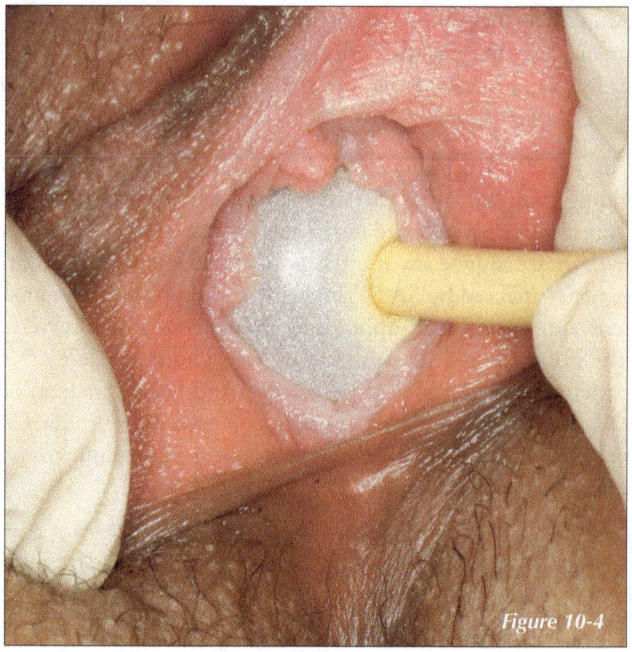

Figure 10-4

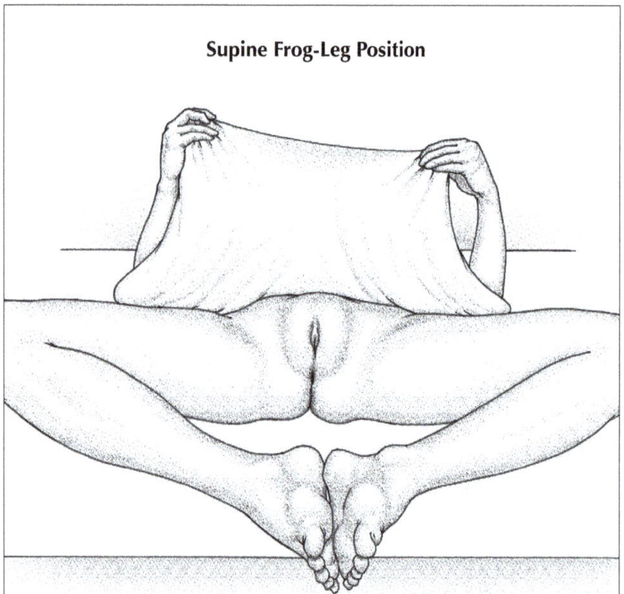

Figure 10-5

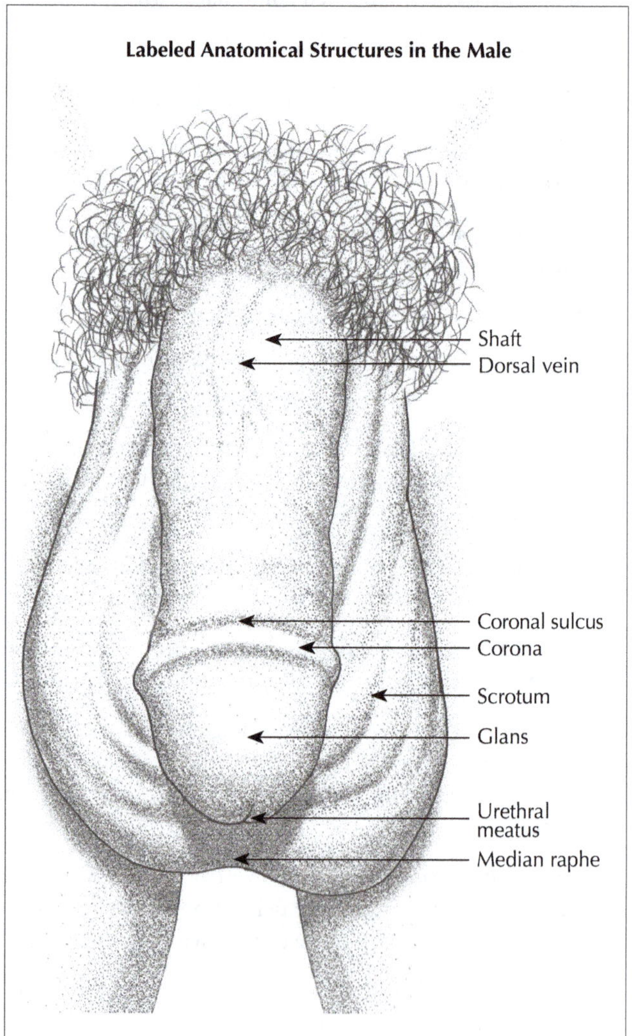

Figure 10-6

Figure 10-3. *Structures of the female genitalia while speculum is in place.*

Figure 10-4. *Utilizing the foley balloon technique to visualize the hymenal rim. The balloon is filled with air.*

Figure 10-5. *Genital examination of the female in the supine frog-leg position.*

Figure 10-6. *Frontal view of the external male genitalia.*

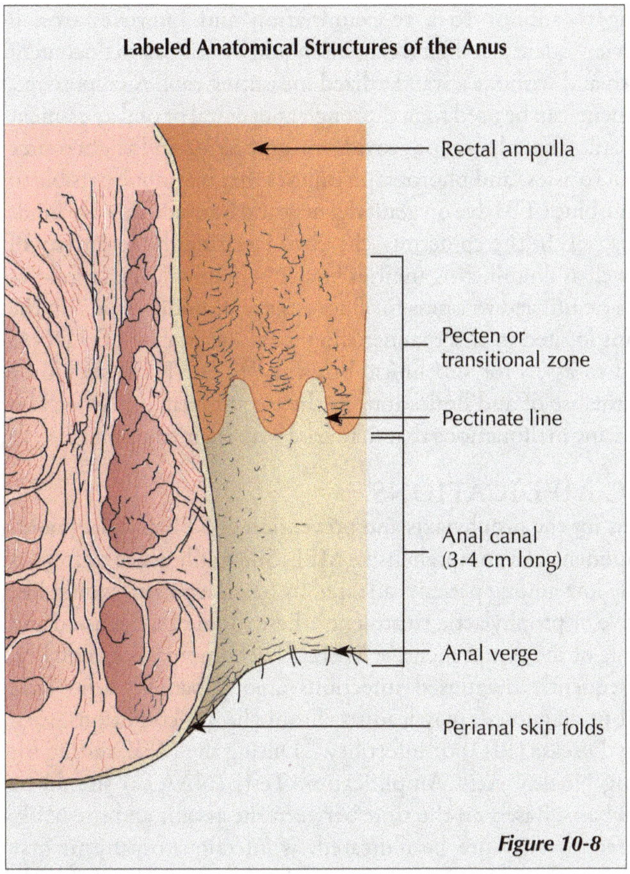

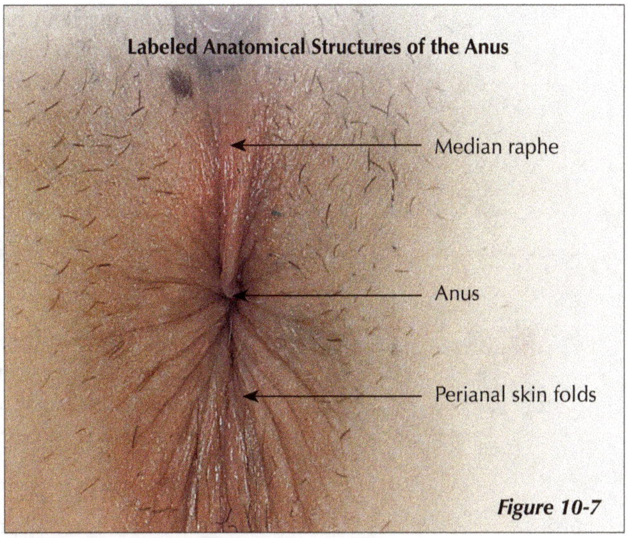

Figure 10-7. *Anal anatomy.*

Figure 10-8. *Cross-sectional view of anus.*

Reporting Options and Maintaining Confidentiality

Reporting options will vary by state jurisdiction, as well as the patient's civilian or military status and age.[10] The most common option across jurisdictions is reporting to law enforcement, which involves a statement given to police by the patient as well as a subsequent investigation. Reporting options may also be affected by mandatory reporting statutes for that state, such as in cases of elder or child abuse where they must be reported to law enforcement and child or adult protection. HCPs should always educate patients about their available reporting options to make an informed decision regarding their case. HCPs performing an MFE must remain in compliance with the Health Insurance Portability and Accountability Act (HIPAA) and follow all policies and guidelines for the management of Protected Health Information (PHI). HCPs may share PHI with law enforcement if a court order is produced by a judge, if an administrative request or attestation form is produced by law enforcement officials, if it is to comply with mandatory reporting, or if the patient signs an authorization form to release PHI.[10] However, if the HCP is providing information in situations that do not include a signed release by the patient, the scope of PHI divulged should be limited to the minimum necessary to fulfill the obligation. The same provisions apply to the PHI of a suspect who has undergone an exam. It is crucial for the clinician to understand HIPAA policies and rely on their risk and legal departments for further guidance.[10]

Equipment and Other Supplies

HCPs must document the presence or absence of injury. Documentation can be completed with various photographic equipment, which reduces the likelihood of the patient having to submit to a re-examination and improves overall documentation and review quality. A digital camera should be utilized to document any bodily injuries with and without a standardized measuring tool. A colposcope, or colposcope replacement, can be used for a thorough anogenital or oral assessment based on the type of assault. The colposcope provides magnification and a light source that allows the clinician to assess and photograph injuries that may not be visible to the naked eye. Toluidine blue (TB) dye on genitalia may also be used. This dye binds to nucleated squamous cells in the epidermis, thereby increasing the sensitivity of visual assessments, as well as illuminating injuries for photography.[10] An alternative light source (ALS) can be utilized to assess for fluorescence of bodily fluids on the body or clothing. Stains located in this manner should also be swabbed for DNA. It may also be utilized to assess for subclinical bruising.[18,19] The HCP should be knowledgeable about the use of and limitations to their equipment and must also be able to troubleshoot any malfunctions that may arise with their equipment.

Prophylactic Medications

Pharmaceutical options for the prophylaxis and prevention of STIs and pregnancy are an important component of a comprehensive MFE. Since adherence to follow-up visits is traditionally low among patients affected by SA, if a patient would like to pursue any preventive or prophylactic treatments, these should be discussed and administered at the time of the comprehensive MFE.[10] Trichomoniasis, gonorrhea, and chlamydia are frequently diagnosed infections among patients who have experienced SA and if undiagnosed, may lead to chronic health conditions, such as Pelvic Inflammatory Disease (PID) or infertility.[20] During the MFE, testing for current infection using Nucleic Acid Amplification Tests (NAATs) should be made on an individual basis. Based on the time between the assault and the MFE, testing for current infection may not be indicated, as infectious organisms may not have reached sufficient concentrations detectable by current testing methods. Instead, prophylactic treatment is recommended for chlamydia, gonorrhea, and trichomoniasis for women and chlamydia and gonorrhea for men.[21] If initial testing is negative and prophylactic treatment is not provided, testing should be repeated in 1 to 2 weeks. If prophylactic treatment is provided, the patient does not need to repeat testing unless they are experiencing symptoms related to infection. If infection in the perpetrator cannot be ruled out, serologic testing for syphilis should be performed. This test should be repeated at 4 to 6 weeks and at 3 months.[21]

Although infrequent, cases of HIV transmission after SA have been described.[21] Multiple characteristics of SA increase the risk of HIV transmission, including genital or anal trauma leading to bleeding, presence of STIs or genital lesions in the assailant or patient, the number of assailants, and risk-taking behaviors of the assailant such as using intravenous drugs. Post Exposure Prophylaxis (PEP) is a 28-day course of highly active antiretroviral therapy that, when initiated soon after a high-risk exposure, can reduce the risk of HIV infection significantly. If the assailant's HIV status is unknown, HCPs should evaluate the risks and benefits of PEP on a case-by-case basis. If indicated, PEP should be initiated as soon as possible but no later than 72 hours after potential exposure to HIV.[21] A serum HIV sample, pregnancy test, and labs to assess liver and kidney function should be drawn prior to commencing treatment. HIV testing should be repeated at 6 weeks and 3 months.[21] Extensive discussion with the patient regarding risks and benefits, adverse side effects, compliance, and follow-up is required. The CDC[21] provides guidance surrounding the decision to start PEP, as well as patient education on PEP usage. In addition, postexposure hepatitis B vaccination is recommended if the hepatitis status of the assailant is unknown.[21] Hepatitis B Immune Globulin (HBIG) is recommended in addition to vaccination if the assailant is known to be positive for hepatitis B or if the patient has not been previously vaccinated. If the patient has been vaccinated, a booster dose can be administered. After the initial vaccination is administered at the time of examination, 2 follow-up doses should be administered at 1 to 2 months and at 6 months to complete the series.[21]

Patients affected by SA are also at risk for acquiring Human Papillomavirus (HPV). Vaccination for HPV is recommended for all patients 26 years or younger. As some patients may not have been adequately vaccinated for HPV previously and fall outside of this age range, shared clinical decision making is recommended to assess the benefits of vaccination between 26 and 45 years of age. If HPV vaccination is administered during an MFE, education must be provided to the patient regarding follow-up appointments at 1 to 2 months and at 6 months to complete the series.[21]

Although the risk of pregnancy after a single instance of vaginal intercourse varies during the menstrual cycle, EC should be offered, given the uncertainty in the timing of ovulation. This requires the availability of EC in hospitals and facilities where patients affected by SA are treated.[20] ECs are used to prevent pregnancy and therefore are ineffective in cases where pregnancy is already established. EC should be offered to all people capable of pregnancy, and while confirmed pregnancy is the only absolute contraindication to EC use, EC does not cause abortion.[1] It is equally important to conduct a thorough assessment on nonbinary and female to male (FTM) transgender patients as unwanted pregnancy post-SA is possible. Gender-affirming hormone therapy is not effective contraception, therefore, if the patient has an intact uterus and ovaries, EC must be discussed during the MFE. The HCP must recognize that these topics may be sensitive and difficult for the patient to discuss. Providing an inclusive and welcoming environment and a thorough explanation regarding the medical need of such assessments is necessary to ease potential distress in gender diverse patients.[22] There are currently 3 EC options available in the United States, including ulipristal acetate, levonorgestrel, and combined estrogen and progestin. Studies published regarding timing of the first dose show varying degrees of efficacy between the options but conclude that EC should be started no later than 3 to 5 days from the time of unprotected intercourse for maximum efficacy.[23] Insertion of a copper intrauterine device (IUD) is a highly effective method of EC that may also be considered.[1] When determining the best option for EC, financial and logistical barriers should be discussed with the patient to decrease issues with medication compliance and follow-up. Utilization of patient assistance programs can also help mitigate costs associated with medications.

Supplemental Assessments

As a part of the comprehensive MFE, other assessments should be considered based on the history the patient provided and the assessment completed by the HCP. For example, exposure to trauma, including SA, increases suicidal ideation and behavior as well as depressive symptoms.[23,24] Therefore, TJC's 2019 National Patient Safety Goals reaffirmed the use of validated suicide screening tools (eg, PHQ-9, ASQ Suicide Risk Screening Tool, The Columbia-Suicide Severity Rating Scale, TASR Adolescent Screener, ED Safe Secondary Screener, the Patient Safety Screener) to identify suicide risk.[25] Patients identified as having high suicidality risk should be further evaluated following facility protocols, though it should be noted that the screening tool selected should be appropriate for the individual undergoing the assessment.[25]

For patients whose SA was committed by an intimate partner, a lethality screen should be considered. There are 5 assessments that have been validated for use in IPV risk lethality assessments. These are the Danger Assessment (DA), the Domestic Violence Screening Inventory (DVSI, DVSI-R), the Kingston Screening Instrument for Domestic Violence (K-SID), the Spousal Assault Risk Assessment (SARA), and the Ontario Domestic Assault Risk Assessment (ODARA). An analysis comparing the 5 tools found ODARA to have the greatest predictive validity followed by the SARA, the DA, the DVSI, and the K-SID.[26]

If strangulation or head trauma is present in the patient's history, a comprehensive strangulation evaluation and concussion screening should be considered. Strangulation is a form of asphyxia with profound health consequences, including hypoxia, anoxia, and death. Studies show that nonfatal strangulation is common in SA, which highlights the importance of screening all patients presenting post-SA for strangulation.[27] A concussion is a form of traumatic brain injury (TBI) that can be serious and have long-term health implications. Concussions may lead to changes in the brain affecting how a person thinks, learns, feels, acts, and sleeps. The evaluating HCP should screen for concussions using the CDC's Acute Concussion Evaluation (ACE) or comparable screening tool.[28] Additional interventions, such as imaging studies, may be advisable based on the results of strangulation and concussion screenings.

Psychosocial Issues and Safety Planning

Many studies have examined the link between SA and its profound long-term health implications for an individual. This can include not only physical and mental health implications, but also implications regarding economic wellbeing. Advocacy groups that specialize in SA can help with support, connection to resources, and navigation of any barriers the patient may experience.[29] A comprehensive MFE should also include an assessment of the patient's discharge and safety needs. In addition to ensuring the patient's medical and mental health needs related to the assault have been addressed, the HCP should help facilitate the development of a discharge safety plan. This includes but is not limited to where the patient will go upon discharge; if this arrangement could result in exposure to further violence; what to do if the patient feels unsafe; and identification of support persons and resources.

Case Study

Case Study 10-1

A 28-year-old, cisgender female presented to the ED complaining of vaginal and anal pain. She told the triage nurse that she met a man on a dating app, had been talking to him for several days, and finally agreed to meet him for dinner last night. She stated that after dinner, they agreed to get into her car and go for a drive. She reports she pulled over to a scenic overlook to watch the sunset and began consensual kissing, but she then reported that following the kissing, the man began to initiate sexual activities that were not consensual. She requested an SA evidence kit and confirmed the SA occurred 12 hours prior to ED arrival. The ED triage nurse placed the patient in a treatment ED room and consulted the FNE. The FNE responded to the patient's room and, after introductions and an explanation of their role and the MFE, discussed reporting options and obtained a medical history. The FNE reported to law enforcement and obtained a case number based upon the patient's reporting decision, as directed by state statutes, and offered support if the patient decided to collaborate or speak with law enforcement. Applicable consents and paperwork for the MFE were reviewed and signed. A victim advocate was notified, and all efforts were made to ensure the exam would be conducted in a private, secure, and safe environment. The MFE began with a thorough history, for the purposes of medical diagnosis and treatment and to guide evidence collection. The patient confirmed that oral penetration took place, so the FNE immediately collected swabs, knowing that if they waited too long, the patient's salivary enzymes would degrade the evidence. After oral swabs were obtained, the FNE offered food and beverage, as well as other comforts such as warm blankets. Clothing collection was discussed, and the patient agreed to disrobe over a drop cloth, which would also be collected as evidence. The FNE was mindful to bag each item of clothing in a separate paper bag, seal the bags, and label them per protocol. The patient was then assisted into a patient gown and a thorough and complete head-to-toe examination was performed, with photographs taken of each injury finding. Each finding included 3 photos: 1 far away to demonstrate anatomical location, 1 up close, and 1 up close with a measurement tool such as an American Board of Forensic Odontology (ABFO) photomacrographic scale. Evidence swabs from the body, such as breasts, fingernails, and neck were collected based on the patient history. ALS was used as indicated and guided the FNE to collect swabs from additional areas of the body. The exam continued with a detailed anogenital examination, using a colposcope, and genital evidence collection. TB dye and a foley catheter were also utilized. See **Figures 10-9-a, b,** and **c** and **Figure 10-10** for anogenital assessment findings.

The FNE then discussed pregnancy risk and EC, prophylactic treatment for STIs, immunizations, and HIV risk assessment. After education was provided, including risks, benefits, and the possible side effects of all medications, the FNE administered the applicable pharmaceutical therapies per standing orders or other facility protocols. The patient reported hitting her head on the dashboard of the car during the SA, so she was screened for concussion, a form of TBI. To identify potential strangulation, the patient was asked if anything was applied with pressure to her neck at any time, but the patient denied this. Safety planning and crisis interventions were discussed, assisted by the victim advocate and the ED

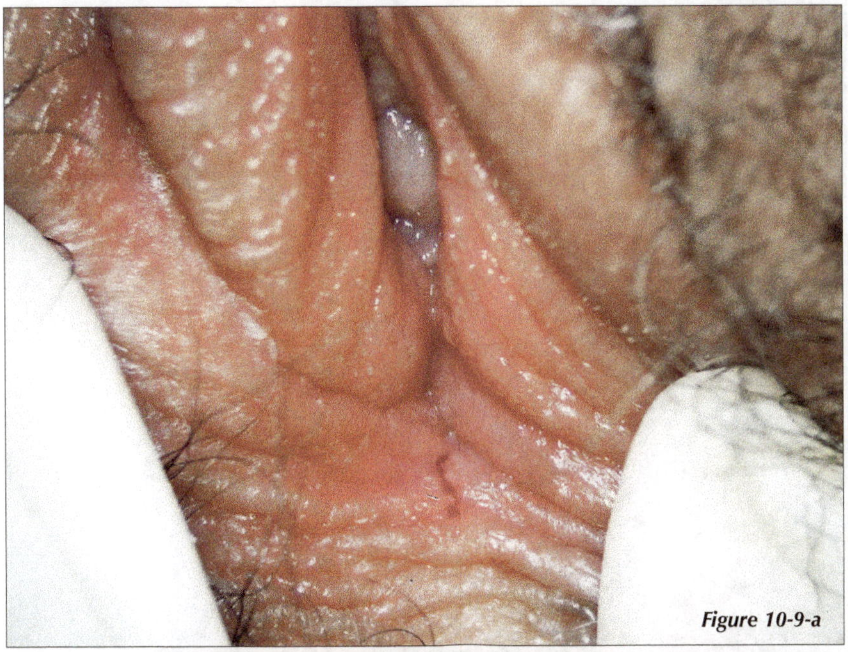

Figure 10-9-a

Figure 10-9-a. *Laceration noted to 6 o'clock of the fossa navicularis.*

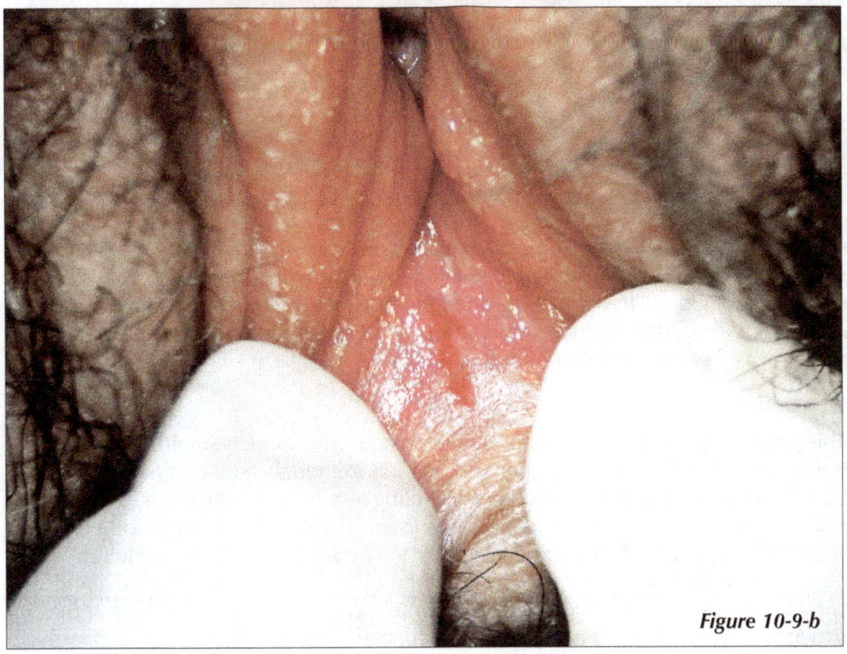

Figure 10-9-b

Figure 10-9-b. *Clearer view of laceration with gentle separation and traction.*

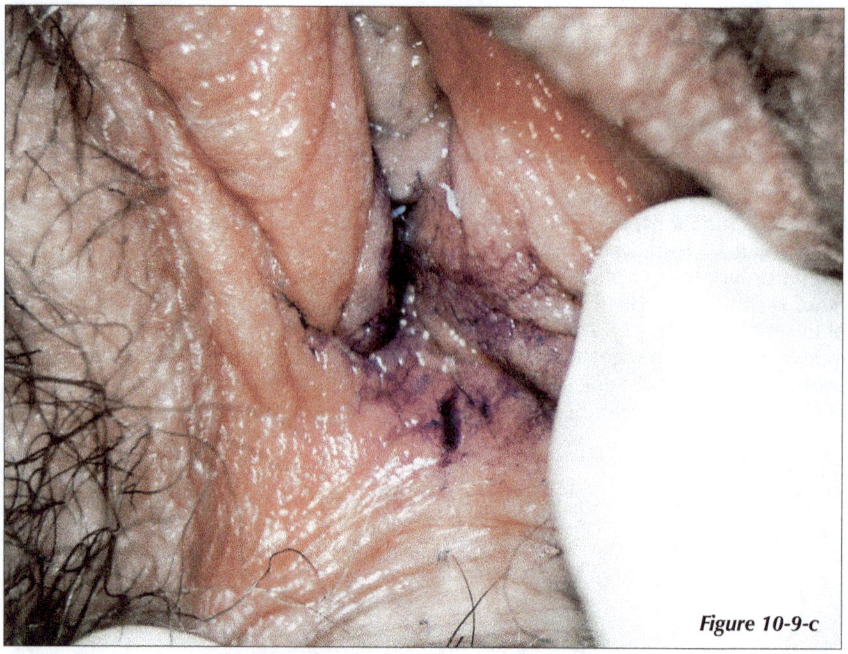

Figure 10-9-c. *View of laceration after the application of TB dye.*

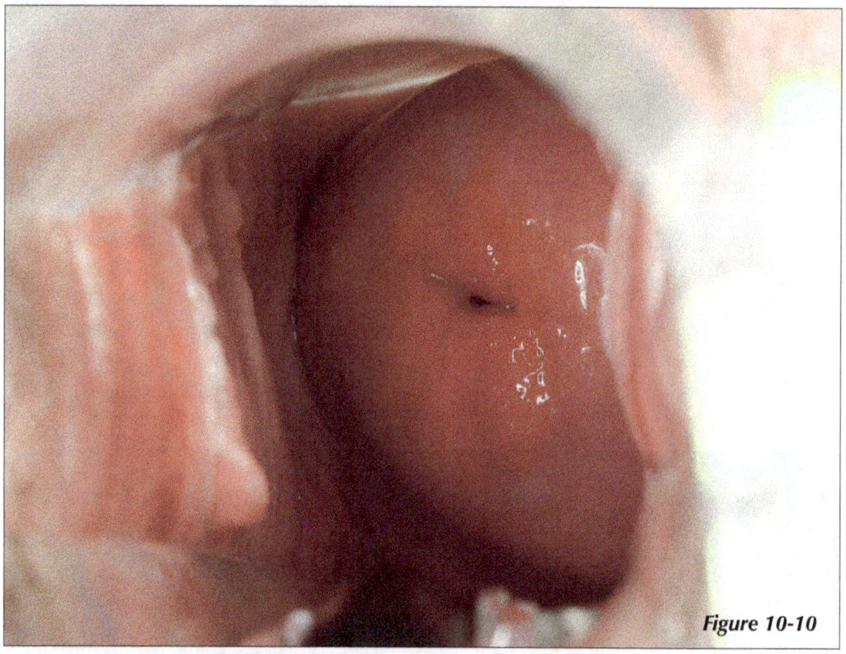

Figure 10-10. *Cervical ectropion.*

social worker as necessary. Appropriate patient education, referrals for medical and psychological care, and community resources were provided. A follow-up visit was scheduled to address injury healing and emotional wellbeing, as well as to reinforce community resources and safety planning. After obtaining a set of vital signs, the patient was discharged with a friend.

Discussion

This patient reported sexual violence and was quickly connected with a forensic nurse who specializes in this patient population. Although genital injury findings are not common, this patient did have a finding at her fossa navicularis, which is a common location when findings are present. The patient was appropriately screened for STIs, high-risk exposure to HIV, TBI, and strangulation. Health education, including teaching on body autonomy, as well as safety planning and community resources were provided, and a follow-up was scheduled so that the patient's continued health and psychosocial needs can be addressed.

Summary

SA is prevalent and may result in physical, emotional, and psychological trauma. This can include genital and extragenital trauma, contraction of STIs, general health risks, pregnancy, substance abuse, sexual dysfunction, depression, anxiety, fear, post-traumatic stress disorder, self-blame, and shame. All HCPs who encounter patients who have been affected by SA should understand these acute and chronic health issues, as well as the applicable legislation in their jurisdiction. While an MFE cannot prove or disprove SA, it provides an opportunity for the HCP to mitigate the psychological impact, restore a sense of control and power to the patient, validate the patient's concerns, ensure all medical needs are met, collect forensic evidence, and promote healing.

References

1. Buchanan JA. Evaluation and management of adult and adolescent sexual assault victims in the emergency department. UpToDate. 2023. Accessed August 11, 2023. https://www.uptodate.com/contents/evaluation-and-management-of-adult-and-adolescent-sexual-assault-victims-in-the-emergency-department

2. Standards for joint commission accreditation and certification. The Joint Commission. Accessed August 27, 2022. https://www.jointcommission.org/standards/

3. Chandramani A, Dussault N, Parameswaran R, et al. A needs assessment and educational intervention addressing the care of sexual assault patients in the emergency department. *J Forensic Nurs*. 2020;16(2):73-82. doi:10.1097/JFN.0000000000000290

4. National crime victimization survey (NCVS). Bureau of Justice Statistics, US Department of Justice. 2021. https://bjs.ojp.gov/data-collections/ncvs

5. Scurich N. Introduction to this special issue: underreporting of sexual abuse. *Behav Sci Law*. 2020;38(6):537-542. doi:10.1002/bsl.2491

6. Scheim AI, Baker KE, Restar AJ, Sell RL. Health and health care among transgender adults in the United States. *Annu Rev Public Health*. 2021;43(1). doi:10.1146/annurev-publhealth-052620-100313

7. O'Donohue WT, Schewe PA. *Handbook of Sexual Assault and Sexual Assault Prevention*. Cham Springer International Publishing Imprint, Springer; 2019.

8. Dole P. Sequelae of sexual assault. In: Lynch VA, Barber Duval J, eds. *Forensic Nursing Science*. 2nd ed. Mosby, Inc; 2011:397-413.

9. Yesodharan R, Shehata SA, Jose TT, et al. Medico-legal history taking from the victims of sexual assaults: the role of nurse examiners. *Egypt J Forensic Sci*. 2022;12(24). doi:10.1186/s41935-022-00284-4

10. *Evaluation and Management of the Sexually Assaulted or Sexually Abused Patient.* American College of Emergency Physicians; 2013.

11. Wilson C, Lonsway K, Archambault J. Understanding the neurobiology of trauma and implications for interviewing victims. Justice Information Resource Network. 2019. Accessed August 27, 2022. https://justiceresearch.dspacedirect.org/items/f59faffd-a136-4c3d-b60c-2ff8c0749650

12. Jänisch S, Meyer H, Germerott T, Albrecht UV, Schulz Y, Debertin AS. Analysis of clinical forensic examination reports on sexual assault. *Int J Legal Med*. 2010;124(3):227-235. doi:10.1007/s00414-010-0430-z

13. Ferrell J, Caruso C. Sexual assault evidence recovery. In: Lynch VA, Duval JB, eds. *Forensic Nursing Science*. 2nd ed. Mosby, Inc.; 2011:144-154.

14. Adams JA, Kellogg ND, Farst KJ, et al. Updated guidelines for the medical assessment and care of children who may have been sexually abused. *J Pediatr Adolesc Gynecol.* 2016;29(2):81-87. doi:10.1016/j.jpag.2015.01.007

15. Foote-Lucero C, Tsu L. Sexual violence. In: Faugno D, Mitchell S, Sievers V, Pederson S, Volz J, Speck P, eds. *Introduction to Forensic Nursing: Principles and Practice.* STM Learning Inc.; 2022:201-205.

16. Sommers MS, Fargo JD. Discriminating between consensual intercourse and sexual assault: genital-anal injury pattern in females. *J Forensic Leg Med.* 2021; 79:102138. doi:10.1016/j.jflm.2021.102138

17. DuMont J, Saad M, Kosa S, Kia H, Macdonald S. Providing trans-affirming care for sexual assault survivors: an evaluation of a novel curriculum for forensic nurses. *Nurse Educ Today.* 2020;93:104541. doi:10.1016/j.nedt.2020.104541

18. Scafide KN, Sheridan DJ, Downing NR, Hayat MJ. Detection of inflicted bruises by alternate light: results of a randomized controlled trial. *J Forensic Sci.* 2020;65(4):1191-1198. doi:10.1111/1556-4029.14294

19. Scafide K, Ekroos R, Mallinson R, et al. Improving the forensic documentation of injuries through alternate light: a researcher-practitioner partnership. *J Forensic Nurs.* 2023;19(1):30-40. doi:10.1097/JFN.0000000000000389

20. Sexual assault. The American College of Obstetricians and Gynecologists. 2019. Accessed August 5, 2022. https://www.acog.org/clinical/clinical-guidance/committee-opinion/articles/2019/04/sexual-assault

21. STI treatment guidelines. Centers for Disease Control and Prevention. 2021. https://www.cdc.gov/std/treatment-guidelines/toc.htm

22. Health care for transgender and gender diverse individuals: ACOG committee opinion, Number 823. *Obstet Gynecol.* 2021;137(3):e75-e88. doi:10.1097/AOG.0000000000004294

23. Dworkin ER, DeCou CR, Fitzpatrick S. Associations between sexual assault and suicidal thoughts and behavior: a meta-analysis. *Psychol Trauma.* 2022;14(7):1208-1211. doi:10.1037/tra0000570

24. Gilmore AK, Flanagan JC. Acute mental health symptoms among individuals receiving a sexual assault medical forensic exam: the role of previous intimate partner violence victimization. *Arch Womens Ment Health.* 2020;23(1):81-89. doi:10.1007/s00737-019-0947-1

25. National patient safety goal for suicide prevention. The Joint Commission. 2019. https://www.jointcommission.org/-/media/tjc/documents/standards/r3-reports/r3_18_suicide_prevention_hap_bhc_cah_ 11_4_19_final1.pdf

26. Messing JT, Campbell J, Sullivan Wilson J, Brown S, Patchell B. The lethality screen: the predictive validity of an intimate partner violence risk assessment for use by first responders. *J Interpers Violence.* 2017;32(2):205-226. doi:10.1177/0886260515585540

27. Cannon LM, Bailey JM, Ernst SD, et al. Examining trends in non-fatal strangulation among sexual assault survivors seeking Sexual Assault Nurse Examiner care from 2002 to 2017. *Int J Gynaecol Obstet.* 2020;149(1):106-107. doi:10.1002/ijgo.13058

28. Gioia G, Collins M. Acute Concussion Evaluation (ACE) - physician/clinician office version. Centers for Disease Control and Prevention. 2015. https://www.cdc.gov/headsup/pdfs/providers/ace_v2-a.pdf

29. Examination process – discharge and followup. SAFEta.org. Accessed August 27, 2022. https://www.safeta.org/page/examprocessdischarge/

Chapter 11

Intimate Partner Violence and Sexually Transmitted Infections

Christina Hall, MSW
Mitzy D. Flores, PhDc, MSN, RN, AHN-BC, CHSE, COI, Caritas Coach®, Introspective Hypnosis Practitioner

Key Points

1. *Human immunodeficiency virus (HIV) and acquired immunodeficiency syndrome (AIDS) disproportionately impact marginalized communities,[1] including victims/survivors of intimate partner violence (IPV).*
2. *IPV can increase the likelihood of contracting a sexually transmitted infection (STI).[2]*
3. *Trauma-informed practices at the individual, organizational, and clinic levels are vital in ensuring that people living with HIV (PLWH) do not experience bias during their care.*

Background and Significance

Historically, there has been stigma and secrecy around the topic of IPV. There is also shame around sexual health, including the prevention and treatment of STIs in general and HIV in particular. Although IPV is still a topic that is often difficult to talk about, with the assistance of media and public discourse, there is a greater awareness of IPV as a serious public health issue. IPV does not occur in a vacuum, and it is often not the only challenge that a person experiences at a given time. The intersection of IPV and other health, social, and financial challenges puts further strain on victim-survivors, making IPV difficult to address. This is especially

Figure 11-1. Prevalence of STIs in the United States, 2018.

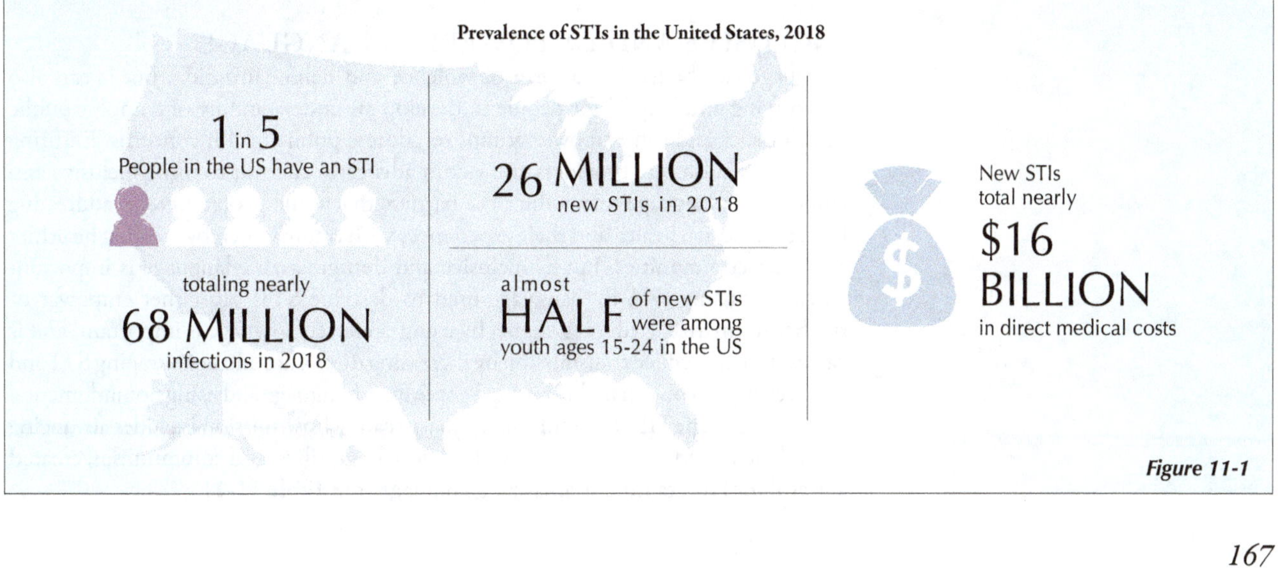

Figure 11-1

true when advocates attempt to address IPV without addressing the co-occurring challenges that impact the victim-survivor's overall wellness. In this chapter, the authors will be examining the intersections of IPV and STIs and some best practices for addressing public health concerns without ignoring or diminishing either issue.

STIs are a major public health concern that can impact anyone. In 2018, it was estimated that 20% of the United States population had an STI (see **Figure 11-1**).[3] To address these 2 major public health issues, one must understand how both issues have historically been marginalized and ignored, often due to stigma, discrimination, and disparities based on race, sexual orientation, and socioeconomic status. The history of HIV and AIDS highlights how a serious public health issue can be ignored and mishandled because it primarily impacts a marginalized community. The first instances of what would become HIV were identified in men who have sex with men (MSM), people who inject drugs, and people who engage in transactional sex.[1] Due to the affiliation with specific groups of people, public health messages about HIV focused on "fixing" personal behavior, which further fueled the blaming of these marginalized communities and resulted in discrimination in medical care, housing, and employment. Despite concerted advocacy efforts by grassroots organizations, many of which were founded by the LGBTQIA+ community, public health interest and intervention was incredibly slow to respond, even as more people were suffering and dying.[4]

Eventually, because of the persistent advocacy of the HIV community and scientific breakthroughs regarding how the virus impacts the immune system, how it is spread, and how it can be treated, there have been some incredible improvements in HIV care. Today, HIV can be managed so that people living with it can lead long and healthy lives. However, there are still disparities in the response and treatment of HIV in the most marginalized communities. For example, Black Americans in the United States, who are impacted by structural racism and inequality, are disproportionately affected by the HIV pandemic and often do not receive the care that they need.[1] In 2018, Black people made up 13% of the general population but accounted for 42% of new HIV diagnoses, and in 2019, Black Americans had the highest rate of new HIV diagnoses, which was 8.5 times the rate for White Americans.[1] In addition, in 2020, only 65% of Black people in the United States were virally suppressed within 6 months of diagnosis, compared to 71% of Hispanic/Latinx people and 68% of White people.[1] This shows that there are health disparities in HIV prevention, care, and treatment by race, and that the intersection of multiple identities (eg, LGBTQIA+ individuals, people who inject drugs, and people who engage in transactional sex) further compounds these disparities. The same structural inequality and racism that marginalized communities experience throughout our social systems also show up in the health care system, as well as within HIV care.

Inclusive and Empowering Language

Language can be used as a form of violence and dehumanization, but it can also be unifying and helpful for people to develop an understanding of complex public health issues and can empower groups to address public health concerns. Ensuring that both health care providers and victim advocates commit to using inclusive and empowering language may reduce the barriers that some people have to addressing both their sexual health and their experiences with trauma, thereby creating healthier and safer communities. Just as inclusive and destigmatizing language is important when discussing IPV, the language used to describe STIs can either empower or further stigmatize. Reducing stigma by using preferred language is important, and it can even "help reduce transmission by increasing disclosure and encouraging STI and HIV testing."[5] This can include using People First Language and using nonjudgmental terminology. The HIVE, a multidisciplinary team whose mission includes advancing reproductive and sexual wellness for individuals, families, and communities, created a useful tool to examine stigmatizing language (see **Table 11-1**).[5]

Table 11-1. Stigmatizing vs Preferred Language

Stigmatizing	Preferred	How this can avoid stigma
HIV-infected person HIV patient, AIDS patient Positives or HIVers AIDS or HIV carrier	Person living with HIV (PLWH), Stage 1 HIV (acute), Stage 2 HIV (clinical latency), or Stage 3 HIV (AIDS)	By using person-first language, we reinforce that their identity as a person is more important than their diagnosis. They are no longer only identified by their diagnosis.
Died of AIDS, to die of AIDS	Died of AIDS-related illness, AIDS-related complications, or end stage HIV	By using this terminology, incorrect assumptions about the progression of AIDS are challenged.
Unprotected sex	Condomless sex, sex not protected by condoms or antiretroviral prevention methods such as TasP or PrEP	The preferred language is more precise and refers to actions, instead of using words that have value statements attached.
Victim, innocent victim, sufferer, contaminated, infected	Person living with HIV (never use the term "infected" when referring to a person), survivor	By using this terminology, we avoid the incorrect connotation that a crime has been committed.
To catch HIV/AIDS	To contract HIV, diagnosed with HIV, develop AIDS, diagnosed with AIDS; AIDS is a diagnosis and not a virus, AIDS cannot be transmitted or "passed" to someone else	By using this language, it avoids feeding into incorrect assumptions about how HIV is contracted and how it can progress to AIDS.
Death sentence, "HIV is not a death sentence anymore," "HIV does not have to be a life-threatening/fatal condition"	HIV, chronic health condition, manageable health condition	This language equates HIV with other chronic and manageable health conditions, instead of unnecessarily sensationalizing it.
Prostitute or prostitution	Sex worker, sale of sexual services, transactional sex	This language separates the person's identity from the sex work that they engage in, making it less stigmatizing.

Public Health Issues: IPV

When addressing a public health concern such as IPV, it is important to understand that IPV crosses all experiences and identities and can be found at every socioeconomic level and in all types of relationships. While there has been higher awareness of IPV in recent years, it is often discussed in the context of heterosexual relationships. Yet, recent reports estimate that 43.8% of lesbian women and 61.1% of bisexual women have experienced rape, physical violence, or stalking by an intimate partner at some point in their lifetime; and that 26% of gay men and 37.3% of bisexual men report that they have experienced these same behaviors by an intimate partner in their lifetime.[6]

Additionally, a 2019 report noted that IPV is occurring outside of heterosexual relationships, however, some medical providers, social service providers, and IPV organizations may be unlikely to identify it.[7] Power imbalances may show up differently in an LGBTQIA+ relationship compared to a heterosexual relationship, and standard IPV measurement tools often do not include IPV against transgender individuals.[8] This may be because many IPV services are not specific to the LGBTQIA+ community. Many IPV organizations may spend 1 session of their training on IPV within LGBTQIA+ relationships, but do not go beyond this surface level understanding. Advocates should always strive to increase their knowledge about how IPV dynamics show up in all kinds of relationships. The Power and Control Wheel, created by the Domestic Abuse Intervention Project, is a useful tool for advocates and victim-survivors to understand the dynamics of power and control that can be present in abusive relationships.[9] Advocates should also familiarize themselves with the Power and Control Wheel for Lesbian, Gay, Bisexual and Trans Relationships as a starting place to understand the unique ways power and control can show up in non-heterosexual relationships.[10] For example, an abuser might use isolation by telling their partner that no one will believe them, especially not if they are LGBTQIA+, or by reinforcing internalized homophobia, biphobia, or transphobia as another way to use emotional abuse.[10] Advocates should also consider that the LGBTQIA+ community may face additional barriers to reporting and healing from IPV, such as: internal conflict or embarrassment, fear of not being believed or taken seriously, varied legal protections, and loss of community.[6]

While recognizing that IPV crosses all experiences and identities, people of Black, American Indian and Alaska Native, and multiracial identities experience the highest percentage of IPV compared to other races and ethnicities.[11] This shows that people of marginalized communities are disproportionately impacted by both of these major public health concerns. Since both IPV and HIV are still associated with stigmas, this can further impact access to resources, equitable housing and financial opportunities, and comprehensive health care. Advocates and health care professionals can work to combat this by engaging in lifelong learning and cultural humility, as well as examining their established policies, procedures, and protocols for any intentional and unintentional barriers to accessing equitable services for marginalized identities.

Public Health Issues: STIs

While the impacts of each individual STI will vary for each person depending on the severity and type of infection, in 2018 the monetary impact from the United States health care system was nearly $16 billion in health care costs alone.[3] The 8 most common types of STIs can be found in **Table 11-2.**[3] This chart can be a useful tool for advocates when discussing sexual health as part of a larger safety plan with clients who are experiencing IPV. While it should not be used for medical diagnosis, it can be a useful way to open the conversation about the possibility of STIs when working with clients.

Table 11-2. Common STI Signs, Symptoms, and Treatment

Name	Description	Symptoms	Treatment
Chlamydia[12]	A common STI that can cause permanent damage to a woman's reproductive system. This can make it difficult or impossible to get pregnant later.	There are often no symptoms, but the infection can cause serious health problems to a woman's reproductive system even without symptoms. Symptoms can include: — Abnormal vaginal discharge — A burning sensation when peeing — Discharge from the penis — Pain and swelling in 1 or both testicles	If treatment is taken correctly when prescribed by a doctor, it will stop the infection and could decrease a patient's chances of having problems later. Although treatment will stop the infection, it will not undo any permanent damage already caused.

(continued)

Table 11-2. Common STI Signs, Symptoms, and Treatment *(continued)*

Name	Description	Symptoms	Treatment
Gonorrhea[13]	A common STI that can cause infection in the genitals, rectum, and throat. It is most common among people aged 15 to 24 years.	There are often no symptoms, but the infection can cause serious health problems even without symptoms. Symptoms can include: — Painful or burning sensation when peeing — Increased vaginal discharge — Vaginal bleeding between periods — A white, yellow, or green discharge from the penis — Painful or swollen testicles	If treatment is taken correctly when prescribed by a doctor, it will stop the infection and could decrease a patient's chances of having problems later. Although treatment will stop the infection, it will not undo any permanent damage already caused. It is becoming harder to treat, as drug resistant strains of gonorrhea are increasing. If symptoms continue, notify your health care provider.
Hepatitis B Virus (HBV)[14]	A vaccine-preventable liver infection caused by the hepatitis B virus. It is spread by bodily fluids.	Hepatitis B does not always cause symptoms, but symptoms of acute hepatitis B can include: — Fever — Fatigue — Loss of appetite — Nausea — Vomiting — Abdominal pain — Dark urine — Clay-colored bowel movements — Joint pain — Jaundice	While some people with acute hepatitis B can fight the virus without treatment, for some it can lead to lifelong infection known as chronic hepatitis B. There is no treatment for chronic hepatitis B, but there are several medications approved to treat chronic hepatitis B. There is currently no cure.
Herpes Simplex Virus Type 2 (HSV-2)[15]	This is a common STI caused by a virus that is spread by having vaginal, anal, or oral sex with someone who has the infection.	Most people do not have symptoms or have very mild symptoms with HSV-2, but symptoms can include: — Blisters around the genitals, rectum, or mouth — Fever — Body aches — Swollen glands	There is currently no cure, but there are medicines that can prevent or shorten outbreaks, and daily anti-herpes medicine can make it less likely to pass the infection on to sexual partner(s).

(continued)

Table 11-2. Common STI Signs, Symptoms, and Treatment *(continued)*

Name	Description	Symptoms	Treatment
Human Immunodeficiency virus (HIV)[16]	A virus that attacks the body's immune system. If not treated, it can lead to acquired immunodeficiency syndrome (AIDS). There are 3 stages of HIV: acute HIV infection, chronic HIV infection, and AIDS.	Though the best way to know if HIV is present is to get tested, there are also symptoms that indicate HIV infection. Symptoms can include: — Flu-like symptoms 2 to 4 weeks after infection during stage 1, acute HIV infection. — There are often no symptoms during stage 2. — Stage 3 symptoms can include a wide range of opportunistic infections due to damaged immune systems.	There is currently no cure for HIV, but with medical care, HIV can be controlled. HIV treatment can slow or prevent progression of the disease, and progression to stage 3 (AIDS) is less common today. PrEP (pre-exposure prophylaxis) is medicine that reduces your chances of getting HIV from sex or injection drug use. When taken as prescribed, PrEP is highly effective for preventing HIV.[17] PEP (post-exposure prophylaxis) means taking medicine to prevent HIV after a possible exposure. PEP must be started within 72 hours of possible exposure to HIV.[18]
Human Papillomavirus (HPV)[19]	HPV is the most common STI. There are many varieties of the infection, some of which can cause health problems.	Most people with HPV do not know they have the infection, and never develop symptoms or health problems from it. Some people find out they have HPV when they experience: — The presence of genital warts — Abnormal pap test results during a cervical cancer screening — Development of cervical cancer	There is currently no test for HPV, except for ones that can screen for cervical cancer. The HPV vaccine is a safe and effective way to protect against diseases, including cancers, caused by HPV.
Syphilis[20]	An STI that can cause serious health problems without treatment. It develops in stages (primary, secondary, latent, and tertiary).	The 4 stages each have different symptoms. These can include: — Primary: single or multiple (often painless) sores in or around the penis, vagina, anus, rectum, lips, or mouth — Secondary: rash or sores in the mouth, vagina, or anus, fever, swollen lymph glands, sore throat, patchy hair loss, headaches, weight loss, muscle aches, fatigue — Latent: no visible symptoms — Tertiary: potentially deadly damage to internal organs, including the heart, blood vessels, brain, and nervous system	If treatment is taken correctly when prescribed by a doctor, syphilis is curable. Treatment may not undo any damage already caused by the infection, and having syphilis once does not protect a patient from getting it again, so regular testing is recommended.

(continued)

Table 11-2. Common STI Signs, Symptoms, and Treatment *(continued)*

Name	Description	Symptoms	Treatment
Trichomoniasis[21]	A common and treatable STI caused by a protozoan parasite called *trichomonas vaginalis.*	Most people do not have symptoms, but symptoms may develop between 5 and 28 days after infection. Symptoms can include: — Itching, irritation, and burning of the penis or genitals — Burning or discomfort when peeing or ejaculating — Discharge from the penis or vagina — Sex feels unpleasant	If treatment is taken correctly when prescribed by a doctor, trichomoniasis is curable. Treatment does not prevent reinfection.

The Intersection of IPV, STIs, and HIV

While many of the health impacts of experiencing trauma are well-known, the link between experiencing IPV and increased risk for contracting STIs is often overlooked. Research has consistently shown a correlation between IPV and elevated STI risk for victim-survivors.[2,22,23] Research specifically shows that female victim-survivors of IPV have a higher STI prevalence than women in nonviolent relationships, possibly due to a higher prevalence of STI risk behaviors.[2] The main way that the sexual health field has addressed the prevention of STIs is through risk reduction strategies. Risk reduction usually refers to behaviors that are expected to reduce the likelihood of contracting an STI.[24] This can include the promotion of the following: abstinence, vaccination, reducing one's number of sexual partners, mutual monogamy, condoms, and regular STI testing.[24] While these methods can contribute to the prevention of STIs, public health messages need to be careful that this does not lead to the stigmatizing message of "fixing" personal behavior, or assigning harmful value judgements, as discussed previously in this chapter. In addition, traditional risk reduction strategies may be difficult, if not impossible, to engage in for someone experiencing IPV.[25]

Some of the STI risk behaviors that are more likely to be present in an IPV relationship include higher instances of unprotected vaginal sex, unprotected anal sex, and injection drug use.[23,26] Many studies examining STI risk behaviors identified that victim-survivors of IPV often reported fears around negotiating condom use with abusive partners, a reported inability or fear to refuse sex, and reported being more likely to have a sexual partner that engages in risky sexual behaviors that can increase the likelihood of contracting an STI than women who have not experienced IPV.[23] Women experiencing IPV may also be experiencing reproductive coercion, which is behavior intended to maintain power and control in a relationship related to reproductive health. Often, this behavior interferes with contraception use, including condom use, and pregnancy.[27] In one study examining reproductive coercion, only 19% of participants who were experiencing IPV reported using condoms consistently.[28]

MSM and transgender individuals who experience IPV are also at increased risk for STI contraction.[29] While research around the LGBTQIA+ community and IPV is limited, especially research specifically on the transgender community, some research suggests that rates of IPV are higher for transgender individuals in particular. 57% of transgender women reported experiencing IPV, and transgender women reporting recent IPV were more likely to have a diagnosed STI than transgender women without recent experiences of IPV.[29,30] This may be due to a higher prevalence of STI-risk behaviors among individuals experiencing IPV, including group sex, commercial sex, and sexualized drug use.[31]

At the same time, research suggests that abusers/perpetrators of IPV have an increased risk for STIs.[31] Physical/sexual IPV perpetration was associated with past-year infidelity, sex worker patronage, refusal to wear a condom, and unprotected sex. These high STI-risk behaviors result in abusers being more likely to have and transmit STIs.[32,33] This demonstrates that victim-survivors of all gender identities are at an increased risk for STIs because they are dealing with an abusive intimate partner that may be more likely to engage in STI risk behavior, and the victim-survivor is unable to engage in these behaviors safely. This research shows that 1 intersection between IPV and STIs is that IPV victim-survivors and abusers both have an increased risk for contracting an STI.

IPV Impacts on HIV Health Outcomes

As stated in the previous section, IPV is associated with increased risk for STIs, including HIV. Similarly, IPV prevalence among PLWH is also elevated, with estimates of IPV prevalence up to 53.1% in a sample of men and women living with HIV.[34,35] Given this high prevalence, IPV can also impact STI/HIV health outcomes, starting with regular testing. Only 53% of persons accessing services for IPV also request an STI/HIV test.[36] There could be many reasons survivors may not be as likely to get tested, including apprehension to undergo additional trauma during medical care, fear of escalated violence from their partner due to being diagnosed with HIV, and lack of resources (eg, money or transportation) to undergo regular STI/HIV testing because those resources are being controlled by their harm doer. Regular testing is one of the ways to address STI/HIV in a way that will promote positive health outcomes, and for these reasons, regular testing may be difficult if not impossible for people experiencing IPV.

Another way in which IPV can impact STI health outcomes is by decreasing the chances that someone might engage in medical care and stay in medical care. This happens in a couple of different ways. First, it is important to understand that there are 3 major HIV measures that are used to determine HIV health outcomes through the HIV Care Continuum, pictured below (**Figure 11-2**).[37]

Figure 11-2. *HIV Care Continuum.*

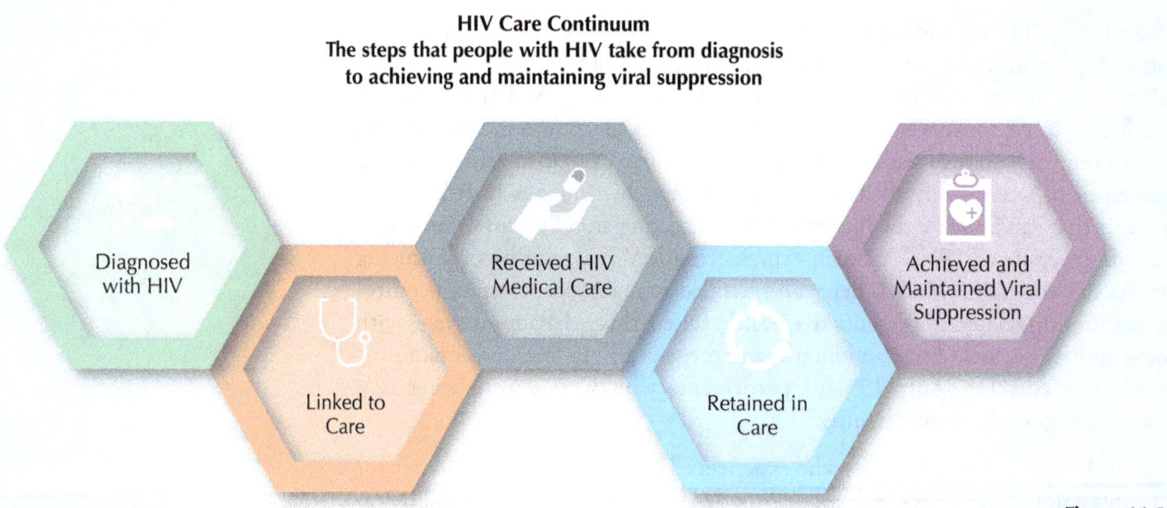

Figure 11-2

These measures are CD4 count, HIV viral load, and engagement in care. CD4 count measures the amount of CD4 cells in the body, which is an indication of the health of the immune system. A CD4 count of less than 200 is an indication of a compromised immune system that is vulnerable to opportunistic infections that can lead to serious illness.[38] HIV viral load refers to the amount of the HIV virus in the body, and is used to guide treatment decisions, including whether different HIV treatment is needed if the HIV viral load is not decreasing.[39] Finally, engagement in care refers to PLWH who have had 2 or more clinic visits at least 3 months apart. Engagement in care has been shown to increase positive health outcomes for PLWH.[37]

It is well-documented that IPV is associated with worse HIV outcomes.[40] Experiencing multiple traumas including trauma associated with IPV is associated with an increase in AIDS-related mortality, increased opportunistic infections, progression to AIDS, and decreased engagement in care.[40] In particular, the experience of being threatened by a partner was associated with low CD4 count, detectable viral load, and low engagement in care.[40] The reasons for low engagement in care could be the same as the reasons for lack of HIV testing, including fear of violence and a lack of resources to be able to attend clinic appointments.

Best Practices for Advocates and Health Care Professionals

In other sections of this book, trauma-informed care is discussed in the context of how to apply key concepts to a provider's response to IPV. The same guiding principles should be applied when working with victim-survivors who are living with HIV. By striving toward a trauma-informed approach to HIV care and treatment, providers center the individual autonomy of each person, seeing each client as the expert in their own experiences and further empowering them by providing information and resources that will support the survivor as they work towards meeting their needs.

For Anti-Violence Advocates Working with People Living with HIV

Other chapters of this text will go into depth on the philosophy and practice recommendations for each of the steps in the role of the advocate, and they should be followed when working with clients who are living with HIV as well. Special considerations for anti-violence advocates and medical providers who are working with people experiencing IPV while living with HIV are listed below. These processes are intended to elevate a client's right to make the choices that are the best choice for them, with the foundational assumption that victim-survivors are the experts in their own lives.

1. *Notify the client of confidentiality prior to inviting client disclosures of violence.* First, providers should make sure they understand their individual state and agency laws and policies around mandated reporting, including limits to confidentiality. Many states have specific requirements for confidential advocates, so all employees of an agency need to understand whether they are protected by confidentiality. When working with a client who is interested in STI testing, let them know that health providers are often mandated reporters as well. In some states, laws require people with HIV who are aware of their status to disclose to their sexual partners.[41] For a client experiencing IPV, this partner notification can be a major safety concern and can lead to an escalation of violence. Medical providers should be aware of this possibility and connect the client to a local IPV agency in order to engage in safety planning and supportive measures for when their partner is notified.
2. *Ensure client's immediate physical and emotional safety.* Advocates should assess physical and emotional safety with all clients, including continuing clients, since

IPV situations can evolve in between meetings. For a client who is considering being tested for HIV, the advocate should work with the client prior to testing to assess any safety concerns that might be present if their partner becomes aware of their HIV status.

3. *Provide emotional support.* Advocates should always be ready to provide emotional support or hold space for clients who are experiencing IPV. For clients who are also living with HIV, advocates should understand that the client is also navigating the realities and impacts of having a chronic health condition. Advocates can also provide emotional support around navigating stigma and misconceptions around HIV, including connecting the client with an HIV peer support group, as well as integrating HIV health and psychological impacts into their case management plan.

4. *Examine client needs and possible resources.* For a client who is living with HIV, there may be additional needs and resources to navigate. For someone living with HIV and who is experiencing IPV-related challenges, such as housing insecurity and basic safety concerns, their HIV treatment may not be the most salient need at the moment. Understanding this and helping the client identify their most pressing safety and housing needs so that they can later address their HIV care needs can be helpful. Once the client is ready to address their needs related to HIV care, advocates can empower clients in the difficult process of finding a provider and navigating the health care and insurance system in partnership with local health departments and organizations that specialize in HIV care.

5. *Create a personalized safety plan.* As discussed above, when an abusive partner finds out about an HIV diagnosis, this can lead to an escalated threat of violence to the victim-survivor. Anti-violence advocates should create safety plans with the client and consider possible ramifications to the client's HIV care. Advocates could discuss safe medication storage and access and plans around attending doctor's appointments with clients, considering the client's unique IPV concerns.

6. *Obtain a commitment.* When obtaining a commitment from a client who is experiencing IPV and is living with HIV, it is important to use consensus-driven questions that empower the client to make commitments and deadlines that are feasible and safe. Advocates should avoid commitments or questions that evoke shame and embarrassment, whether in relation to their HIV care or IPV situation. Avoiding shame-based language may help the client feel more comfortable with continuing to receive further support, even if commitments are not met. Advocates can then work with the client to adapt plans to evolving situations and create plans that are more feasible for the client to meet.

For Health Care Providers Working with People Experiencing IPV

This section is meant for health care providers, especially in a sexual health setting such as a sexual health clinic. The following are recommended practices when working with people living with HIV or other STIs and who are also experiencing IPV.

1. *Create the space.* When creating a safe space for a patient who may be experiencing IPV, it is important that the health care provider ensures that the conversation is private and will not be overheard or disrupted. Providers can also create sample scripts to use when requesting to meet privately with a patient when they are accompanied by another person. This is helpful when a provider is concerned that the abuser has accompanied the client to the

appointment. This way, the provider can ask questions about a relationship that they may be concerned about.

2. *Train all staff.* All health care staff should be trained on the impacts and signs of trauma, the various forms of IPV and what they can look like, and the unique health concerns of PLWH who are also experiencing IPV. This can be done by offering continued education opportunities to staff through partnering with local anti-violence agencies.
3. *Notify of confidentiality.* It is crucial that providers notify patients of their limits to confidentiality (including responsibilities for mandated reporting) **before** asking questions about their relationships or doing any assessments. If a report does need to be made because the information disclosed falls under mandatory reporting, this should not be a surprise to the patient, since the provider explained their role as a mandated reporter. Any reports can be made in partnership with the patient, to preserve as much autonomy as possible for the patient. Health care providers should weigh the risks of involving state authorities before making a mandated report by being critical about when mandatory reports are required versus recommended.
4. *Ask the right questions.* While some questions are necessary to assess the health and safety of the patient, providers should avoid asking questions that satisfy curiosity by asking only the necessary questions to assess health and safety. This will help avoid unintentionally invading the privacy of the patient. Providers should also avoid asking "why" questions, as they can feel accusatory.
5. *Educate to empower.* While health care providers are not expected to be an expert on IPV, they can empower their patients with resources, such as local anti-violence agencies, to connect clients with confidential advocates. They can also have educational materials available from trustworthy sources about healthy relationships and power and control tactics.
6. *Offer meaningful interventions.* Health care providers are not expected to engage in long-term safety planning or victim advocacy for patients who are experiencing IPV. However, they can make sure all trained clinic and health care staff have access to and are familiar with needs assessments and resource guides so that each resource and option can be given to the patient.

Earlier in this chapter, it was recognized that IPV does not occur in a vacuum, and that the presence of other health, social, and financial challenges intersect with the impacts of IPV. Because of this, the response to IPV cannot occur in a vacuum. Anti-violence agencies, health care providers, public health departments, social justice advocates, and more will be required to truly move the mark. By following all 6 of these steps, health care providers can be prepared to recognize and respond appropriately to patients who disclose experiences of IPV and co-occurring health conditions such as STIs and HIV. Most of these steps require partnership with and knowledge of local resources, including anti-violence agencies.

Case Studies

Case Study 11-1

A patient who was a 27-year-old, Black, heterosexual female presented at the OBGYN for a prenatal visit and was accompanied by her husband. During routine testing, it was discovered that she was living with HIV. The client was pregnant with her first child and was not previously aware that she was living with HIV. In order to inform the client, the nurse practitioner asked to speak to the client alone. The husband was very reluctant to leave, but eventually complied, stating that he would wait outside. The nurse practitioner noticed that as the client was left alone, she looked much more comfortable. As the nurse practitioner explained the diagnosis, and how medication can help manage it and even prevent the unborn child from being diagnosed with HIV, the client became more and more withdrawn and upset, especially when hearing that she would need to be able to take medication regularly and have multiple visits to the HIV clinic in order to monitor her and the baby's health.

The client then explained that while her husband had never been physically violent, he was incredibly controlling and did not let her leave the house alone and monitored everything she did. When asked about barriers to HIV care, she explained that her husband did not believe that HIV existed, that it was a government conspiracy, and that he would refuse to allow her to take medication, come to medical appointments for checkups, or to pick up medication. This worried the client, as she understood that this could lead to her child being diagnosed with HIV.

Discussion

In this scenario, it could be easy for the nurse practitioner to miss the reaction of the client to the husband leaving the room or assume that the reaction of the client to the diagnosis and explanation of treatment is only shock at hearing about this previously unknown medical condition. However, if the nurse practitioner has the training to notice and respond to these signs, it could open the opportunity to assess the needs and barriers to treatment. The nurse practitioner could make some observations followed with open-ended questions, such as: "I noticed that when your husband left the room that you seemed to become more comfortable. Is there something that is making you feel unsafe?" and "I realize that this is a huge thing to process, and it is okay to feel a lot of feelings right now. I did notice that you got particularly upset when I was explaining the treatment and follow-up appointments that will be needed. Is there something that might prevent you from taking the medication and coming to follow-up appointments for HIV care?"

Once the nurse practitioner is aware of the safety concerns and barriers to care, they could work with the client to assess the safest way possible to overcome the client's barriers to care. The husband will allow the client to come to prenatal visits, and the OBGYN office can work with the local clinic to coordinate prenatal visits with picking up HIV medication and completing testing, resulting in a healthy birth for the mother and child. The clinic then can continue to work with the client for continued HIV treatment and care.

Case Study 11-2

A patient who was a 20-year-old Latinx presented in the local STI clinic for regular STI testing and was diagnosed with chlamydia. This was the third STI that the patient had been diagnosed with in the past 5 months. The nurse practitioner began to discuss safe sex practices with the client, when the client suddenly bursted out, "I know!" and was visibly upset.

Discussion

In this scenario, a non-trauma-informed approach would be to be offended by the outburst and to label the patient as "difficult." A trauma-informed response would recognize that anger is often related to a trauma reaction, not a personal attack on the practitioner. In this response, the nurse could calmly respond to the emotional reaction with compassion and curiosity, saying, "I see that you are frustrated in hearing these safe sex practices again. Is there something that is making it difficult for you to engage in these practices?" The client then began to explain that he knows that wearing condoms would help to prevent future STIs, but that he does not feel safe negotiating condom use with his partner. Last time he tried to ask for his partner to wear a condom, the partner yelled, "What, you don't trust me?" and it led to a big argument that included physical violence and his partner kicking him out of their apartment, forcing him to sleep in his car. This opened the opportunity for the practitioner to connect the patient to IPV services if willing, and to discuss alternative options to prevent STIs, including PrEP, which can reduce the chance of getting HIV and does not require negotiation with a partner. PrEP is highly effective for preventing HIV through sex or injection drug use.[17]

Summary

This chapter discussed the intersections of IPV and STIs, including the special safety considerations for a PLWH who is also experiencing violence. Topics covered also included empowering and inclusive language to be used in practice, the historical context of HIV, and the intersections of IPV and STIs. Finally, this chapter proposed some best practices for both anti-violence advocates and health care practitioners when working with clients or patients that are living with STIs and experiencing IPV. Best practices for anti-violence advocates should have special considerations for clients living with HIV, including notifying the patient of confidentiality, ensuring safety, providing emotional support, examining needs and possible resources, making a plan, and obtaining a commitment. Special considerations for health care providers working with patients experiencing IPV include creating the space, training all staff, notifying the patient of confidentiality, asking the right questions, educating to empower, and offering meaningful interventions.

References

1. State of the HIV epidemic. Gilead HIV. 2022. Accessed December 9, 2022. https://www.gileadhiv.com/landscape/state-of-epidemic/?gclid=CjwKCAiAjs2bBhACEiwALTBWZRN1W5JGSiudP5ofGCpG45TPoXvery3XPKu-79b_jHT_Gvz3pR2TuhoC1eIQAvD

2. Hess KL, Javanbakht M, Brown JM, Weiss RE, Hsu P, Gorbach PM. Intimate partner violence and sexually transmitted infections among young adult women. *Sex Transm Dis*. 2012;39(5):366-371. doi:10.1097/olq.0b013e3182478fa5

3. At a glance. Centers for Disease Control and Prevention. January 25, 2021. Accessed December 9, 2022. https://www.cdc.gov/std/statistics/prevalence-2020-at-a-glance.htm

4. Shilts R. *And the Band Played on: Politics, People, and the AIDS Epidemic*. Serpent's Tail; 2021.

5. HIV #LanguageMatters: addressing stigma by using preferred language. HIVE. 2022. Accessed December 9, 2022. http://www.hiveonline.org/wp-content/uploads/2016/01/Anti-StigmaSign-Onletter1.pdf

6. Domestic violence and the LGBTQ community. NCADV: National Coalition Against Domestic Violence. 2018. Accessed December 9, 2022. https://ncadv.org/blog/posts/domestic-violence-and-the-lgbtq-community

7. Miltz AR, Lampe FC, Bacchus LJ, et al. Intimate partner violence, depression, and sexual behaviour among gay, bisexual and other men who have sex with men in the proud trial. *BMC Public Health*. 2019;19(1). doi:10.1186/s12889-019-6757-6

8. Peitzmeier SM, Hughto JM, Potter J, Deutsch MB, Reisner SL. Development of a novel tool to assess intimate partner violence against transgender individuals. *J Interpers Violence*. 2019;34(11):2376-2397. doi:10.1177/0886260519827660

9. Home page. Domestic Abuse Intervention Programs. Accessed December 9, 2022. https://www.theduluthmodel.org/

10. Roe, Jagodinsky. Power and control wheel for lesbian, gay, bisexual and trans relationships. Love is Respect. https://www.loveisrespect.org/lir-files/LGBT-Power-and-Control-Wheel.pdf

11. 2018 NCVRW resource guide: intimate partner violence fact sheet. Office for Victims of Crime. 2018. Accessed December 9, 2022. https://ovc.ojp.gov/sites/g/files/xyckuh226/files/ncvrw2018/info_flyers/fact_sheets/2018NCVRW_Stalking_508_QC_v2.pdf

12. STD facts—chlamydia. Centers for Disease Control and Prevention. April 12, 2022. Accessed December 9, 2022. https://www.cdc.gov/std/chlamydia/

stdfact-chlamydia.htm#:~:text=Chlamydia%20is%20a%20common%20STD,that%20occurs%20outside%20the%20womb

13. STD facts—gonorrhea. Centers for Disease Control and Prevention. August 22, 2022. Accessed December 9, 2022. https://www.cdc.gov/std/gonorrhea/stdfact-gonorrhea.htm#:~:text=What%20is%20gonorrhea%3F,people%20ages%2015%2D24%20years
14. Hepatitis B. Centers for Disease Control and Prevention. October 12, 2021. Accessed December 9, 2022. https://www.cdc.gov/hepatitis/hbv/index.htm#:~:text=Hepatitis%20B%20is%20a%20vaccine,someone%20who%20is%20not%20infected
15. STD facts—genital herpes. Centers for Disease Control and Prevention. January 3, 2022. Accessed December 9, 2022. https://www.cdc.gov/std/herpes/stdfact-herpes.htm
16. About HIV/AIDS. Centers for Disease Control and Prevention. June 30, 2022. Accessed December 9, 2022. https://www.cdc.gov/hiv/basics/whatishiv.html
17. Prep. Centers for Disease Control and Prevention. June 3, 2022. Accessed December 12, 2022. https://www.cdc.gov/hiv/basics/prep.html
18. PEP. Centers for Disease Control and Prevention. July 12, 2022. Accessed February 15, 2023. https://www.cdc.gov/hiv/basics/pep/about-pep.html
19. STD facts—human papillomavirus (HPV). Centers for Disease Control and Prevention. April 12, 2022. Accessed December 9, 2022. https://www.cdc.gov/std/hpv/stdfact-hpv.htm
20. STD facts—syphilis. Centers for Disease Control and Prevention. February 10, 2022. Accessed December 9, 2022. https://www.cdc.gov/std/syphilis/stdfact-syphilis.htm
21. STD facts—trichomoniasis. Centers for Disease Control and Prevention. April 25, 2022. Accessed December 9, 2022. https://www.cdc.gov/std/trichomonas/stdfact-trichomoniasis.htm
22. Spiwak R, Afifi TO, Halli S, Garcia-Moreno C, Sareen J. The relationship between physical intimate partner violence and sexually transmitted infection among women in India and the United States. *J Interpers Violence*. 2013;28(13):2770-2791. doi:10.1177/0886260513487992
23. Decker MR, Miller E, McCauley HL, et al. Recent partner violence and sexual and drug-related STI/HIV risk among adolescent and young adult women attending Family Planning Clinics. *Sex Transm Infect*. 2013;90(2):145-149. doi:10.1136/sextrans-2013-051288
24. How to prevent STIs. Centers for Disease Control and Prevention. Updated April 9, 2024. Accessed December 12, 2022. https://www.cdc.gov/sti/prevention/?CDC_AAref_Val=https://www.cdc.gov/std/prevention/default.htm
25. Laughon K, Sutherland MA, Parker BJ. A brief intervention for prevention of sexually transmitted infection among battered women. *J Obstet Gynecol Neonatal Nurs*. 2011;40(6):702-708. doi:10.1111/j.1552-6909.2011.01305.x
26. Seth P, Wingood GM, Robinson LSS, Raiford JL, DiClemente RJ. Abuse impedes prevention: the intersection of intimate partner violence and HIV/STI risk among young African American women. *AIDS Behav*. 2014;19(8):1438-1445. doi:10.1007/s10461-014-0940-7
27. Reproductive and sexual coercion. The American College of Obstetricians and Gynecologists. 2022. Accessed December 12, 2022. https://www.acog.org/

clinical/clinical-guidance/committee-opinion/articles/2013/02/reproductive-and-sexual-coercion

28. Wilson K, Caplon A, Willie T, Alexander KA. 37. 'Safety with my life or my freedom is real to me': sexual safety strategies among young black women experiencing reproductive coercion. *J Adolesc Health.* 2019;64(2):S19-S20. doi:10.1016/j.jadohealth.2018.10.051

29. Passaro RC, Segura ER, Gonzales-Saavedra W, et al. Sexual partnership-level correlates of intimate partner violence among men who have sex with men and transgender women in Lima, Peru. *Arch Sex Behav.* 2020;49(7):2703-2713. doi:10.1007/s10508-020-01682-2

30. Wang L, Barile JP, Simoni JM, et al. Intimate partner violence among Chinese transwomen: associations with sexual risk behaviors and HIV testing. *Sex Transm Dis.* 2020;48(5):362-369. doi:10.1097/olq.0000000000001317

31. Zhang Y, Best J, Tang W, et al. Transgender sexual health in China: a cross-sectional online survey in China. *Sex Transm Infect.* 2016;92:515-519. doi:10.1136/sextrans-2015-052350

32. Decker MR, Seage GR, Hemenway D, Gupta J, Raj A, Silverman JG. Intimate partner violence perpetration, standard and gendered STI/HIV risk behaviour, and STI/HIV diagnosis among a clinic-based sample of men. *Sex Transm Infect.* 2009;85(7):555-560. doi:10.1136/sti.2009.036368

33. Raj A, Reed E, Welles SL, Santana MC, Silverman JG. Intimate partner violence perpetration, risky sexual behavior, and STI/HIV diagnosis among heterosexual African American men. *Am J Men's Health.* 2008;2(3):291-295. doi:10.1177/1557988308320269

34. Campbell JC, Baty ML, Ghandour RM, Stockman JK, Francisco L, Wagman J. The intersection of intimate partner violence against women and HIV/AIDS: a review. *Int J Inj Control Saf Promot.* 2008;15(4):221-231. doi:10.1080/17457300802423224

35. Leserman J, Pence BW, Whetten K, et al. Relation of lifetime trauma and depressive symptoms to mortality in HIV. *Am J Psychiatr.* 2007;164(11):1707-1713. doi:10.1176/appi.ajp.2007.06111775

36. Gonzalez-Guarda RM, Williams JR, Williams W, Lorenzo D, Carrington C. Determinants of HIV and sexually transmitted infection testing and acquisition among female victims of intimate partner violence. *J Interpers Violence.* 2019;36(13-14). doi:10.1177/0886260519827662

37. HIV care continuum. HIV.gov. Accessed December 12, 2022. https://www.hiv.gov/federal-response/policies-issues/hiv-aids-care-continuum

38. CD4 count (or T-cell test). US Department of Veterans Affairs. June 21, 2005. Accessed December 12, 2022. https://www.hiv.va.gov/patient/diagnosis/labs-CD4-count.asp

39. HIV viral load: MedlinePlus medical test. MedlinePlus. Accessed December 12, 2022. https://medlineplus.gov/lab-tests/hiv-viral-load/

40. Schafer KR, Brant J, Gupta S, et al. Intimate partner violence: a predictor of worse HIV outcomes and engagement in care. *AIDS Patient Care STDs.* 2012;26(6):356-365. doi:10.1089/apc.2011.0409

41. HIV and STD criminalization laws. Centers for Disease Control and Prevention. October 24, 2022. Accessed December 12, 2022. https://www.cdc.gov/hiv/policies/law/states/exposure.html

Chapter 12

Safety Planning

Kathy Bell, MS, RN, AFN-C, SANE-A, SANE-P, IVSE-C, DF-AFN

Key Points

1. *It is important to include patients in the safety planning process because they will know what could work and what is not feasible.*
2. *Assessment of danger and lethality is a good way to begin safety planning because it provides interaction and establishes the risk a patient is experiencing.*
3. *Patients experiencing violence need to feel supported and safe when planning for their safety.*

Background and Significance

Patient safety is the cornerstone of high quality health care.[1] While there is very little research that addresses the effectiveness of safety planning,[2] in the studies that have been done, there is evidence that safety planning can promote the increased safety of patients experiencing intimate partner violence (IPV).[1] There is a wide variety of practices associated with safety planning, often associated with the availability of resources and education. There is minimal attention to emotional safety needs.[1] In a focus group study, IPV service provider participants described their perceptions of the safety risks of victims and domestic violence in the community, timing, and personnel involved in safety planning, training, and adherence to safety planning.[1] Future research will continue to support the development and effectiveness of safety planning strategies. Safety is a basic concept in nursing, and, therefore, also in forensic nursing. Nurses regularly assess the risk to patients and their environments. Nurses play a key role in the communication and coordination of many aspects of addressing safety. Discharge planning typically includes discussing precautions with any new medications victims are being prescribed, wound care, follow-up appointments, where they will go, making sure they have an emergency cell phone, and whether they want to involve law enforcement. Safety planning should include specific information, not just giving them a phone number for an advocacy program. The victim may not have the strength or wherewithal to make that call, thus missing an opportunity to get education and resources that will allow them to be safer.

Safety is 1 of the 5 basic needs of humans as described by Maslow, just above the physiological need for things like food and water (see **Figure 12-1**). It is difficult to move to higher-level needs until the previous level is met. For example, a patient who has little to eat and has no idea where their next meal is coming from or how they are going to feed their children, will have difficulty focusing on or caring about where they can find a safe environment, unless it comes with food too. Safety is different from one patient to another. For one person it might be having a place to live and for another, it might be sleeping soundly in that place. Identifying what safety means to an individual is the first step in developing a safety plan.

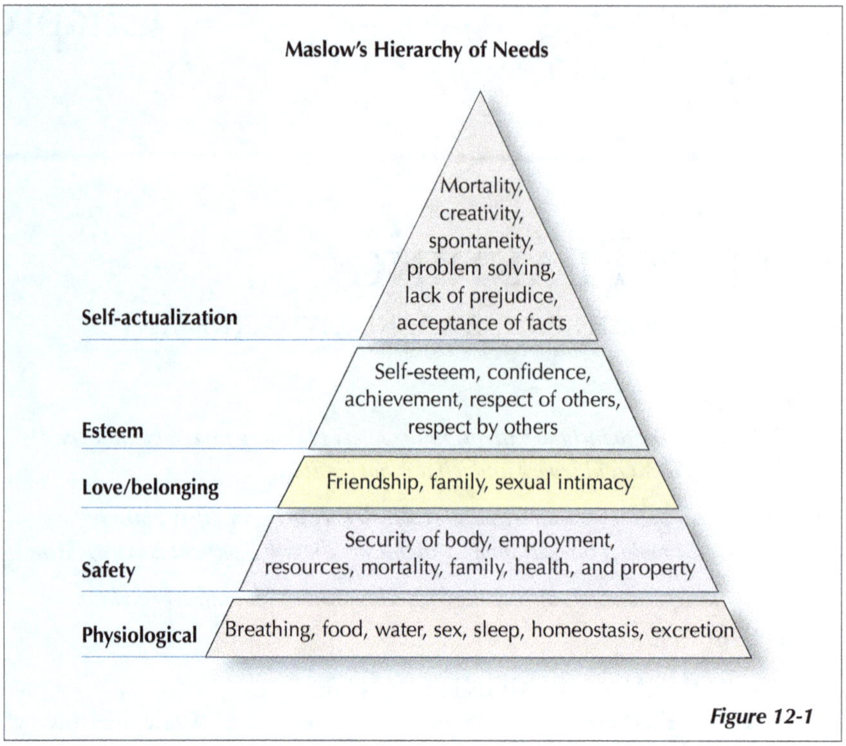

Figure 12-1. Maslow's hierarchy of needs.

Health care typically gives discharge planning instructions to make sure patients are safe in relation to health needs and include things like when to make a follow-up exam, medications, what to watch for, and what activity is appropriate. When reviewing the discharge instruction sheets that have been given to patients when seen in health care settings prior to coming for a forensic medical examination, there is very little discussion and virtually no practical information about how to be safer in whatever violent situation they are in.

Each individual's definition of safety is unique. Safety planning is more effective when an individual's specific needs are assessed and their wishes are considered. Self-management was the specific area addressed in one research study on safety planning. The study built on current research that explored the lived experiences of women affected by IPV and their self-management strategies to improve health outcomes.[3] The operational definition of self-management that was used in Clemmons' study was the ability to perform tasks that increased quality of life. This was chosen based on other studies that outline a link between health literacy skills and health outcomes for women affected by IPV. Health literacy was defined as the degree to which women affected by IPV possessed the capacity to obtain, process, and understand basic health information needed to make appropriate health decisions.[3] Clemmons[3] stated that research indicated that symptom management, adherence to treatment regimes, commitment to appropriate behavioral changes, and the ability to deal with the psychological and physical consequences improved health decisions. Although limiting factors such as low literacy and difficulty in completing and comprehending forms have an impact, the use of self-management strategies to create behavioral changes empowered and prepared individuals experiencing IPV to manage their health, improve their quality-of-life outcomes, and enhance their understanding of the discharge planning processes.[3]

Approaches to safety planning have evolved as domestic violence advocates have worked at changing the vision and practice.[4] Historically, the approach has been to get the patient out of the violent situation. What professionals have found is that this approach is not feasible or even desired for some individuals and their children.

The approach that is now being discussed is to listen carefully to what the victim is saying and identify how to reduce violent behavior. These patients will also need to know resources to help them meet their basic needs.

Judith Hermann's *Trauma and Recovery* states that recovery from traumatic events occurs in 3 stages, with Safety being the first stage, followed by Remembrance and Mourning, then Reconnection and Integration. Hermann defines personal safety and environmental safety as they pertain to individuals who have experienced a traumatic event.[5] Personal safety involves control of the body, such as sleep, eating, and control of self-destructive activities.[5] Environmental safety will add social support such as family, friends, and self-help organizations.[5] When discussing safety, the risks to be aware of are important to address. Just as important is discussing the atmosphere in which the patient can regain control and begin to heal from the trauma. Immediately after an assault, many individuals experience a wide variety of feelings and emotions. Hermann[5] suggests that a person will be far less frightened by these feelings if they are prepared with education about how to cope with them. Without alternative options for how to manage those reactions, some victims will resort to unhealthy activities, such as isolating oneself from others or self-medicating with drugs or alcohol. The patient may think these activities will help them through a difficult time, but they can actually put them at a higher risk. As part of the safety planning process, the nurse can help them find more positive coping methods that will promote better health and safety. It is important to use a nonjudgmental approach when discussing unhealthy behaviors.

Risk Assessment

Safety planning is an opportunity for the abused individual to gain information to strategize their response to their current situation.[6] Leaving has been identified as one of the most dangerous times in ending a relationship, and therefore should be carefully orchestrated unless an extreme emergency exists. Whether someone stays or leaves a violent relationship, they might be killed or injured, their children could be hurt, they could become depressed, they could lose credibility with family and friends, and their health could be impacted.[7]

Research has identified the following as risk factors in the most dangerous situations, with strangulation being added to this list[8]:

— Access to or ownership of guns

— Use of a weapon in prior abusive incidents

— Threats with weapons

— Threats to kill

— Serious injury in prior abusive incidents

— Threats of suicide

— Drug or alcohol abuse

— Forced sex

— Possessiveness/extreme jealousy/extreme dominance

Combining victim perception of their situation and a validated instrument with the assessment of a skilled clinician may be the best method to identify the risks of an individual patient and use that information as the basis of an individualized safety plan.[8] The 2019 version of the Danger Assessment (DA)[9] assesses victim education and awareness for education, safety planning, and service provision (see **Figure 12-2**). It is designed as a patient interview to be administered by health care professionals or victim advocates. The assessment consists of 20 yes/no questions

DANGER ASSESSMENT

Jacquelyn C. Campbell, PhD, R.N. Copyright, 2003; update 2019; www.dangerassessment.com

Several risk factors have been associated with increased risk of homicides (murders) of women and men in violent relationships. We cannot predict what will happen in your case, but we would like you to be aware of the danger of homicide in situations of abuse and for you to see how many of the risk factors apply to your situation.

Using the calendar, please mark the approximate dates during the past year when you were abused by your partner or ex-partner. Write on that date how bad the incident was according to the following scale:

1. Slapping, pushing; no injuries and/or lasting pain
2. Punching, kicking; bruises, cuts, and/or continuing pain
3. "Beating up"; severe contusions, burns, broken bones
4. Threat to use weapon; head injury, internal injury, permanent injury, miscarriage or choking* (use a © in the date to indicate choking/strangulation/cut off your breathing- example 4©)
5. Use of weapon; wounds from weapon

(If **any** of the descriptions for the higher number apply, use the higher number.)

Mark **Yes** or **No** for each of the following. ("He" refers to your husband, partner, ex-husband, ex-partner, or whoever is currently physically hurting you.)

_____ 1. Has the physical violence increased in severity or frequency over the past year?
_____ 2. Does he own a gun?
_____ 3. Have you left him after living together during the past year?
3a. (If you have *never* lived with him, check here: __)
_____ 4. Is he unemployed?
_____ 5. Has he ever used a weapon against you or threatened you with a lethal weapon? (If yes, was the weapon a gun? check here: __)
_____ 6. Does he threaten to kill you?
_____ 7. Has he avoided being arrested for domestic violence?
_____ 8. Do you have a child that is not his?
_____ 9. Has he ever forced you to have sex when you did not wish to do so?
_____ 10. Does he ever try to choke/strangle you or cut off your breathing?
10a. (If yes, has he done it more than once, or did it make you pass out or black out or make you dizzy? check here: __)
_____ 11. Does he use illegal drugs? By drugs, I mean "uppers" or amphetamines, "meth", speed, angel dust, cocaine, "crack", street drugs or mixtures.
_____ 12. Is he an alcoholic or problem drinker?
_____ 13. Does he control most or all of your daily activities? For instance, does he tell you who you can be friends with, when you can see your family, how much money you can use, or when you can take the car? (If he tries, but you do not let him, check here: __)
_____ 14. Is he violently and constantly jealous of you? (For instance, does he say: "If I can't have you, no one can.")
_____ 15. Have you ever been beaten by him while you were pregnant? (If you have never been pregnant by him, check here: __)
_____ 16. Has he ever threatened or tried to commit suicide?
_____ 17. Does he threaten to harm your children?
_____ 18. Do you believe he is capable of killing you?
_____ 19. Does he follow or spy on you, leave threatening notes or messages, destroy your property, or call you when you don't want him to?
_____ 20. Have you ever threatened or tried to commit suicide?

_____ Total "Yes" Answers

Thank you. Please talk to your nurse, advocate, or counselor about what the Danger Assessment means in your situation.

Figure 12-2

Figure 12-2. *The Danger Assessment, as updated in 2019.*

about risk factors and is scored 1 point per question for items 1 through 19. Question 20 is not given a score but identifies the risk of suicidal ideation potential and offers an opportunity to discuss a safety plan should the patient develop self-harm thoughts or activities. The score results may present as variable, increased, severe, or extreme danger.

The 2019 DA also incorporates a calendar that plots the dates of abuse events according to severity over a period of time. The calendar is an effective tool for the patient to be able to see and acknowledge the trajectory of violence that has been occurring. It validates that what they are experiencing is really happening and that it is dangerous. When presented in this manner, many patients have said, "I knew it was bad, but I didn't realize it was this bad."

The DA-5 was developed as a short form of the DA for use in health care settings, including emergency and urgent care settings.[10] It is recommended that the DA-5 be used for a quick assessment of homicide or near-homicide risk among IPV survivors once it is stated or suspected that violence is occurring. Four of the 5 questions are also included on the DA. The addition of strangulation was added to acknowledge the potential lethality and long-term consequences of multiple strangulations. In addition to safety planning, a protocol for immediate referral and examination for further injury should be adopted for individuals experiencing strangulation.

Figure 12-3. *Danger Assessment-5.*

DANGER ASSESSMENT-5

Jacquelyn C. Campbell, PhD, RN. Copyright, 2015; www.dangerassessment.com

The brief risk assessment identifies women who are at high risk for homicide or severe injury by an intimate partner.
Mark **Yes** or **No** for each of the following questions.
("He" refers to your husband, partner, ex-husband, ex-partner, or whoever is currently physically hurting you.)

_____ 1. Has the physical violence increased in frequency or over the past year?
_____ 2. Has he ever used a weapon against you or threatened you with a weapon?
_____ 3. Do you believe he is capable of killing you?
_____ 4. Does he ever try to choke you?
_____ 5. Is he violently and constantly jealous of you?

Figure 12-3

Safety Plan

Basic safety behaviors that are typically discussed with patients include activities such as hiding money, having an extra set of keys to the house and car, letting neighbors know to call the police if violence begins, hiding weapons, and having a bag packed. If children are in the family, the bag should include toys and childcare items. Important documents should be available and readily accessible or copied and kept at an easy-to-access separate location (eg, a place of employment, a friend's house). Documents include social security numbers, driver's licenses, rent and utility receipts, bank account numbers, birth certificates, and important phone numbers.

Copies of insurance policies and numbers or marriage licenses should also be considered. If a protective order is in place, keeping a copy on one's person is recommended. Safety words are another basic safety behavior to put in place. This word is an alert that help is needed; the receiver knows not to come forward but to leave and get help. It is especially important that children know how to use the safety word. Often, they want to help, but they need to be educated that they are helping in the best way possible by reaching out for help and that they are liable to get hurt if they intervene directly. Even in nonviolent family situations, safety words are recommended for preteens or teens to alert parents if they are feeling uncomfortable in a social situation.

Approaching a Patient

Engaging the patient in the process is quite possibly the most important step of safety planning. Victims are often most open to change immediately after a crisis event (the severity of an event needed to deem it a crisis varies from person to person), beginning to minimize and deny the details of their victimization quickly thereafter. This means that providers should begin safety planning conversations as early as possible in a patient interaction. Trauma impacts the brain of both the listener and the speaker, making it difficult to stay in the present.[11]

It is not easy to listen to the histories of trauma that patients describe. Manning[11] describes listening as the greatest gift that can be given because it aids in their healing and shows respect for them and for what they have experienced. However, at the same time, it can impact a health professional in physical and emotional ways. It may even be more difficult to respond to these patients in a supportive way, making effective communication a key ingredient to effective safety planning. A patient who feels accepted and noticed no matter the situation will be more likely to participate in developing a trusting relationship with the person performing the safety planning. Professionals have a short time to establish trust with patients. *Blink*, by Malcolm Gladwell,[12] gives multiple examples of how a situation or person is sized up in the blink of an eye. That evaluation can be right or wrong depending on factors such as stress, emotions, other interests, and attitudes.[12] The development of some level of trust is a key component of effective communication. There is not a clear, clinical definition of trust, but it clearly has a major influence on patients' acceptance of care and treatment from health care professionals.[13]

The stress response of the listener can show up as disbelief, anger, or disgust.[11] To defuse the possibility of the patient sensing this stress in the listener, actions such as breathing, curling one's toes, or engaging all 5 senses about the environment around them (eg, the smell, the feel of the air, the sound of the heating or air conditioning) are recommended. Employing empathy is another way to defuse the patient's awareness of their stress response.

To show the patient acceptance and care, providers must stay engaged. Manning[11] describes using encouragement, eye contact, mirroring, looping, using clarification, and asking open-ended questions as effective means of staying engaged in the conversation. Brief words such as "go on" could encourage a person talking to continue with the conversation. Eye contact lets the patient know that the listener is paying attention to what they are saying. Mirroring can demonstrate that the listener is engaged and listening to them and can be used to subconsciously calm and relax a tense patient. An example of mirroring may be taking slow deep breaths and releasing them from the abdomen or consciously dropping the shoulders to a more relaxed position.[11] Looping is repeating back to the patient what they just said to show the speaker that the listener is hearing and engaged with what they are saying. Clarifying within the conversation assures the patient that the practitioner hears what they are saying and wants to be sure they have it correct. Asking open-ended questions allows the patient to describe their event and feelings without any extraneous information interjected by the listener.

For communication about safety to be useful, the conversation should be done where the person is comfortable and safe. A private, calm, quiet area free of noise and bright lights is ideal, and distractions should be minimized. If children are present, a safe place nearby, preferably where the patient can still see them, will allow the patient to better focus on the conversation. Setting up a safe environment where the patient is alone, in a calm, comfortable setting to have a conversation about safety planning involves offering choices and not telling the person what they should or should not do. Maintaining a safe and trusting environment also means that a provider should never touch a patient without permission.

Communication can be broken down into 3 elements: nonverbal, tone, and words. The interaction of tone of voice, body language, and the words used influence the impact of messages.[14] The senses of hearing, sight, and touch are important in communication, and in particular, the listening aspect of communication. Betts[15] states that the International Listening Association defines listening as "the process of receiving, constructing meaning from, and responding to spoken and/or nonverbal messages," whereas hearing is specifically the receiving of speech. Hearing is critical because it is the first element of the listening process.[16] Safety planning conversations can be difficult to initiate, but some strategies include building from the information that has been provided by the patient before that point, sharing concerns about the patient's danger assessment, or the provider can begin by telling the patient that they want to talk about some ways to keep them and their family safe.[17]

Key concepts to keep in mind[18]:

— Providers should never let a visitor know that the assessment was done, as this could put the patient in more danger.

— Some perpetrators will not let the patient be alone. Providers should think about ways to separate the patient from the perpetrator without raising red flags.

— Some patients are volatile, angry, or belligerent, which can be signs of intoxication or drug use. Providers should also consider that strangulation may have occurred if there are no other obvious signs of drug and alcohol ingestion.

— Providers must keep in mind that this patient is already at risk, so they should be looking for ways to minimize that risk.

— Providers should focus on giving the patient knowledge, which is the power to make their own decisions.

— It can take several abusive incidents before a person is willing and able to change.

— Family or friends should not be used as interpreters.

Coming up with the right words at the right time can sometimes be difficult in these situations, especially if it is not a situation you often find yourself in or when beginning to work with victims that have experienced IPV. Although this reference is somewhat dated, it gives a few examples of effective means of talking to a patient[19]:

— Communicating: "I see the bruising around your eye. Are there other injuries that you can show me?"

— Reflecting: "Is it difficult to talk about your relationship with your partner?"

— Active listening: "Could you explain for me what you mean by your partner 'freaked out'?"

— Congruence: "You seem uncomfortable when I ask you about the cause of your injury. Would it be okay to ask you a few questions?"

— Empathy: "You look frightened when you talk about your partner. Do you feel frightened?"

— Empowerment: "You have a choice about your safety and whether you remain in your relationship. There are various resources available to assist you in attaining safety."

— Validation: "Abuse is unacceptable. You deserve to feel free from violence."

— Acceptance: "It is understandable that you feel sad about your relationship with your partner."

— Honesty: "Would you mind if I discuss your situation with___________? I feel that we can assist you more effectively by combining our different areas of expertise."

Another way to open the conversation about safety planning could be "What is your biggest concern when you leave here today?" Depending on the unique history that each patient gives will guide the development of each individual plan. Potential issues, topics, and suggestions for discussion follow.

In an Emergency

In an emergency, encourage a patient to[20]:

— Stay away from the kitchen

— Stay away from the garage

— Stay away from bathrooms

— Get to a room with a door

— Get to a room with a phone

— Call 911

Kitchens and garages have many items that can be used as a weapon. Bathrooms often have only 1 way out, and a victim can get trapped with no way out. Individuals that are living in a violent situation should try to always keep a phone near them.

If Living with the Abuser

All documents should be photocopied and kept at a separate location, and safety words should be established with those that are able to summon help. In this situation, it is necessary for the victim to have a safe location to keep documents and other essential items when it is necessary to leave. It is important that the offender does not know there is a safety plan, and it can therefore be helpful to use apps and online safety plans.[11] Some sites and apps such as the MyPlan app have secure exit options and do not indicate that the site has anything to do with safety information. If a decision is made to leave, individuals may feel they "owe it" to their partner to tell them in person that they are leaving. However, leaving is known as one of the most dangerous times in a relationship, and person-to-person encounters provide the offender with the opportunity to control, injure, or kill the victim.[8] Providers should assist the patient in identifying other safe ways for a partner to discover that information.

When Living Separately

Actions can be taken to eliminate the possibility of an abuser gaining access to the patient once the patient has left the relationship. Limited access to resources will hinder some of these options. The local advocacy center may be able to help with accessing resources to help with changing locks and protective orders.

Many states have address confidentiality programs that a person can enroll in. Information about these programs can often be accessed through a website or discussing with the local advocacy program. These programs often offer an alternate address and mail forwarding services. If resources are available, wooden doors could be replaced with stronger or steel doors. Safety instructions that suggest installing security systems and outside lighting are good advice but may not be feasible because of the financial situation many victims are in. When children are involved, anyone caring for them needs to know who can and cannot pick them up. Additionally, there needs to be a plan for what to do if there is any alteration to that plan, for any reason. Family, friends, clergy, and neighbors need to know that the abuser no longer lives there and to call the police if they see the abuser on the victim's property when a protective order is in place.

When Outside the Home

Although inconvenient, it may be necessary to change travel, shopping, and errand habits. If a person is walking to their car alone, they should be aware of their surroundings and carry a cell phone programmed for 911. Many women carry purses or other items with them when going to their car and situate those items in the seat next to them before securing the door. When getting into a car, it is best to get in, shut the door, lock it, and then situate the items. Many organizations and companies that have security employees encourage escorts to cars if there are safety risks. Thinking ahead and having a plan to respond in a particular situation will provide confidence in moving around the community. If a protective order is in place, it should always be kept on the person that has the order issued to them. If a victim's employer, coworkers, or security do not know what the offender looks like, it is recommended to give or show them a picture and ask that if they see that person, they call the police.

Emotional Safety and Use of Drugs and Alcohol

Judith Hermann's seminal work mentioned earlier also talks about how someone will be less frightened by being prepared for common emotional responses following a violent event.[5]

The following are considerations to include in safety planning discussions:

— Awareness of drug and alcohol use

— What to do when feeling down

— What to do when communicating with an abuser on the phone

— Use of "I can" statements

— Support groups

— Numbers to call if not emotionally safe

Technology Safety

Technology today is so common that most people do not think about how it can make them vulnerable. For example, tracking systems can be difficult to notice on phones and watches, social media can be used to locate someone or give personal information, baby monitors can be used to listen in on conversations, and computer usage can give clues as to what a patient may be planning, just to name a few. Offenders regularly use access to common technology to gain access to the individuals. There are many resources that are available surrounding technology safety and IPV. Many of the technology safety plans include items such as:

— Trusting one's instincts

— Staying off social media

— Using a computer that the offender does not have access to

— Getting a new email account

— Keeping emails and text messages that detail the abuse; these records should be shared with the police if a report has been made

— Checking cell phone settings to make sure that tracking cannot occur

— Changing passwords and pin numbers to ones that could not be guessed by the offender; any password that has been used in the past should be avoided

— Minimizing the use of cordless phones and baby monitors

— Using a donated or new cell phone

— Getting a private PO mailbox

Children

The following is a list of things to think about and address during safety planning when children are involved. If talking directly to the child, it is important to consider their age and development.

— Do they have a safe place?

— Do they know who is safe to tell if they feel unsafe?

— Do they know how to call 911?

Children are often aware of the violence around them even when parents think they have been shielding it from them. Telling children that the violence they witness is not their fault is important. Research shows that there are negative effects of exposure to witnessing violence. Supportive nurses can minimize the trauma in many cases. Including children in safety planning and empowering them with knowledge of what they can do is important to promote protective factors that will enhance resiliency.

Children need to know to stay out of adult conflicts and that their job is to be safe, not to protect their parents.

Other Considerations

Documenting Events

During trauma, the brain may not remember events accurately. It may be helpful to suggest a patient keep a diary with the relevant names, dates, and times of conversations. These items could include conversations with medical personnel about follow-up appointments, conversations with law enforcement about the next steps in the process of the investigation, or it could be about the violent experience. Keeping this documentation may be helpful in eliminating some confusion that is often experienced. As mentioned previously, it is important to keep this type of information in a safe location that the offender does not have access to.

Pets

Pets are another important consideration. Some victims are more concerned about their pets than their own safety. Some domestic violence shelters now have the option of housing pets. The person that owns the pet needs to establish ownership of the pet (eg, obtain an animal license, proof of vaccinations, or veterinary receipts in the victim's name to help prove they own the pets). Law enforcement or animal care and control officers can assist in reclaiming pets if left behind.

Resources and Services for Safety Planning

Knowing the resources available in the community and having them readily available is a key component of safety planning. Being able to give the patient the specific information they need to be safe will go a long way in helping someone that has just experienced a traumatic event and has little strength and knowledge to find the information on their own. Without this information, some victims may find it easier to return to the violent environment.

The following services are regularly needed by individuals that have experienced violence. Practitioners should keep a list of contact information to these organizations so that they can refer patients to appropriate services.

— Domestic violence shelter

— Child Protective Services

— Adult Protective Services

— Health services

— Free or sliding scale clinics

— Pharmacy

— Law enforcement

— Counseling

— Protective order

— Animal shelter

— Food assistance

— Childcare assistance

Case Study

Case Study 12-1

Janice was a 32-year-old woman that came for an IPV exam following an incident that happened 2 days before her appointment. She stated that she and Jason, aged 37 years, had been together for the last 8 years. Assaults have been happening for the entire length of the relationship. She stated that she only vaguely remembers the incident 2 days previously, but she thought he was going to kill her. She reports that, "He was hitting, kicking, and choking me. He put his arm across my neck." Janice stated that Jason owned a gun and had threatened her with it in the past but did not this time. She talked slowly, her speech was somewhat slurred, and she had difficulty staying focused. She had contusions and abrasions to her face, abdomen, chest, under her chin, and to both upper arms and legs. Her past medical history includes 3 pregnancies with 2 live births. She was in a methadone treatment program and was positive for hepatitis C. She had a recent pilonidal cyst removal that was healing. Her blood pressure was 110/72 P 72 and R 16. Pulse oximeter was 98%. Her current medications were methadone, clonazepam, levothyroxine, and hydrocodone. She had an old scar on her forehead from a previous incident with the same partner where he slammed her head into a dresser, knocking her unconscious and lacerating her forehead.

When the provider performed a DA-5 assessment, Janice scored 5 of 5 points.

On a subsequent full DA, she responded yes to the following numbered items:

1. Has the physical violence increased in severity or frequency over the past year?
4. Is he unemployed?
5. Has he ever used a weapon against you or threatened you with a lethal weapon? (If yes, was the weapon a gun?)
6. Does he threaten to kill you?
10. Does he ever try to choke/strangle you or cut off your breathing? 10a. (If yes, has he done it more than once, or did it make you pass out or black out or make you dizzy?)
12. Is he an alcoholic or problem drinker?
13. Does he control most or all of your daily activities? For instance, does he tell you who you can be friends with, when you can see your family, how much money you can use, or when you can take the car?
14. Is he violently and constantly jealous of you? (For instance, does he say: "If I can't have you, no one can.")

16. Has he ever threatened or tried to commit suicide?

18. Do you believe he is capable of killing you?

20. Have you ever threatened or tried to commit suicide?

The offender was arrested before Janice's arrival at the Emergency Department and was put in jail with a bond of $10 000. Janice did not have a car.

Discussion

A score of 5 out of 5 indicates that Janice is at risk of being killed or experiencing a severe injury. She has many medical needs that will require attention, especially because of her history of strangulation and the current symptoms she is displaying. While Jason is in jail, she will have some time to think and plan. Addressing her immediate safety needs would involve a safe place to stay. Where is she going (eg, shelter, friend) once she leaves the facility that is treating her? What about her children? What is her support system without him? What are the support options for her children? She should be given the number to a domestic violence crisis line. Ideally, before she leaves the facility, she would be given a phone and put on the line with that agency to be made aware of the services that they could provide for her and at the same time develop a safety plan. What is her risk for drug use? Has she already used? Is that the reason for her slurred speech and lack of focus? Or is it due to her strangulation? How will she access her methadone services with no transportation? Does she have money or resources for food? Does she want to get a protective order? Does she have a phone? If not, does the local advocacy center have emergency cell phones available? The patient would only be able to call 911, but when a high danger and lethality score is present, the reassurance that they could get help if needed would likely calm to a great extent.

As Janice has had suicidal ideation or attempts in the past, the provider should inquire into her support and what her plan would be if she did develop those thoughts. Whom can she call? See that she has the phone number for those services that are readily and easily accessible such as local mental health organizations or 988, the Suicide and Crisis Lifeline. Continued conversation with this patient will identify other safety and medical needs she might have.

Summary

IPV as a public health issue affects millions of women, men, and children each year. Over the years, it has been estimated that the cost of domestic and sexual violence to society exceeds $8 billion in medical, mental, and lost productivity costs and kills at least 1500 individuals a year.[8,21] Only approximately 4% of victims who die have contact with domestic violence programs, and 40% to 60% sought some type of health care the year before their death.[8] Every patient encounter, no matter the setting, is an opportunity for developing a safety plan when someone is experiencing violence.

Not all health care organizations have social service employees who can address the safety needs of a patient once they leave the facility, so other professionals need to be able to ensure that patients leave with the resources that will allow them to be safe in whatever environment they decide to go to. Due to the limited research on the effectiveness of various safety planning practices, it may be no more than planting a seed by asking about abuse or showing a patient that someone cares.[2,22] There is not just 1 method of safety planning, so spending time with a patient and finding out what their specific needs are regarding safety is important. Common sense discussions are valuable and are not put into place to frighten or scare patients, but to calm them and give them confidence that they will know what to do if something like their most recent incident of abuse happens again. It is important to never give up on patients in a violent relationship. They need to know they can return for help as many times as needed and that they will not be judged.

Additional Resources

Table 12-1. 48-Hour Safety Plan

1. It appears you are in danger now. I'd like to talk with you about your safety.
   a. Is there anything else you would like to tell me?
   b. DVIS/Call Rape has a shelter. Would you like to go to the shelter? Yes No
2. DVIS offers free counseling for you and your children. Walk-in crisis counseling is available without an appointment M-F 8:30am-5pm at 4300 S. Harvard. The 24-hour crisis line is available 7 days a week at 918-7HELPME. (918-743-5763)
3. What are the plans for the night?
   a. Where will you be staying?
   b. Do you have a safe place to go/be right now?
   c. Who can you call for support?
   d. If you are going to stay in your home:
      i. Has it been secured?
      ii. Have you thought about the quickest way to get out of the house in an emergency?
      iii. Call 911 immediately if the person who harmed you returns.
4. If you have to leave your house quickly, is there a safe place you could go?
   a. Friend/Relative/Neighbor?
   b. Can you talk to that person and let them know that in case of an emergency you are considering going there?
5. Can you pack a bag and put it where you could get to it quickly if you need to leave because of your safety?
   a. Include important documents, medicine, money, etc.
   b. Leave it by the door, in the trunk of a car, or with a neighbor, friend, or relative.
6. Are you planning to return to work in the next 48 hours?
   a. Can you let your supervisor, security staff, or coworkers know that you might be in danger?
   b. Walk with someone to and from parking lot/have someone screen calls/move office.
7. Did you know that you can apply for a protective order?
   a. Protective order paperwork can be done at the Family Safety Center, Monday-Friday at 9am, at 3010 S. Harvard.
   b. Advocates are there to provide additional safety planning and provide resources for you whether you want a protective order or not.
   c. If you receive a protective order, keep a copy on your person at all times and give copies to your supervisor at work, your children's school, and your landlord.
8. Is it okay if we get a safe telephone number to call and follow-up with you?

Adapted from Domestic Violence Intervention Services, 48-Hour Safety Plan. Tulsa, OK.

References

1. Mitchell PH. Defining patient safety and quality care. In: Hughes RG, ed. *Patient Safety and Quality: An Evidence-Based Handbook for Nurses*. Agency for Healthcare Research and Quality; 2008.

2. Murray CE, Horton GE, Johnson CH, et al. Domestic violence service providers' perceptions of safety planning: a focus group study. *J Fam Violence.* 2015;30(3):381-392. doi:10.1007/s10896-015-9674-1

3. Clemons YM. *Safety Planning: Self-Management Approaches for Intimate Partner Violence in Ohio.* Dissertation. Walden University; 2021.

4. Davies J. Victim-defined advocacy beyond leaving: safer through strategies to reduce violent behavior. VAWnet. 2019. https://vawnet.org/sites/default/files/assets/files/2020-05/NRCDV_VictimDefinedAdvocacyBeyondLeaving-Oct2019.pdf

5. Herman JL. *Trauma and Recovery: The Aftermath of Violence—From Domestic Abuse to Political Terror.* Basic Books; 1993.

6. Campbell JC. Safety planning based on lethality assessment for partners of batterers in intervention programs. *J Aggress Maltreat Trauma.* 2001;5(2):129-143. doi:10.1300/J146v05n02_08

7. Davies J. Victim-defined safety planning: a summary. VAWnet. 2017. Accessed June 22, 2024. https://vawnet.org/material/victim-defined-safety-planning-summary

8. Campbell JC, Messing J, eds. *Assessing Dangerousness: Domestic Violence Offenders and Child Abusers.* Springer Publishing Company; 2017.

9. Danger assessment. The Danger Assessment. Accessed December 31, 2022. https://www.dangerassessment.org/

10. Messing JT, Campbell JC, Snider C. Validation and adaptation of the danger assessment-5: a brief intimate partner violence risk assessment. *J Adv Nurs.* 2017;73(12):3220-3230. doi:10.1111/jan.13459

11. Manning K. *The Empathetic Workplace: 5 Steps to a Compassionate, Calm, and Confident Response to Trauma on the Job.* HarperCollins Leadership; 2021.

12. Gladwell M. *Blink.* Little, Brown and Company; 2005.

13. Belcher M, Jones LK. Graduate nurses' experiences of developing trust in the nurse–patient relationship. *Contemp Nurse.* 2009;31(2):142-152. doi:10.5172/conu.673.31.2.142

14. Mehrabian A. *Silent Messages.* Wadsworth; 1971.

15. Betts K. Lost in translation: importance of effective communication in online education. *Online J Distance Learn Adm.* 2009;12(2):1-4.

16. Tubbs SL, Moss S. *Human Communication: Principles and Contexts.* 10th ed. McGraw-Hill; 2006.

17. Campbell JC. Helping women understand their risk in situations of intimate partner violence. *J Interpers Violence.* 2004;19(12):1464-1477. doi:10.1177/0886260504269698

18. Bell K. Safety Planning. Webinar presented at: Academy of Forensic Nursing; October 27, 2021.

19. Weber T, Levin LK. *Medical Providers' Guide to Managing the Care of Domestic Violence Patients within a Cultural Context.* Mayor's Office to Combat Domestic Violence, New York City; 2004. 2nd ed. https://www.nyc.gov/html/ocdv/downloads/pdf/Materials_Medical_Providers_DV_Guide.pdf

20. Woods-Littlejohn B, Brown S, Furr C. *Domestic Violence Homicide in Oklahoma: A Report of the Oklahoma Domestic Violence Fatality Review Board 2006.* Oklahoma Criminal Justice Resource Center, Oklahoma Domestic Violence Fatality Review Board; 2006. https://www.oag.ok.gov/sites/g/files/gmc766/f/dvfrb_2006_annual_report.pdf

21. The health care costs of domestic and sexual violence. Futures Without Violence. March 2010. Accessed January 2, 2023. https://www.futureswithoutviolence.org/userfiles/file/HealthCare/Health_Care_Costs_of_Domestic_and_Sexual_Violence.pdf

22. Wood SN, Glass N, Decker MR. An integrative review of safety strategies for women experiencing intimate partner violence in low- and middle-income countries. *Trauma Violence Abuse.* 2021;22(1):680-82. doi:10.1177/1524838018823270

Chapter 13

Economic Implications of Interpersonal Violence: *Analyzing the Cyclical and Lifetime Costs of Interpersonal Violence*

Holly Ramella, MA
Kelsey Arias, Peer Support Specialist, MSW
Bibiana Lopez, BA

Key Points

1. *There is a lifetime cost associated with interpersonal violence and victims/survivors are often footing the bill.*
2. *When interpersonal violence is based on power and control, the economic implications of violence create a cyclical experience for victims/survivors struggling to access basic needs.*
3. *The current approach to the economic implications of interpersonal violence is focused on short-term solutions and is not effective in addressing the holistic, long-term, and generational implications.*

Background and Significance

The impacts of interpersonal violence can show up in every aspect of a victim-survivor's life and last for generations. This chapter will explore the economic implications of interpersonal violence on the individual, familial, community, and societal level. Often, when discussing economic implications and interpersonal violence, the focus is on financial abuse in domestic violence situations. While this is a disturbingly common occurrence that will be discussed, this chapter will also focus on all forms of interpersonal violence. For the purposes of this chapter, interpersonal violence refers to an umbrella term for power-based violence including sexual violence, relationship violence, and stalking. Intimate partner violence (IPV) in this chapter will replace the terms domestic violence and relationship violence. This may include financial abuse, sexual abuse, stalking, harassment, physical abuse, etc, between romantic partners. The authors also use the term victim-survivor in reference to anyone who has or is experiencing interpersonal violence. The term "victim-survivor" was coined in 2014 by Régine M. Jean-Charles[1] to highlight a both/and approach to experiences of violence, particularly by Black women. A both/and approach acknowledges the fluidity of identity and is inclusive of those who have experienced violence in the past and those who continue to experience violence. Rather than referring to someone as an abuser or perpetrator, this chapter will use the term "harm-doer" in an attempt to allow space for transformation and restoration while continuing to acknowledge the impact of power and control dynamics and the systemic implications at play. Intentional language allows literature to mirror the complexities of interpersonal violence and its implications.

According to a 2018 American Journal of Preventive Medicine study,[2] the estimated lifetime cost of IPV, not including non-IPV sexual violence or stalking, for 43 million United States adult victim-survivors was $3.6 trillion. Of that cost, government resources pay approximately $1.3 trillion. These costs include both immediate and long-term medical costs, mental health services, legal services, loss of work, childcare, housing, and transportation. Such costs illuminate that interpersonal violence does not occur in a vacuum and is a global epidemic.[2] While the immediate costs of interpersonal violence are often addressed by service providers such as crisis advocates, who provide bus passes or emergency funds for crisis counseling, there is no fund to support a victim-survivor throughout their lifetime in the United States. Yet, the physical and psychological impacts of trauma caused by interpersonal violence often create exorbitant costs following the victim-survivor and their dependents for their entire lives. Victim-survivors can face higher lifelong health costs than those who have not experienced interpersonal violence. In fact, a 2022 study on the lifetime economic burden of interpersonal violence among United States adults found that the health care costs of women who experienced abuse were 42% higher than those who did not.[3] Studies also suggest that victim-survivors are also likely to experience chronic pain[4] and other perpetual health problems, leading to high medical bills throughout their lifetime. The chronic physical and psychological impacts are incredibly costly and include gastrointestinal disorders, depression, post-traumatic stress disorder, anxiety, and autoimmune disorders. These costs can be devastating to individuals, families, and communities, which begs the question, what happens when they cannot pay the cost? For victim-survivors impacted by intersecting forms of oppression who often cannot access the limited financial aid resources available, the inability to pay for medical costs leads to a loss of safe housing, food security, and other basic needs, putting them at a greater risk of revictimization. A scoping review on the risk factors of chronic pain in victims of violence, published in 2017, documented the correlation between economic insecurity and rate of sexual violence. The review found that people experiencing higher levels of economic insecurity were more likely to have experienced forms of sexual violence than people who reported having more economic security.[5] Therefore, the economic implications of interpersonal violence create a cyclical experience of violence, but access to support and resources can halt that cycle.

Violence and all its implications can affect anyone, regardless of their socioeconomic status and identities. However, similar to the way trauma's impact can be minimized with protective factors, economic implications are less destructive for victim-survivors that hold privileged identities. Generational wealth, the ability to be believed, and identity-affirming services are some of the protective factors that can offset the damage of interpersonal violence on an individual's finances. Victim-survivors with these protective factors may still face devastating financial impacts, but their ability to recover increases, and their time to recover shrinks.[6] A person who can go to their family or friends and receive free housing, extended financial support, and guidance in accessing the criminal justice system or other governmental assistance resources is much more likely to avoid recurring costs and revictimization. On the other hand, someone who is the provider for their family, whose family, friends, or community have limited resources to share, and who cannot access an identity-affirming service is much more likely to experience revictimization and feel the economic impacts of interpersonal violence throughout their lifetime.[6] Even free resources such as shelters or crisis hotlines can pose barriers and indirectly incur costs. Victim-survivors may not have access to reliable transportation, childcare to meet with an advocate, or a work schedule that fits the requirements of a shelter.

Those victim-survivors who experience multiple forms of marginalization such as racism, homo/transphobia, or xenophobia may be turned away from services or fear reaching out in the first place. Domestic violence shelters that can provide free and immediate housing may also have screening procedures or requirements that disproportionately impact sex workers, victim-survivors struggling with substances, and LGBTQIA+ victim-survivors. Fear of deportation, long-standing police violence, language barriers, and overt and covert racist experiences are all barriers that victim-survivors of color face when attempting to access resources.[7]

Figure 13-1. *Financial insecurity is greatest among Black and Brown women survivors.[8] Year of the study was 2021.*

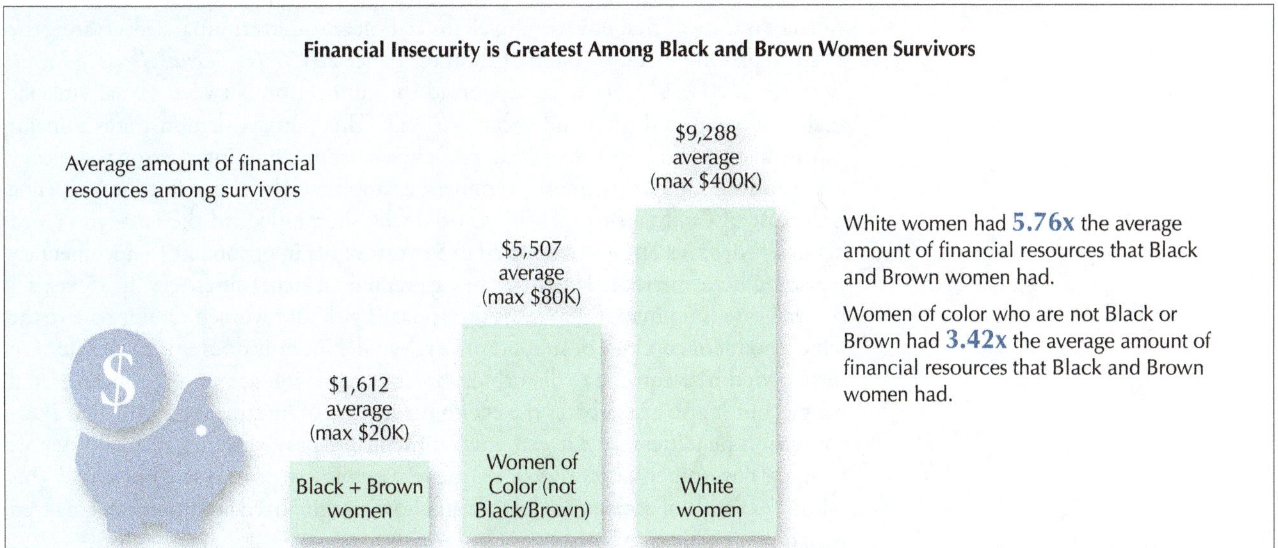

Figure 13-1

Despite the lifetime and systemic economic implications of interpersonal violence, most service providers focus on the immediate needs of the victim-survivor instead of using a holistic approach. For example, many victim advocates are trained to identify and support a client with financial abuse, which occurs in 99% of IPV cases.[8] They may offer short-term shelter stays, a one-time emergency grant, or financial literacy programs that ignore the reality and cyclical nature of poverty. They also ignore how victim-survivors are showing up to their services. As shown in **Figure 13-1**, White women on average have a significantly higher amount of financial resources than Black and Brown women. Therefore, a resource like a one-time emergency grant may do very little for a victim-survivor who is unable to afford their day-to-day basic necessities. It may even cause panic or stress to try and calculate the most effective use for a one-time grant when there are several other competing financial priorities. In recent years, with the attention to economic disparities coming to light due to COVID-19, there has been a slow paradigm shift across the anti-violence movement to focus on financial empowerment.[9] Initiatives have been created, like the AllState Foundation that provides victim-survivors and providers with financial education and tools, or the creation of FreeFrom, a nonprofit organization that works to support survivors' collective economic and community power and prioritize the financial safety and wellbeing of victim-survivors. Collectively, the focus is moving from an intervention lens to a prevention approach to truly achieve economic liberation for victim-survivors.

Historical Institutional Response to Economic Violence

Interpersonal Versus Institutional

Victim-survivors of interpersonal violence may experience economic implications directly from their harm-doer and from institutions. While the initial costs are a direct result of the harm-doer's violence, such as legal fees, moving fees, medical fees, etc, the compounding effects of these costs are typically due to institutions. For example, if a victim-survivor is not able to afford their medical costs upfront, they may incur substantial medical debt down the line. They may also face an increase in their insurance premiums due to pre-existing conditions, exorbitant credit card debt due to a lack of protected employment leave, or other debilitating costs exacerbated by a lack of or gap in federal policies that protect people's financial stability. This chapter uses the term "economic violence" as a reference to the institutional or systemic actions that cause economic hardship. A common instance of economic violence is the way that poverty and victimization are often criminalized, creating the abuse to prison pipeline.[10] Numerous studies since 2015's *The Sexual Abuse to Prison Pipeline: The Girls' Story* have supported the connection between sexual violence against women and girls and incarceration.[10] This pattern demonstrates a major gap in institutional and societal approaches to addressing interpersonal violence intervention. One of the most prominent examples of the abuse to prison pipeline is the case of Cyntoia Brown, a 16-year-old who shot and killed the man who raped her in self-defense. She was sentenced to 51 years of life in prison until a documentary capturing her experience led to her being granted clemency after serving 15 years.[10] Brown's case is unique in that most incarcerated girls and women do not receive the same amount of coverage or support once released. Not only does this pattern lead to further victimization due to disturbing rates of sexual violence amongst incarcerated people, but it also exacerbates the economic impact of interpersonal violence. Post-conviction penalties make it extremely difficult for previously incarcerated people to access governmental assistance, permanent employment, and safe housing.[11] This is just 1 example of economic violence and how marginalized communities are faced with disproportionate costs.

Policing's Role in Economic Violence

Financial support for victim-survivors is extremely limited and the resources that exist often require interacting with systems of policing. Crime victim compensation programs in each state throughout the United States provide funding to victim-survivors through fees and fines charged against those convicted of crime. Most programs require victim-survivors to report their experience to police and cooperate with police and prosecutors through the duration of any potential investigation or court case. This funding can be vital to those experiencing a loss of employment, large medical bills, and mental health treatment as the average maximum payout across the United States is $25 000.[12] However, reporting to and working with law enforcement can retraumatize victim-survivors and potentially lead to more harm. A 2021 law enforcement experience report conducted by The Hotline reports that 39% of victim-survivors surveyed felt less safe after contacting police. Out of those that contacted police, 55% shared they felt discriminated against in some way.[13] These barriers can be exasperated for those whose harm-doers are law enforcement. According to 2 studies from the 1990s by Johnson & Neidig, at least 40% of police officer families experience IPV. When victim-survivor help looks like a harm-doer's group of friends, filing a police report can be terrifying and lethal.[14] States such as Connecticut have removed the requirement of reporting to police in order to access their victim compensation program, allowing victim-survivors to work with a confidential advocate or mental health provider instead. For those in other states, the inability to work with law enforcement continues to prevent them from accessing critical emergency funding.

Offering victim-survivors the opportunity to work with confidential advocates instead of law enforcement can decrease significant barriers. However, advocates are not immune to the barriers created by systems of policing. Despite many advocates holding confidentiality that protects them from disclosing crimes to law enforcement, most are required to report instances of child or elder abuse. Fear of involving Child Protective Services (CPS) or Adult Protective Services (APS) can prevent victim-survivors from disclosing their experience and accessing crucial support, including emergency funding opportunities. Older adults and vulnerable people as determined by state statutes must decide whether to risk starting an investigation with APS and sharing their experience in order to access resources and support. CPS involvement in particular can be costly, in addition to traumatizing for the children and parent/victim-survivor. If CPS is notified of violence in the home, even if the violence occurred in the past and the children are now in a shelter, for example, they must still investigate. That investigation can turn into separating children from the victim-survivor, exorbitant legal fees, and, in the case of 1 particular example shared by the National Institute for Children's Health Quality, a loss of shelter and future employment.[15] Gloria's story, a case of a Black woman having her children removed from her care due to recreational marijuana usage and losing access to the shelter while avoiding a violent home, is not a standalone event. CPS impacts Black families at higher rates than White families, with over 50% of Black children experiencing a CPS investigation by 18 years old.[16] Thus, bringing attention to violence occurring in the home by working with an advocate or even a therapist can be an even greater risk for Black victim-survivors. While the national conversation on mandated reporting's impact on those most marginalized continues, it is essential for those serving victim-survivors to consider best approaches to remove as many barriers to accessing support as possible.

Generational Costs of Interpersonal Violence

The family and dependents of victim-survivors who cannot afford the enormous costs of violence and its impact are not immune from these economic implications. These costs become generational until someone can break the cycle. Predatory loans, overdraft fees, and compounding expenses from unaddressed physical health issues create unending cycles of poverty. Children growing up in low-income households often face an insurmountable financial barrier that bleeds into every aspect of their life. Children who grow up in poverty are less likely to have access to basic needs, as well as educational opportunities that allow them to grow their income. For those that are able to access higher education, they are often saddled with debt that can follow them through their life.[17] Ending the cycle of poverty is not about work ethic, but instead luck or community intervention. It is also generational due to the difficulty of getting out from the debilitating grip of poverty.

How Did it Get Here?

Interpersonal violence, sexual violence in particular, has been used as a tool to oppress marginalized people for far longer than federal regulations to support victim-survivors have been in place. In the United States, sexual violence was used as a tactic to control and traumatize enslaved African women and Indigenous women. Rape was originally considered a property crime against the male head of household. Many attribute the second wave feminist movement that birthed rape crisis centers as the origins of the anti-violence movement. While much of how the anti-violence movement exists today stems from the work of the second wave, anti-violence organizing in the United States began much earlier by Black women. In the 1860s, Frances Thompson, a Black trans woman, became a vocal anti-rape activist after the Memphis Massacre.[18] Ida B. Wells documented the lynchings of Black men and women in the South as well as the rape of Black women in the 1870s.[19] And in the 1940s, Rosa Parks led the investigation of the gang rape of Recy Taylor by a mob of White men. Taylor and Parks cofounded the Alabama Committee for Equal Justice that worked to reclaim Black women's bodies against sexual violence.[20] These accolades are often brushed over during conversations of the anti-violence movement. Instead, focus falls on the 1970s when one of the first rape crisis centers was founded in Washington and the first Take Back the Night rally was held.[21]

While documented organizing to address sexual violence in the United States goes back to the 1800s, it took the federal government until the 1980s to provide funding for the cause as well as domestic violence, with the Preventive Health and Health Services Block Grants.[22] From there, the Victims of Crime Act (VOCA) was passed by Congress in 1984 and uses federal criminal fines, fees, penalties, and special assessments to fund support services for victim-survivors of crime, not just interpersonal violence.[23] VOCA funding helps to cover finances for service organizations such as domestic violence shelters and rape crisis programs. It also helps cover state crime victim compensation programs, service grants, victim witness coordinators, Federal Bureau of Investigation victim specialists, the Federal Victim Notification System, and more.[23] Ten years later, in 1994, then Senator Joseph Biden passed legislation that is still aiding victim-survivors to this day through the Violence Against Women Act (VAWA). VAWA allows for service providers to receive more substantial financial support for the creation and continuation of services for victim-survivors, as well as rape prevention and education funding. Unlike VOCA, which broadly provides federal funding for all forms of violent crime, VAWA's sole focus is on domestic violence, sexual assault, dating violence, and stalking. By acknowledging domestic violence and sexual assault as crimes on a federal level, this legislation encouraged community-coordinated responses with collaboration of advocates, medical providers, courts, and law enforcement. Federal funding allowed services tied by a lack of funding the ability to prioritize anti-violence efforts.

Community-coordinated responses provided more streamlined services for victim-survivors and stronger referrals from one agency to the other. Rather than stumbling upon each resource by chance, victim-survivors were able to receive information on their options whether they went to the hospital first, law enforcement, a rape crisis program, or shelter. Funding was also provided to services that focused on underserved populations such as Indigenous victim-survivors. This increase in funding also allowed services to expand and support an increasing number of victim-survivors.[24]

Since 1994, VAWA has been reauthorized 4 times, in 2000, 2005, 2013, and 2022. Each reauthorization has expanded the foundation of the 1994 act to provide more services, include more victim-survivors, and enhance protections for victim-survivors of marginalized identities. Agencies across the country are able to apply annually for VOCA and VAWA grants to help expand their services such as obtaining space to provide shelter to families, cover expenses for rape kits, or implement 24/7 crisis hotline services. The 2000 reauthorization of VAWA specifically focused on creating legal assistance programs for victim-survivors. Legal assistance grant funds could be used for adding a court advocate to an agency's staff, a trainer to facilitate vital educational workshops and training to courts and law enforcement on the needs of victim-survivors, or legal representation for victim-survivors in need of immigration status support.[25] Essentially, this funding decreased barriers for victim-survivors to accessing vital resources they may not have been able to afford on their own or incurred significant financial duress in accessing. Most recently, in 2022, the VAWA reauthorization under President Joseph Biden increased services for marginalized communities, in particular LGBTQIA+ victim-survivors, by prioritizing culturally specific services in funding applications.[25] In many ways, these funds have been crucial to the anti-violence movement; however, gaps still remain.

According to the National Network to End Domestic Violence's (NNEDV) 17th annual report, the Crime Victims Fund, which is funded by criminal fees and fines, has significantly decreased, impacting the VOCA funds.[26] At the same time, demand for services has increased, which places anti-violence agencies in an impossible spot of doing more with less. On one day in 2022, 30% of emergency shelter requests, 20% of transitional or other housing, 3% of hotel stays, and 47% of non-residential supportive services went unmet in the United States.[26] These unmet requests create a compounding effect on each victim-survivor's physical, emotional, and financial safety.

For more than 20 years, IPV and sexual violence service providers have received direct funding from the federal government. With the exception of VOCA's victim of crime compensation programs, most of this money has not been directed into the pockets of victim-survivors, despite their need for lifetime financial support. For services that do attempt to redirect funding into the hands of victim-survivors, they often face mounds of red tape. VOCA's allowables and disallowables for expenses are incredibly specific and highly limited, based on the government's perspective of what is permissive. Repairing damage committed by an abuser is a common need of victim-survivors.[27] However, VOCA will not cover replacements or repairs unless to ensure safety, forcing victim-survivors to access victims of crime compensation,[14] which may require a police report, which creates an additional barrier that some victim-survivors are not able to maneuver. These regulations create a dynamic of mistrust with victim-survivors, ensuring that every cost is approved by the agency and grantors. For example, grantees must create a credit or charge procedure with vendors or provide a gift card in limited situations. Gift card usage must be tracked by the agency and they must ensure it is used for authorized purposes only.[27] Strict monitoring of spending is a common tactic in IPV relationships and thus, the replication of this in VOCA funding can make it difficult for victim-survivors to request funds in addition to the limitations of what they may use the funds on. Requiring victim-survivors to provide documentation of reporting an assault, being over the age of 18, having an ID available in order to cash a check, and receiving notifications of bank activity that may be intercepted by their harm-doer, are all additional barriers to accessing financial safety.

In order to create a relationship of trust with victim-survivors and provide sustainable and flexible funding for financial wellbeing, agencies are often forced to utilize alternative funding such as donations or fundraising. While this can create a flexible spending account to cover short-term and long-term needs unmet by federal and state grants, it can require a lot of time and energy to maintain. Rural agencies or those competing with similar services nearby may find it difficult to obtain or sustain donations or fundraising efforts. Decreasing the number of barriers to receiving access to emergency funds through grants such as VOCA increases victim-survivors' financial safety, empowers agencies to build trusting relationships with the community they serve, and creates more time and energy for service providers to focus on a multitude of other urgent needs.

Best Practices: Empowerment-Based Approach

In recent years, terms such as "trauma-informed," "person-centered," and "empowerment-based" have picked up momentum in the social services world. Ultimately, these terms share a common purpose of centering victim-survivors as the experts of their own experiences and working to remove systemic and individual barriers to create safe and holistic opportunities.[28] Empowerment-based approaches lead to trust-building, allowing service providers to gather more information and create safety plans that are unique and specific to each client. Ripple effects of interpersonal violence are shown to decrease when the relationship between victim-survivor and service provider is one of strong alliance.[29] Financial support that requires proof of purchase or refuses to disburse money directly into the hands of victim-survivors can be interpreted as telling victim-survivors that they cannot be trusted with money or are incapable of making smart decisions. As 1 participant of FreeFrom's safety fund shared, "Receiving a grant [from FreeFrom] no questions asked was like being looked at and received by people who trusted me unconditionally. That's extremely important for a survivor who has often been shamed, had to deal with people gaslighting and creating false stories about their integrity and believability."[30] Too often, the harmful dynamics that service providers work to help victim-survivors dismantle (eg, distrust, controlling of finances, etc) are foundationally embedded into service provider practices through regulations, policies, and procedures. Restrictions on who can apply for funding, how much, what it can be used on, and documentation of usage can all create distrust between victim-survivors and service providers. A report on economic empowerment and career counseling highlighted this distrust in one of the survivors' interviews. When asked to reflect on their experience with a public assistance welfare-to-work program, the survivor shared that it was disempowering and felt abusive and coercive.[31] Providing victim-survivors with cash that they can use without an agency or organization tracking how they spend it or limiting what they can purchase and when helps to establish a relationship of trust. Another finding from the FreeFrom Safety Fund analysis reports that 73% of their participants identified cash without restrictions as their number one need.[32] An empowerment-based approach means trusting victim-survivors and empowering them with financial literacy, emergency funding, and support while following their lead. One method of disbursing cash directly to victim-survivors is implementing an emergency fund.

The Care Survivor Fund

The Care Survivor Fund was created in 2015 at the University of Nevada, Las Vegas (UNLV) through a collaboration between a registered student organization, The Care Advocates, and a campus department called the Care Center. Originally created with and sustained by community donations and fundraisers, the emergency fund expanded with a yearly stipend from UNLV's student government. Clients seen by the Care Center, limited to those who are active students, can apply for an emergency grant of up to $1000. Funds are disbursed virtually into the client's bank account or via check if needed. There are no receipts required, and clients are only asked to work with an advocate to address immediate safety concerns and identify both current and future short-term uncovered costs before submitting an application. Students impacted by interpersonal violence may apply to the fund multiple times up until they receive $1000. They may also re-apply (even if they have previously received the full amount of funds) if they experience interpersonal violence again in the future. Once the application has been submitted and reviewed by the registered student organization board and 1 full-time staff member, in a timeline of less than 72 business hours, the funds can be disbursed immediately via Zelle (ie, an online cash transfer app).[33] Clients are asked to check off what general needs their emergency funding request falls under in order to identify trends and

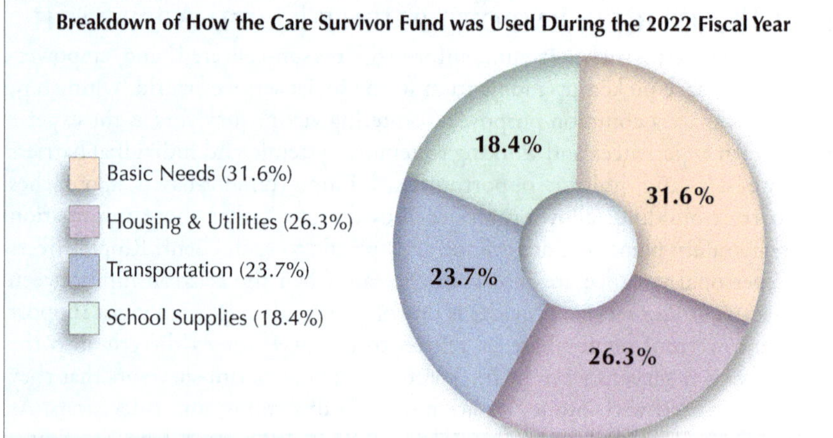

Figure 13-2

Figure 13-2. Breakdown of how the Care Survivor Fund was used during the 2022 fiscal year.[33]

advocate for systemic change, such as emergency campus housing. As seen in **Figure 13-2**, the data collected from clients accessing The Care Survivor Fund demonstrates the general financial needs covered by the fund. 31.6% of clients stated that they utilized the emergency funds for basic needs. This category is purposely broad in order to honor clients' privacy. However, this data correlates with other similar data such as the FreeFrom Safety Fund analysis that shows participants noting essentials as their top need.[32]

This fund is unique in the anti-violence movement and amongst other advocacy programs.

Creating an Emergency Fund

Campus and community organizations may decide that implementing an emergency fund or cash assistance program is a feasible and pertinent project. In order to establish a successful emergency fund, organizations should consider the importance of funding, applications, disbursements, and tracking and reporting processes in their advocacy for financial support for victim-survivors.

Funding

In the UNLV Care Center's case, they had the advantage of accessing a reliable funder with limited restrictions. Other campus or community organizations may face hurdles to identifying funding sources that provide the quantity necessary with few strings attached. Some possible funding sources identified by the National Alliance for Safe Housing include a private sponsor such as a foundation, charity, business, or community fundraising plan that focuses on long-term and sustainable success, or creatively utilizing local, state, or federal funding.[34] Building and maintaining a relationship with a funder and tracking budgeting needs can require a lot of time and energy. Hiring an additional staff member to prioritize funding can help ensure it does not fall through the cracks, funds are accurately documented, and gaps in funding are avoided.

Obtaining support from victim-survivors, partner agencies, volunteers, staff, etc through letters, petitions, or reports may help encourage funders to participate. It may also be beneficial to gather data on current services provided, unmet needs, and national data, such as from the Cost of Intimate Partner Violence report by the International Center for Research on Women.[35] Agencies should also consult the Internal Revenue Service (IRS) and their legal consults if available to ensure the funding follows important tax requirements while ensuring confidentiality.[36] If using grant funds to implement an emergency fund, agencies may contact their grantor for additional guidance.

Application Process

The application process for the emergency fund should have low-barrier access, swift dissemination of funds, flexibility, and include victim-survivor-led safety planning with support of an advocate. Restrictions on who can apply, how to apply, and documentation to apply all create barriers that impact marginalized victim-survivors.[34] Creating a short application that can be completed in-person or virtually allows victim-survivors with disabilities, transportation barriers, and more to access this vital service. Removing requirements of evidence or documentation of interpersonal violence and restrictions based on when the violence happened opens the fund to victim-survivors who are unable to safely access police reports and reiterates that the organization believes survivors.[30] Creating an efficient and quick application and disbursement process also allows victim-survivors to avoid compounding interest or debt, which can lead to evictions, loss of a vehicle, course removal for students, and more. Agencies can use research to identify the needs and timelines of the population they serve; however, 24 to 48 hours may be an effective start. In addition to the application form, service providers should work collaboratively with the victim-survivor to identify and address financial and physical safety concerns. Receiving funds may pose a threat to victim-survivors if intercepted by their harm-doer. Using funds for situations like leaving a violent relationship or moving out of a job where they are being sexually harassed could escalate violence and increase risk of lethality.

While victim-survivors should not be forced to create a plan, it is essential that service providers offer to review safety concerns and create a holistic safety plan that addresses the unique needs of the victim-survivor.[37] For guidance on creating safety plans, service providers should connect with appropriate technical assistance contacts such as the National Network to End Domestic Violence[38] and the National Sexual Violence Resource Center.[39] Finally, requirements on how victim-survivors can utilize the funds should be limited or nonexistent. Questions about the general categories of how the funds were spent may be collected for grant or funding purposes but should be explicitly optional. Information gathered from applicants should be limited to confirming a safe method of disbursement, amount needed, contact information for safety, acknowledgement that these funds are for victim-survivors of interpersonal violence, and optional demographic data.

Disbursement

Due to safety concerns, disbursement of funds should be flexible with a variety of options. For example, in the FreeFrom Trust Survivor's report, participants provided differing responses to the safest methods of applying for and receiving funds. The top choice was through federal governments like stimulus payments, which typically are deposited directly into a bank account or mailed. The second choice was bank or credit union despite many participants sharing that banks posed a number of access and safety barriers. Victim-survivors who are homeless, have a harm-doer who monitors their bank activity, lack transportation, etc may not be able to utilize a bank to receive funding. Therefore, providing funds only through cash or checks can create barriers. Direct deposits, such as with Venmo or Paypal, can be more accessible for those who cannot physically make it to the bank but still require some kind of bank account.[30] Providing multiple options that victim-survivors can choose from based on their access and safety needs breaks down unnecessary barriers and enhances the impact of an emergency fund.

Tracking and Reporting

Sustaining funds typically requires accurate tracking and reporting of incoming funds and disbursements. When working with victim-survivors, confidentiality obligates agencies to maintain the anonymity of their clients. It is essential that agencies convey this need to funders upfront to ensure that they are able to provide redacted documentation in order to continue to receive funding. Information such as the amount of funding provided per client, demographic information, needs that went unmet, etc will help meet requirements of funders but also provide helpful data for strategizing enhancements to the fund or services in general, and encouraging future funders to participate.

While emergency funds can be a powerful tool for economic empowerment of victim-survivors, it is not without its shortfalls. Despite their innovative efforts, many clients of The Care Center were left with continued financial emergencies that could not be addressed by a one-time grant of only $1000. For example, a client who had lost their regular income due to the shutdown associated with COVID-19 needed funds for re-housing due to experiencing interpersonal violence in their dorm room. In addition, their car was in jeopardy of being repossessed, they had medical and psychological appointments required for chronic issues associated with childhood trauma, and academic costs that were tied to their housing. Even with other community funds and a coordinated campus response, the financial needs of this client were too extensive for the limited capacity of all agencies and organizations involved. In FreeFrom's 2020 Survivors Know Best report, survey participants shared that on average, they needed $730 to stay safe.[30] This estimate does not include additional support services nor does it include a timeframe. Meaning, victim-survivors may need $730 to access safety immediately but long-term safety and financial security likely requires a much higher number. Unfortunately, a one-time emergency fund, budgeting, and financial safety planning cannot replace systemic economic oppression.

Victim-survivors are often faced with the decision of what basic necessity they should use their emergency funds to cover and what necessities they may need to go without.

Better Practices: Economic Empowerment

Similar to approaches to service provisions, economic empowerment services should be holistic and expand beyond 1 resource. Service providers and their agencies should consider implementing a multi-pronged approach to supporting victim-survivor's immediate and long-term financial wellbeing.

Employment Support

Employment attainment is a key aspect of economic empowerment for victim-survivors. Safe and sustainable employment ensures that victim-survivors have access to steady income to help cover current and long-term financial needs. Health insurance, paid time off, and investment opportunities that come with employment can help victim-survivors build wealth, navigate difficult processes like court, and access medical and mental health care.[31] When victim-survivors have access to a living wage, health benefits, time-off, and flexible schedules, they are less likely to encounter serious credit card debt, long-term physical and mental health issues or at least the medical debt associated with the inability to pay those costs upfront, and unsafe or unstable housing. Livable wages also empower people with options. While there are many reasons someone may stay in an abusive relationship, stable income not tied to their harm-doer breaks down a multitude of barriers to leaving.[31] Additionally, for victim-survivors who are employed, they may be in need of workplace accommodations or legal options to address harassment at work.

Employment advocacy is a form of advocacy that supports victim-survivors in exploring their employment needs in a holistic way. Advocates and other service providers working directly with victim-survivors can open the conversation around employment needs and work collaboratively to create an action plan. Researching the rights of employees, specifically victim-survivors of interpersonal violence, and having that information easily accessible is one way to implement employment advocacy. Building relationships with legal resources and attorneys to refer victim-survivors for pro bono services is another example of employee advocacy.[40] Warm referrals to important resources helps reduce barriers and create a more trauma-informed experience.[41] Another warm referral process could include career-ready services, community colleges for certification or training opportunities, and other job prep resources. These resources should include options that address the specific needs of victim-survivors who have been incarcerated, are undocumented, or are at other intersections of marginalization. Advocates may also engage in mock interviews or help hold resume workshops to provide victim-survivors with a trauma-informed space to practice their skills.

College campuses often have career services that could provide training on current interview and resume skills in exchange for a workshop on supporting victim-survivors. Lastly, accompanying victim-survivors either physically or virtually to meetings with their employer or contacting their employer on their behalf is another option for employment advocacy. Addressing safety needs and workplace concerns as a victim-survivor may be overwhelming; advocates can help reduce some of that stress by showing up with or for their clients.[41]

Housing Support

IPV and sexual assault are some of the leading causes of homelessness.[42] Fleeing violent homes and navigating ruined credit can force victim-survivors out of stable housing.

Victim-survivors also experience housing discrimination by landlords who evict them due to tenant complaints or property damage caused by their harm-doer.[42] A lack of safe and stable housing can cause cyclical financial insecurity due to impacts such as disruptive schedules that make it difficult to attend work on time, inability to apply for assistance due to a lack of permanent address, etc. Emergency shelters can provide immediate safety for victim-survivors and their children. However, shelters can have many restrictions that prevent LGBTQIA+ and male victim-survivors, sex workers, those using substances, and disabled victim-survivors from using their services. In the National Network to End Domestic Violence's 2022 Domestic Violence Counts report, of the 9 444 domestic violence services unmet requests, 33% were emergency shelter.[43] For those who successfully accessed emergency shelter, permanent housing is not always the outcome.

According to a 2019 study, approximately 75% of those who utilized domestic violence emergency shelters left without housing in place.[43] Research like this has encouraged many organizations to implement the Domestic Violence Housing First (DVHF) model. The DVHF focuses on working collaboratively with victim-survivors in obtaining safe and stable housing. This may include immediate emergency shelter for safety concerns before identifying more permanent housing. Signing a new lease is often only a small component of a victim-survivor's needs when it comes to safe and stable housing. Ensuring that the housing location is safe, the landlord is supportive of victim-survivors, and providing consistent flexible funding to avoid missing payments are all essential components of the DVHF model.[44] The Washington State Coalition Against Domestic Violence launched a 5-year pilot project for DVHF in 2010. They provide a toolkit for organizations to implement their own DVHF that includes 7 components: Preparing your Organization, Implementing Survivor-Driven, Trauma-Informed Advocacy, Implementing Mobile Advocacy, Implementing Flexible Financial Assistance, Implementing Community Engagement, Evaluating and Revising, and Sustaining.[45] Agencies that serve victim-survivors should review this toolkit and connect with other DVHF programs for guidance. Additional programs using this model are Violence Free Colorado, The California Office of Emergency Services, The Minnesota Coalition for Battered Women, and The District Alliance for Safe Housing.[34]

Starting Over: Repairing and Building Credit

Coerced debt and credit damage are common instances of financial abuse for victim-survivors of IPV.[46] Harm-doers may overuse credit cards, hide missed payments, or coerce victim-survivors into taking out loans, which create a significant financial barrier to leaving.

According to a Financial Abuse Fact Sheet by NNEDV, 50% of sexual assault victim-survivors either voluntarily left their jobs or had their employment terminated.[47] As discussed in previous sections, loss of employment can lead to compounding financial issues such as accumulating debt and credit damage. These issues can prevent victim-survivors from securing permanent housing, pursuing or completing academic degrees or certifications, starting a business, or even landing a new job.[48] Even when victim-survivors are physically or emotionally able to begin their healing journey after leaving an abusive relationship, which is not always possible, or recovering from sexual assault, they are often unable to start from scratch. Instead, debilitating debt and low credit scores put them behind.

Service providers are in a powerful position to provide resources and support to victim-survivors on repairing and building credit and tackling debt. However, not all service providers are experts or even comfortable in financial literacy. The AllState Foundation's Moving Forward Curriculum is an important tool to help educate service providers and victim-survivors on financial abuse and how to address it. There is a section on mastering credit basics, which may be a helpful start to understanding credit, debt, and how to improve scores. Once a plan is in place and needs are identified, service providers may need to connect the victim-survivors to additional resources.

Victim-survivors may need legal help to dispute charges or credit report activity, file bankruptcy, or file a lawsuit. As of 2010, WomensLaw.org is a project of NNEDV that provides legal information for victims of abuse with a page dedicated to financial abuse.[49] The website also highlights the Identity Theft Resource Center[50] and the National Foundation for Credit Counseling[51] as additional resources for victim-survivors. Regardless of one's position, FreeFrom's Before and Beyond Crisis report documents ways different organizations and institutions can support victim-survivors in maintaining financial safety and repairing their credit.[52] Service providers who work directly with victim-survivors may utilize this tool to encourage local and national organizations to implement change. Ultimately, obtaining education on debt and credit repair, identifying and creating referral processes with resources that can support victim-survivors with debt and credit repair, and educating community and national agencies on how to support the financial safety of victim-survivors are all ways a service provider can address debt and credit damage for their clients.

Building Wealth: Savings and Banking

Once the damage and immediate financial needs of the victim-survivor have been assessed and a plan has been implemented, the focus can shift from survival mode to thriving. As economic implications can last lifetimes, it is essential for victim-survivors to receive support in building their wealth. Creating and expanding savings and providing opportunities for sustainable income provide protective factors against violence.[53] It is important to note that regardless of one's savings, financial planning, or budgeting, violence and harm can still occur. These steps and tools are meant to empower victim-survivors and provide them with options to make informed decisions. It is never a victim-survivor's fault when they experience interpersonal violence, and events such as lay-offs, recessions, and inflation are beyond the control of individuals. Creating budgets, identifying creative ways to grow income, starting a business, investing, and maximizing employee benefits are all ways to build wealth. One approach to building wealth that anti-violence agencies have taken is the use of micro-loans. These small loans, the amount of which is dependent on the source, are given to victim-survivors after meeting with an advocate and determining that a micro-loan could be an effective way to rebuild their credit. The goal is to use small investments to ensure payments are met, and the disbursement of the loan through an anti-violence agency helps those with low credit scores. Coalitions such as NNEDV with the Independence Project[54] and the Nevada Coalition to End Domestic and Sexual Violence with the LIFE microloan[55] have utilized micro-lending. As of Spring 2023, however, neither program is active.

While micro-loans can be effective for some victim-survivors if they are able to maintain the payments, studies suggest that micro-lending may not prove as effective in the United States as it is in other countries. Starting a business in the United States can be extremely difficult and small loans can be less impactful due to rising costs of living.[56] Instead, supporting victim-survivors in obtaining stable employment, degrees, and certifications can ensure more permanent financial stability. From there, service providers may work with victim-survivors to create budgets, open saving accounts, review loan options, connect with a financial planner, and review investment options. NNEDV's Moving Ahead Curriculum also provides a breakdown of why and how to engage in all of the above.[57] A less common approach, identified in FreeFrom's Beyond Crisis report, encourages hiring victim-survivors at a living wage. Nonprofits in particular that work with victim-survivors often have victim-survivors on their staff. Those in leadership can implement best practices for supporting victim-survivors into their own workplace policies, including equitable pay, investment opportunities, and more.[52]

A Macro-Approach: Systems Advocacy

Economic empowerment must occur on a macro level in order to be felt by all victim-survivors. A single service provider or organization prioritizing economic empowerment still leaves countless victim-survivors at the hands of economic violence. While many service providers and nonprofits either do not have the bandwidth for policy support or are prevented from engaging in it, systems advocacy is essential to economic empowerment. Many of the steps and tools listed before, while powerful, are only a bandage to core issues that must be addressed by federal policy.

Systems advocacy focuses on the root of an issue and requires challenging systemic norms. For example, testifying at a legislative hearing in support of a bill to protect victim-survivors is a form of systems advocacy.[58] Despite barriers to engaging in systems advocacy, service providers and organizations can get creative in the ways they support policy change. Collecting ethical data and creating a report identifying the trending needs and gaps of service for victim-survivors is one way to empower legislators to make informed decisions. NNEDV has a list of economic justice policies that impact victim-survivors most, which service providers and organizations can utilize to stay informed and engage in action.[59] Adding a policy person to the team or building relationships with change organizations in the community are options to stay involved in decisions that have deeply profound impacts, especially on the most marginalized victim-survivors. Centering victim-survivors in these decisions is at the core of the anti-violence movement; therefore, they should have access to impacting policy change. Women Against Abuse facilitates programs to get victim-survivors involved through letter-writing campaigns, inviting survivor representatives to legislative meetings, and an advocacy committee that develops a policy agenda.[60] Professionals should reflect on the ways their organization engages in policy work, and ask questions such as: What education or data collected could help inform local and federal policy? How can local organizations empower victim-survivors to be involved in systems advocacy? As Bell Hooks suggests, "the personal is political."[61] How are professionals, as individuals, engaging in systems advocacy in the movement for economic empowerment?

Holistic Approach to Survivor Support

While service providers are encouraged to reflect on these approaches, it is essential to acknowledge that every victim-survivor is unique and their situation should be approached accordingly. Studies show that marginalized victim-survivors, particularly Black, Brown, trans, and disabled victim-survivors, experience significant economic impact from interpersonal violence.[32] Agencies need to consider the barriers the communities they serve may experience when accessing their services and the referrals they make. A holistic approach to advocacy requires service providers to assess all safety needs of clients while collaborating to create unique plans to address those needs. Potential barriers to accessing safety should be discussed, and alternative options should be provided. To understand how service providers can holistically address the safety needs of victim-survivors, consider starting with the Power and Control Wheel.[62]

This tool helps break down the tactics harm-doers utilize to maintain power and control over a victim-survivor(s).[62] These tactics may also be present in sexual assault and stalking cases outside of IPV. A holistic approach addresses the impacts of all of these tactics and the aspects of the victim-survivor's life. **Figure 13-3** below is an example of areas service providers can explore with their clients.

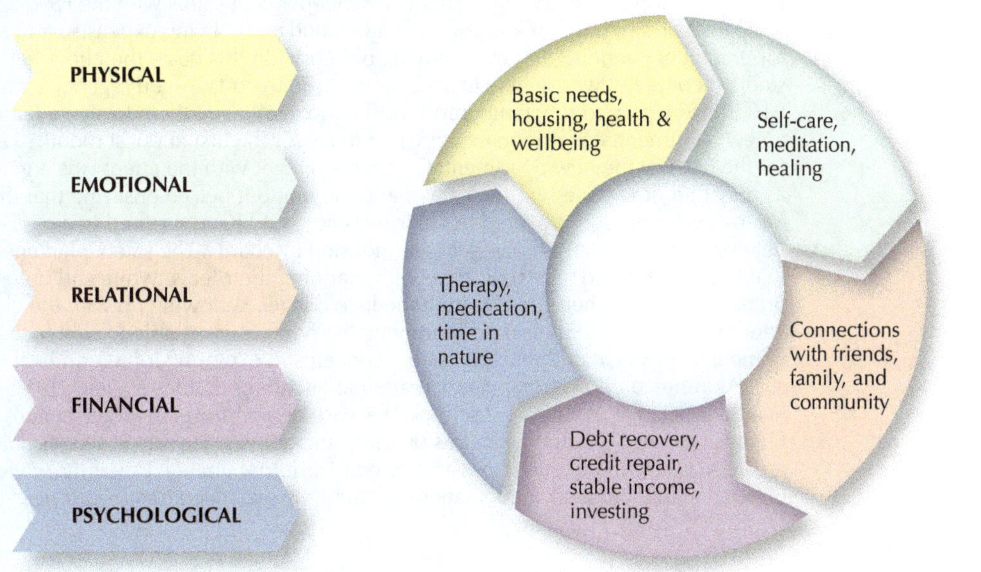

Figure 13-3. *Safety needs.*

Case Study

Case Study 13-1

At the UNLV Care Center, staff and interns primarily serve college-age clients impacted by interpersonal violence. One of the most common cases they deal with is family violence (ie, violence committed by parents or guardians of adult children). An advocate conducted an intake with a student-client who shared that their parents were physically and emotionally abusive: controlling who they talked to, where they went, and using physical violence or verbal harassment when the client tried to set boundaries. The client worked full-time on top of a full load of classes so they could maintain a scholarship and help support their family financially, including their siblings. Their parents were unable to work sustainable jobs due to their immigration status and often used that to guilt the client into overworking and taking out additional loans. On one hand, the client was committed to supporting their family and was happy to help ensure the safety and wellbeing of their siblings. On the other hand, the client was concerned for their mental wellbeing, financial security, and physical safety. The client and advocate worked on ways to save money in a separate bank account and safety plan for if the physical violence escalated. Though the client was emotionally and financially ready to move out, their parents had hidden their personal documents, making it incredibly difficult for the client to sign a lease or apply for student loans. Due to fear of deportation, the client was not able to utilize police assistance for obtaining their documents or filing for a protective order. As the advocate worked with the client over several weeks, it became clear that action was needed to avoid the client completely burning out physically and mentally.

Discussion

While many of the barriers this client faced are similar to those found in IPV between partners or spouses, the need to support one's parents and family financially adds layers of complexity. Often, college-age students need to at least communicate with their parents/guardians in order to apply for financial aid. When communication is a safety risk, students must navigate the messy process of filing for independent status with the Federal Student Aid (FSA) office.[63] In this case, the advocate needs to address the physical, mental, and financial safety of the client. Physical safety is always a priority as it has the most immediate impact on the client. However, decisions that have negative financial implications can create a lifetime cycle of debt or financial insecurity for the client. After assessing physical safety and implementing a plan, the advocate should identify the client's immediate and long-term financial needs. This should include a plan to safely access personal documentation or obtain copies, apply for independent status with the FSA, open a separate and secure bank account, create a budget for living expenses, and apply for emergency funding to cover moving out costs. In this case, the client had a stable income but was unable to save for immediate costs. An emergency grant of $1000 and a plan to stay temporarily with a friend allowed them to sign a lease on a new apartment, cover food expenses, and pay for the first and last month's rent for the lease at the new apartment. Creating a budget with the client was crucial as they had never lived on their own, and moving out before ensuring that their basic needs could be covered by their income could have resulted in a decision between returning home to violence or housing insecurity. The safety plan ensured that the client could take their time with planning their leave while still being prepared to flee if their life was in immediate danger. Following up with the client after they settled into their new apartment, the advocate was able to shift focus from immediate physical and financial safety concerns to exploring long-term healing opportunities such as therapy and academic accommodations to help create a healthier balance of work and school. This case demonstrates the intersections of financial safety with all other forms of safety. In addition, the advocate was able to create a plan with the client that addressed their future financial security, while also understanding that their immediate physical safety may need to take priority.

Summary

After reading this chapter, professionals should consider how they as individuals are currently addressing the economic implications of interpersonal violence. How can they utilize their positionality to leverage improvements at an organizational, community, or federal level? Consider the barriers organizations may unknowingly perpetuate in their service requirements. If none come to mind, identify organizations or resources in the community that serve marginalized populations. Build relationships of trust with these organizations, offering support when appropriate and requesting feedback and guidance on potential gap areas. The more relationships an organization builds, the larger of an ecosystem of safety they can provide to victim-survivors. Organization and agency leaders should reflect on internal policies and procedures and consider how they align with their mission. Are they supporting the financial safety of their staff with equitable pay, protected leave for interpersonal violence, and opportunities for building wealth? What relationships do they have with systems of policing, and have they analyzed that impact on who they serve and who they do not? Finally, in order to truly address the economic implications of interpersonal violence, change must occur on a macro level. What policy changes can individuals or organizations engage in to impact the economic wellbeing of victim-survivors? Economic liberation requires everyone to participate and ensure that the needs of those most marginalized are not only addressed but centered.

Additional Resources

Table 13-1. Additional Resources

Organization	Description	Website
FreeFrom	Federal policy recommendation that prioritizes financial security for victims/survivors	https://www.freefrom.org/2021/01/12/2021-1-11-announcing-our-2021-federal-policy-recommendations/
	Prioritizing financial security in the movement to end interpersonal violence: a roadmap	https://www.freefrom.org/wpcontent/uploads/2021/07/Prioritizing_Financial_Security_Report.pdf
Pennsylvania Coalition Against Domestic Violence	Economic Justice Initiative	https://www.pcadv.org/initiatives/economic-justice/
		https://www.pcadv.org/wp-content/uploads/Economic-Justice-One-Sheeter.pdf
WomensLaw.org	Legal information and support for victim-survivors of interpersonal violence	https://www.womenslaw.org/
New York Coalition Against Sexual Assault	Reimagining VAWA: why criminalization is a failed policy and what a non-carceral VAWA could look like	https://nyscasa.org/wp-content/uploads/2020/09/VAW-Crim-as-failed-policy-1.pdf
NNEDV/AllState Foundation	Financial Empowerment course for victim-survivors and advocates	https://allstatefoundation.org/wp-content/uploads/2020/03/Moving-Ahead-Curriculum_-All_-English.pdf
	Compensation for advocates	https://nnedv.org/wp-content/uploads/2023/04/DV-EJ-Advisory-Council-2023-Recommendations-FINAL.pdf
	Fundraising event toolkit for nonprofits	https://nnedv.org/wp-content/uploads/2021/09/Coalition-Partners-Events-Toolkit-2021 external Final_9.15.2021.pdf
University of Buffalo	Holistic self-care assessment	https://socialwork.buffalo.edu/content/dam/socialwork/home/self-care-kit/self-care-assessment.pdf

References

1. Jean-Charles RM. Toward a victim-survivor narrative: rape and form in Yvonne Vera's Under the Tongue and Calixthe Beyala's Tu t'appelleras Tanga. *Research in African Literatures*. 2014;45(1):39-62. doi:10.2979/reseafrilite.45.1.39

2. Peterson C, Kearns MC, McIntosh WL, et al. Lifetime economic burden of intimate partner violence among US adults. *Am J Prev Med*. 2018;55(4):433-444. doi:10.1016/j.amepre.2018.04.049

3. McLean G, Bocinski SG. The economic cost of intimate partner violence, sexual assault, and stalking. Institute for Women's Policy Research. 2020. Accessed October 3, 2023. https://iwpr.org/the-economic-cost-of-intimate-partner-violence-sexual-assault-and-stalking/

4. Uvelli A, Duranti C, Salvo G, Coluccia A, Gualtieri G, Ferretti F. The risk factors of chronic pain in victims of violence: a scoping review. *Healthcare (Basel).* 2023;11(17):2421. doi:10.3390/healthcare11172421

5. Breiding MJ, Basile KC, Klevens J, Smith SG. Economic insecurity and intimate partner and sexual violence victimization. *Am J Prev Med.* 2017;53(4):457-464. doi:10.1016/j.amepre.2017.03.021

6. Protective factors for intimate partner violence perpetration. Centers for Disease Control and Prevention. 2021. Accessed February 7, 2023. https://www.cdc.gov/violenceprevention/intimatepartnerviolence/riskprotective-factors.html

7. Hulley J, Bailey L, Kirkman G, et al. Intimate partner violence and barriers to help-seeking among Black, Asian, minority ethnic and immigrant women: a qualitative metasynthesis of global research. *Trauma Violence Abuse.* 2023; 24(2):1001-1015. doi:10.1177/15248380211050590

8. Doyle K, Guerra P, Passi S. Prioritizing financial security in the movement to end IPV: a roadmap. FreeFrom. July 13, 2021. https://bit.ly/PFS-report

9. Pappas S. Fighting inequity in the face of COVID-19. American Psychological Association. 2020. Accessed October 3, 2023. https://www.apa.org/monitor/2020/ 06/covid-fighting-inequity

10. Vafa Y, Epstein R. Criminalized survivors: today's abuse to prison pipeline for girls. Rights4Girls. 2023. https://rights4girls.org/wp-content/uploads/2023/04/Criminalized-Survivors_Todays-Abuse-to-Prison-Pipeline.pdf

11. Coordination to reduce barriers to reentry: lessons learned from COVID-19 and beyond. US Department of Justice. 2022. Accessed October 3, 2023. https://www.justice.gov/opa/press-release/file/1497911/download

12. Victim compensation: an overview. National Association of Crime Victims Compensation Boards. 2021. Accessed October 3, 2023. https://nacvcb.org/victim-compensation/

13. Goodmark L, Cook M. Law enforcement experience report - domestic violence survivors' survey regarding interaction with law enforcement. National Domestic Violence Hotline. 2021. Accessed October 3, 2023. https://www.thehotline.org/wp-content/uploads/media/2022/09/2209-Hotline-LES_FINAL.pdf

14. Goodmark L. Who watches the watchers: domestic violence and law enforcement. National Sexual Violence Resource Center. 2023. Accessed July 20, 2023. https://www.nsvrc.org/blogs/saam/who-watches-watchers-domestic-violence-and-law-enforcement-leigh-goodmark

15. Our systems meant to help are hurting black families. NICHQ. 2018. Accessed October 3, 2023. https://nichq.org/insight/our-systems-meant-help-are-hurting-black-families

16. Thomas MMC, Waldfogel J, Williams OF. Inequities in child protective services contact between Black and White children. *Child Maltreat.* 2023; 28(1):42-54. doi:10.1177/10775595211070248

17. New indicators report shows escalating disparities for poor students, students of color [Press release]. University of Pennsylvania Graduate School of Education. 2022. https://www.gse.upenn.edu/news/press-releases/new-indicators-report-show-escalating-disparities-poor-students-students-color

18. Lhant V. HRC honors Frances Thompson, a black transgender hero. Human Rights Campaign. 2021. Accessed October 3, 2023. https://www.hrc.org/news/hrc-honors-frances-thompson-a-black-transgender-hero

19. McShane J. Ida B. Wells called for anti-lynching legislation more than a century ago. Now it's finally law. NBC News. 2022. Accessed July 20, 2023. https://www.nbcnews.com/news/nbcblk/ida-b-wells-pushed-7-presidents-pass-anti-lynching-legislation-now-s-f-rcna23596.38

20. Hunter B. Film detailing Rosa Parks' role in the 1944 Recy Taylor gang rape case debuts in Detroit. Michigan Chronicle. 2019. https://michiganchronicle.com/2019/10/28/film-detailing-rosa-parks-role-in-the-1944-recy-taylor-gang-rape-case-debuts-in-detroit/

21. Friedman D, Lenaerts S, NkengeToure. DC Rape Crisis Center (DCRCC) – early history. DCRCC. 2019. Accessed July 20, 2023. https://www.dcrcc.org/our_history

22. About the PHHS Block Grant Program. Centers for Disease Control and Prevention. 2019. Accessed October 3, 2023. https://www.cdc.gov/phhsblockgrant/about.htm

23. Victims of crime act (VOCA). National Domestic Violence Hotline. 2020. Accessed October 3, 2023. https://www.thehotline.org/resources/victims-of-crime-act-voca/

24. Violence against women act (VAWA). National Domestic Violence Hotline. 2023. Accessed October 3, 2023. https://www.thehotline.org/resources/violence-against-women-act-vawa/

25. Fact sheet: reauthorization of the violence against women act (VAWA). The White House. 2022. Accessed October 3, 2023. https://www.whitehouse.gov/briefing-room/statements-releases/2022/03/16/fact-sheet-reauthorization-of-the-violence-against-women-act-vawa/

26. 17th annual domestic violence counts report. National Network to End Domestic Violence. 2023. Accessed October 4, 2023. https://nnedv.org/wp-content/uploads/2023/03/17th-Annual-Domestic-Violence-Counts-Report-Nat-Summary.pdf

27. Victims of crime act definitions, allowable and unallowable costs and services. Oregon Department of Justice. Updated April 2021. Accessed October 4, 2023. https://www.doj.state.or.us/wp-content/uploads/2017/09/VOCA-Allowable-and-Unallowable-Costs-and-Services-Guiddance-04.2021.pdf

28. Empowerment theory in social work. Virginia Commonwealth University. 2021. Accessed October 3, 2023. https://onlinesocialwork.vcu.edu/blog/empowerment-theory-in-social-work/

29. Cattaneo L, Stylianou A, Hargrove S, Goodman L, Gebhard K, Curby T. Survivor-centered practice and survivor empowerment: evidence from a research–practitioner partnership. *Violence Against Women.* 2021;27(9):1252-1272. doi:10.1177/1077801220935196

30. Durrence A, Doyle K, Passi S. Trust survivors: building an effective and inclusive cash assistance program. FreeFrom. 2021. https://www.freefrom.org/wp-content/uploads/2021/06/TrustSurvivorsReport.pdf

31. Tarshis S, Scott-Marshall H, Alaggia R. An analysis of comparative perspectives on economic empowerment among employment-seeking survivors of intimate partner violence (IPV) and service providers. *Societies.* 2022;12(1):16. doi: 10.3390/soc12010016

32. Support every survivor: how race, ethnicity, gender, sexuality, and disability shape survivors' experiences and needs. FreeFrom. 2022. https://www.freefrom.org/support-everysurvivor

33. The Care Center. Get support. University of Nevada, Las Vegas. 2022. Accessed October 3, 2023. https://www.unlv.edu/carecenter/support

34. Washington State Coalition Against Domestic Violence. Flexible funding for domestic violence and sexual assault survivors. Safe Housing Partnerships. 2019. Accessed October 4, 2023. https://safehousingpartnerships.org/sites/default/files/2019-01/SafeHousingPartnerships-FlexFundingFAQ-Jan2019.pdf

35. Duvvury N, Grown C, Redner J. Costs of intimate partner violence at the household and community levels. International Center for Research on Women. 2016. Accessed October 4, 2023. https://www.icrw.org/wp-content/uploads/2016/10/Costs-of-Intimate-Partner-Violence-at- the-Household-and-Community-Levels-An-Operational-Framework-for-Developing-Countries.pdf

36. Charities and nonprofits. Internal Revenue Service. 2022. Accessed October 3, 2023. https://www.irs.gov/charities-and-nonprofits

37. Sabri B, Tharmarajah S, Njie-Carr VPS, et el. Safety planning with marginalized survivors of intimate partner violence: challenges of conducting safety planning intervention research with marginalized women. *Trauma Violence Abuse*. 2022; 23(5):1728-1751. doi:10.1177/15248380211013136

38. National Network to End Domestic Violence. 2023. Accessed October 3, 2023. https://nnedv.org/

39. National Sexual Violence Resource Center. March 15, 2023. Accessed October 3, 2023. https://www.nsvrc.org/

40. Green L. Finding the path forward: exploring employment advocacy. Resource Sharing Project. 2018. Accessed October 4, 2023. https://resourcesharingproject.org/wp-content/uploads/2021/11/Exploring20Employment20Advocacy_1.pdf

41. Department of Public Health. Tips for making trauma-informed warm referrals. Commonwealth of Massachusetts. 2023. Accessed October 4, 2023. https://www.mass.gov/info-details/tips-for-making-trauma-informed-warm-referrals

42. The intersection of domestic violence and homelessness. Safe Housing Partnerships. 2020. Accessed October 4, 2023. https://safehousingpartnerships.org/sites/default/files/2017-05/SHP-Homelessness%20and%20DV%20Inforgraphic_1.pdf

43. 16th annual domestic violence counts report. National Network to End Domestic Violence. 2022. https://nnedv.org/content/domestic-violence-counts-16th-annual/

44. Sullivan CM, López-Zerón G, Farero A, et al. Impact of the domestic violence housing first model on survivors' safety and housing stability: six month findings. *J Fam Violence*. 2022;38(3):395-406. doi:10.1007/s10896-022-00381-x

45. Toolkit. Washington State Coalition Against Domestic Violence (WSCADV). March 2, 2023. Accessed October 4, 2023. https://wscadv.org/projects/domestic-violence-housing-first/toolkit/

46. Adams AE, Littwin AK, Javorka M. The frequency, nature, and effects of coerced debt among a national sample of women seeking help for intimate partner violence. *Violence Against Women*. 2019;26(11):1324-1342. doi:10.1177/1077801219841445

47. Financial abuse fact sheet. NNEDV. 2019. Accessed October 4, 2023. https://www.nnedv.org/wp-content/uploads/2019/07/Library_EJ_Financial_Abuse_Fact_ Sheet.pdf

48. Brown J, Tarver J. What is a bad credit score? Forbes Advisor. 2021. https://www.forbes.com/advisor/credit-score/what-is-a-bad-credit-score/

49. Financial abuse. WomensLaw.org. 2021. Accessed October 4, 2023. https://www.womenslaw.org/about-abuse/forms-abuse/financial-abuse/getting-your-money-back-and-other-help

50. Help center. Identity Theft Resource Center. Accessed October 4, 2023. https://helpcenter.idtheftcenter.org/s/

51. Non profit credit counseling services: get out of debt. National Foundation for Credit Counseling. 2023. Accessed October 4, 2023. https://www.nfcc.org/

52. Before and beyond crisis: what each of us can do to create a long-term ecosystem of support for all survivors. FreeFrom. 2022. http://freefrom.org/beyond-crisis

53. Risk and protective factors for perpetration. Centers for Disease Control and Prevention. 2021. Accessed October 4, 2023. https://www.cdc.gov/violenceprevention/intimatepartnerviolence/riskprotectivefactors.html

54. Independence project. NNEDV. 2023. Accessed October 4, 2023. https://nnedv.org/content/independence-project/

55. Purple purse challenge. NCEDSV. 2018. Accessed October 4, 2023. https://www.ncedsv.org/news/purplepurse/

56. Matjasko JL, D'Inverno AS, Marshall KJ, Kearns MC. Microfinance and violence prevention: a review of the evidence and adaptations for implementation in the US. *Prev Med.* 2020;133. doi:10.1016/j.ypmed.2020.106017

57. The Allstate Foundation moving ahead curriculum. AllState Foundation. 2019. Accessed October 4, 2023. https://allstatefoundation.org/wp-content/uploads/2020/03/Moving-Ahead-Curriculum_- All_-English.pdf

58. Systems advocacy - improving community safety. DC SAFE. 2023. Accessed October 4, 2023. https://www.dcsafe.org/systems-reform-1

59. Economic justice policy. NNEDV. 2022. Accessed October 4, 2023. https://nnedv.org/content/economic-justice-policy/

60. Public policy & advocacy. Women Against Abuse. 2023. Accessed October 4, 2023. https://www.womenagainstabuse.org/services/public-policy-advocacy

61. Rajah V, Palmer JE, Duggan M. The personal is political and so is discomfort: intersectional, anti-racist praxis in feminist criminology. *Race Justice.* 2022; 12(3):548-568. doi:10.1177/21533687221101793

62. Berg K. The power and control wheel. La Casa de las Madres. 2022. Accessed October 4, 2023. https://www.lacasa.org/blog/2022/3/18/powerandcontrol?locale=en_us

63. Dependency status. Federal Student Aid. 2023. Accessed October 4, 2023. https://studentaid.gov/apply-for-aid/fafsa/filling-out/dependency

Chapter 14

Violence Exposure and Mental Health Outcomes Across the Lifespan

Kaleigh Mancha, MS, LMFT, Certified Full Spectrum Doula
Theresa Fay-Hillier, DrPH, MSN, PMHCNS-BC

Key Points

1. *1 in 15 children are exposed to intimate partner violence (IPV) each year, and 90% of these children are eyewitnesses to this violence.*[1]
2. *Violence is 1 of the top leading causes of death and nonfatal injuries in the United States, especially for young people and socially marginalized or historically oppressed peoples.*[2]
3. *Youth who experience polyvictimization are at an increased risk for drug and alcohol addiction, post-traumatic stress disorder (PTSD), suicide, somatic health problems, and anger as compared to their violence- and adversity-exposed peers.*[3]
4. *Around 1 in 6 people aged 60 years and older experienced some form of abuse in community settings within the span of 1 year, with rates of abuse increasing since COVID-19.*[4]

Background and Significance

Witnessing events of violence and victimization or experiencing them directly is heavily linked to mortality, physical injury, distress, and a myriad of acute and chronic conditions. The range of impact and risk after exposure to violence can be seen in the disproportionate onset of ailments in those exposed, particularly with regards to the expression of physical and behavioral health conditions such as obesity, somatic symptoms, sleep disturbance, alcohol and substance use, anxiety, depression, and impaired socioemotional wellbeing.[2] Violence disproportionally impacts historically oppressed and marginalized communities the most. This compounds the harm of health disparities these populations already experience. The interplay between social, structural, and economic stressors and longstanding inequities warrants closer examination. Health disparity populations as defined by the National Institutes of Health (NIH) include Blacks/African Americans, Hispanics/Latinos, Indigenous Peoples/Alaska Natives, Asian Americans, Native Hawaiians and other Pacific Islanders, socioeconomically disadvantaged populations, underserved rural populations, and sexual and gender minorities (SGM).[2]

One barrier affecting the rate of health disparities in specific populations is structural racism. Structural racism hinders or limits opportunities for adequate housing, and educational and economic opportunities in Black and Latinx communities and on Native reservations, which directly contributes to increased risks for violence perpetuation, victimization, and adverse health conditions.[2]

Exposure to Violence Over the Lifespan

All experiences with violence, whether through direct or secondary exposure, impact the natural and normal development of a person. Children are highly susceptible to violence exposure as was discussed in depth by Mancha & Stewart (see **Chapter 7: The Effects of Violence, Trauma, and Protective Factors on Individuals and Communities**). An isolated traumatic event can impact an individual to varying degrees, while complex or chronic trauma exposure has ongoing negative effects on the progression of development, health, and overall wellbeing. Additionally, a person's likelihood of encountering or experiencing retraumatizing interpersonal or medical care exchanges increases after exposure to trauma due to increased vulnerability. Polyvictimization (ie, exposure to multiple types of victimization) that occurs during formative years of development leads to lifelong biopsychosocial consequences that far surpass specific singular types of adversity or interpersonal stressors.[3] A dose-response relationship is observable in the connection between violence exposure and negative health outcomes, with increasing levels of exposure to violence tied to an increased risk of negative health outcomes. Multiple decades of research have shown a dose-response relationship, whereby physical and mental health challenges are amplified by the cumulative impact of exposure to poly-victimization, particularly those victimizations that have occurred during crucial periods of development. An example of this dose-response relationship includes increased risk for physical, mental, sexual, and reproductive health dysfunction that have been directly linked with IPV. Some of the ailments or consequences observed occurring at higher rates after polyvictimization include adolescent pregnancy, unintended pregnancy, miscarriage, stillbirth, intrauterine hemorrhage, nutritional deficiency, abdominal pain and other gastrointestinal problems, neurological disorders, chronic pain, disability, anxiety, and PTSD, as well as noncommunicable diseases such as hypertension, cancer, and cardiovascular diseases.[2]

Suicide

Younger age groups, specifically those between the ages of 5 and 12 years, are exhibiting rising rates in suicide attempts and completions. There is a clear disparity in suicide rates for young people, especially Black children, who are 2 times as likely to die by suicide compared to their White counterparts.[2] One study conducted in 2019 noted the highest suicide rates were among American Indian/Alaska Native individuals, particularly those between the ages of 15 and 34 years, with a rate of 24.8 for every 100 000 people. Additionally, this group was the only ethnic group to experience a steady and significant increase in suicide by firearm between 2019 and 2020. Adolescent and adult self-directed violence, defined as any form of violence a person commits to or against themselves to cause injury, harm, or death, is reported as occurring most frequently among SGM populations. SGM-identified individuals are at risk for violent victimization at 3.5 times the rate of victimization than those who do not identify as SGM.[2]

Health disparity populations are groups of people at highest risk for exposure and proximity to violent and traumatic experiences, making them more likely to experience heightened rates of dysfunction or chronic ailments, and ultimately more likely to die prematurely by suicide. This data, along with the recommendations for best practices (see **Chapter 3: Trauma- and Violence-Informed Care: Considerations for Providers and Those Who Serve the Community**), further support the case for mandatory trauma- and violence-informed, culturally responsive health care. One such recommendation is that providers are assessing for suicidality, homicidality, IPV, and abuse annually at minimum, especially in pediatric, emergency room, and primary care settings.

Psychological Impact of Trauma

Trauma can be experienced at any point in a person's lifetime, but it most commonly begins during childhood. Of individuals who experience trauma, 74.2% experience their first traumatic event between the ages of 0 and 5 years. By the age of 16 years, more than 2/3 of children have experienced at least 1 traumatic event.[5] Children who experience 1 type of violence, such as physical abuse, are at greater risk for experiencing other forms of violence. In addition to known adverse childhood traumatic experiences, additional traumas that impact childhood development include witnessing violence, living in oppression or underresourced systems (eg, Pair of ACEs Tree: Adverse Childhood Experiences and the social determinants of health), and experiencing severe life-threatening natural disasters.

There is greater risk for negative emotional and psychological consequences when the individual identifies feelings of immobility and helplessness during the trauma or has triggering memories related to the trauma. Although some children are able to recover from traumatic experiences, other children develop maladaptive intrapsychic and behavioral consequences as part of their post-trauma symptoms (see **Table 14-1**). These maladaptive reactions follow patterns of trauma resolution learning, with patterns of reenactment, repetition, and displacement.[5] Developing a trauma resolution learning pattern occurs when repetitive traumatic events are not discovered or disclosed, and the victim lacks the opportunity to process trauma in a

Table 14-1. Expected Responses to Violence Exposure by Chronological Age

Age Ranges	Emotional Signs	Physical/ Behavioral Signs	Provider Interventions	Systemic Interventions
0-12 months	— Unusual fear of certain people or places — Clinging to caregivers — Withdrawn or fearful — Excessive crying — Developmental delays or missed milestones — Delayed or blunted reactions to stimuli, including pain or discomfort	— Bruising, bleeding, burns or redness on the face, lips, genitals, anus, and mouth or on several surface planes at the same time — Tears in the tissue of the gums, possibly because of force-feeding — Consistently dirty or unkept — Extreme changes in weight — Failure to thrive — Discoloration of the skin or loss of hair due to malnutrition — Chronic rashes or infections	— Assess for unusual bruising patterns that reflect the shape of an instrument used to cause injury (eg, belt, wire hanger, hairbrush, hand, human bite marks); injuries on the body where children usually do not get hurt (eg, the torso, back, buttocks, thighs, neck) — Perinatal Mood and Anxiety Disorder Screenings of caregivers — PEdiatric ACEs and Related Life-events Screener (PEARLS) Assessment	— Affordable, accessible childcare — Parenting classes (with multilingual offerings) — Incentives for caregivers to attend infant well visits to increase contact with providers for screening — Insurance reimbursement for violence exposure and mental health screenings of caregivers — Early intervention screenings for delays during routine intakes for social service programs (eg, WIC offices, Medicaid enrollment, etc) — Psychoeducation during perinatal appointments to assist clients in recognizing symptoms of perinatal mood disorders — Efforts made at the national level to strengthen family financial security through wage increases and economic development

Table 14-1. Expected Responses to Violence Exposure by Chronological Age *(continued)*

Age Ranges	Emotional Signs	Physical/ Behavioral Signs	Provider Interventions	Systemic Interventions
1-5 years	— Withdrawn, fearful or extreme behaviors — Change in eating habits — Hyperactivity — Unusual fear of certain people or places — Reluctance to be alone with a certain person/ people — Anger and aggressiveness towards parents, siblings, friends and animals — Sleep disturbances, including nightmares or night terrors — Regression to previously outgrown behaviors, (eg, bedwetting or thumb-sucking) — Abnormal sexual behaviors or knowledge of advanced sexual language and behaviors — Watchful or anxious — Poor concentration/ distractibility	Same as 0-12 months AND — Persistent or recurring pain during urination or bowel movements — Wetting or soiling accidents unrelated to toilet training — Chronic stomach pain — Unexplained or frequent health problems like headaches or stomachaches — Consistently dirty or has severe body odor — Torn, stained, or bloody underclothing — Frequent urinary tract or yeast infections — Feeling threatened by physical contact or closeness — Somatization	Same as 0-12 months	Same as 0-12 months AND — Access to early childhood intervention programs and services — Full-day free kindergarten programs — Free and subsidized food programs (eg, WIC, state-funded food benefits) — Early intervention at first signs of abuse, neglect, or violence exposure not related to punitive social and judicial systems (eg, referrals to community-based programs rather than immediate removal from home when appropriate)

Table 14-1. Expected Responses to Violence Exposure by Chronological Age *(continued)*

Age Ranges	Emotional Signs	Physical/ Behavioral Signs	Provider Interventions	Systemic Interventions
6-12 years	— Change in eating habits — Reluctance to be alone with a certain person — Anger or aggressiveness towards parents, siblings, friends, pets — Lack of interest in friends, sports, or other activities — Change in attitude towards school or academic performance — Rebellion or withdrawal — Anxiety and depression — Poor self-esteem — Self-mutilation — Regression to previously outgrown behaviors — Abnormal sexual behaviors or knowledge including attempts to engage others in sexual activities — Desire to be seen as "perfect" — Overly compliant — Learning problems (or difficulty concentrating) that cannot be attributed to specific physical or psychological causes — Hypervigilant, anxious or nervous — Suicide attempts or threats — Poor concentration/ distractibility	Same as 1-5 years AND — Sexually transmitted diseases — Unexplained or frequent health problems like headaches or stomachaches — Pain or itching in the genital area — Pregnancy — Sleep disturbances, including nightmares or night terrors — Self-harm behaviors, scars or wounds from past self-harm — Frequent visits to the ER — Frequent changes in providers — Substance use/ misuse	Same as 1-5 years AND — Assessments for IPV, abuse, suicide, self-harm — Referrals to mental health resources — Safety planning — Resource sharing — Multi-team collaborations to address areas of vulnerability, resource sharing, skill building, and increase long-term supports (eg, social worker, pediatrician, caregiver and child)	— Increased funding for social emotional programming in schools and increased access to mental health professionals in schools — Accessible and affordable before- and after-school care — Free and subsidized food programs — Annual screening for mental health conditions and IPV/ violence exposure — Peer-led support groups for children and families — Long-term participation in programs that provide recurring or annual follow-ups after program completion to assess recidivism and support families in resecuring resources to stop cycle of violence

Table 14-1. Expected Responses to Violence Exposure by Chronological Age *(continued)*

Age Ranges	Emotional Signs	Physical/ Behavioral Signs	Provider Interventions	Systemic Interventions
13-18 years	Same as 6-12 years AND — Runaway behavior — Anxiety, depression, and other mental health symptoms — Avoidance of relationships — Eating disorders — Lack of motivation or desire to think about the future — Indecisiveness	Same as 6-12 years AND — Defiant towards peers or adults — Interactions with law enforcement or judicial system — Expulsions or school removals — Frequent changes in school placements — Over-identification or engagement with adults	Same as 6-12 years	Same as 6-12 years AND — Comprehensive sexual education programs beyond abstinence, that include components addressing gender diverse identities, consent, and IPV in teen relationships — IPV prevention programs — Access to reproductive centers that offer free STD/ STI testing, pregnancy testing, birth control, and abortion services — College- and job-readiness preparation programs — Allocation of state funds to invest in economic and community enhancements that increase job opportunities, access to social and health care services, and culturally specific resources that enhance community resilience
19-30 years	— Sleep disturbances, including nightmares or night terrors — Mental health conditions or symptoms — Poor self-esteem — Avoidance of relationships — Self-mutilation — Hypervigilant, anxious or nervous — Suicide attempts or threats	— Sexually transmitted diseases — Headaches — Frequent urinary tract or yeast infections — Pregnancy — Feeling threatened by physical contact, closeness — Extreme weight change — Substance use/ misuse — Somatization — Chronic homelessness or job changes	— Routine screenings for IPV, abuse, suicide, self-harm/ suicide — Referrals to mental health resources — Perinatal Mood and Anxiety Disorder screenings (as applicable) — ACEs assessment	Same as 13-18 years AND — Increased access to affordable health care services — Codified legally protected reproductive autonomy and rights — Annual screening for mental health conditions and IPV/ violence exposure covered by insurance — Parenting classes (with multilingual offerings)

Table 14-1. Expected Responses to Violence Exposure by Chronological Age *(continued)*

Age Ranges	Emotional Signs	Physical/ Behavioral Signs	Provider Interventions	Systemic Interventions
31-59 years	Same as 19-30 years AND — Increased fears about loss of autonomy or income — Isolation	Same as 19-30 years	Same as 19-30 years	— Increased access to affordable health care services — Codified legally protected reproductive autonomy and rights — Annual screening for mental health conditions and IPV/ violence exposure covered by insurance
60+ years	Same as 31-59 years AND — Disoriented — Confusion	Same as 31-59 years AND — Torn, stained, or bloody underclothing — Combative or violent behavior — Malnourished, dehydrated — Significant decline in physical health or abilities — Unexplained large bank withdrawals	— Routine screenings — Referrals to mental health resources — Multi-team collaborations to address areas of vulnerability, resource sharing, skill building and increase long-term supports (eg, social worker, primary care provider and caregivers)	Same as 31-59 years AND — Enhanced elder-centered care resources including affordable housing, food security programs, and fiduciary protection education — Respite care for caregivers

supportive environment. Symptoms of anxiety generally appear when there is a lack of trauma resolution or if triggering occurs frequently. Recovery often occurs later in adulthood due to removal from traumatic stimuli, developmental maturation, cultivated resilience, increased autonomy, and sufficient resources to seek out care and support. Resolution of cognitive, behavioral, emotional, or physical symptoms stemming from trauma and violence exposure are not always guaranteed based on maturation or removal from trauma alone. It is not enough to remove oneself from violence if violence exposure has shaped survival and coping strategies that develop into habitual ways of being, in which stunted development has prevented healthful relationship building.[5] The amount and length of exposure to violence over the course of an individual's lifetime, the greater the risk for chronic illness such as diabetes, mental illness, or other health issues. The impact of polyvictimization can have a negative impact on both the mental and physical health of victims across the lifespan. Victims of any age who do not receive treatment and support for their trauma are at the greatest risk for complications.[6]

Children

Because children inherently depend on caregivers to survive and thrive, they are vulnerable when their caregivers are experiencing victimization. Their risk factors for victimization increase when exposed to violence, and this may result in secondary trauma, becoming an intended target of violence or experiencing unintentional injuries as a result of their proximity to violence occurring near or around them. Children may be vulnerable to injury during exposure to IPV as they may[7]:

— Be too small or unable to escape or distance themselves from the violent interactions occurring around them

— Feel compelled to intervene to protect a loved one or animal companion

— Become an object of abuse in order for the abuser to manipulate or harm another person (eg, caregiver threatens to hurt child to intimidate or harm other vulnerable persons including other caregivers and siblings)

— Experience neglect as a result of a caregiver's experience with persistent and chronic mental instability, illness, or substance misuse, rendering the caregiver unable to anticipate, assess, or meet the child's needs

Additionally, due to developmentally appropriate limitations in cognitive development, children may have cognitive distortions or misunderstandings surrounding why violence is happening and what is happening to them or others. Children are more likely to blame themselves, blame victim(s) of violence, and experience intense and inflammatory emotions around authorities who attempt to intervene,[8] especially if intervention involves removal from the home, a caregiver going to jail, or other family system disruption.

Older Adults, 60+

As the global population of people over the age of 60 will more than double between 2015 and 2050, the number of people over 60 years will range from 900 million to 2 billion.[4] There are also significant increases in incidences of abuse by caretakers and in institutions. When studied, 2 out of every 3 nursing home and long-term care facility staff members surveyed disclosed committing acts of abuse in the past year.[4] While 64.2% of staff reported they had committed acts of abuse, there is a gap of studies of self-reported abuse of older adults and their proxies in long-term care facilities.[4] Older adults are at risk for all forms of violence: physical, sexual, psychological, emotional, fiduciary, and material abuse; abandonment; neglect; and a serious loss of dignity and respect. The consequences of abuse that occurs in older age involve long recovery times or an inability to recover from physical injuries, premature death, depression, cognitive decline, financial devastation, and increased chances of placement in long-term care facilities, further increasing chances of multiple victimizations.

A promising factor to decrease the risk of revictimization and the negative health consequences of victims of elder abuse is the quality of social supports received after the initial victimization. Those victims who receive the necessary supports after the initial victimization is reported are more likely to have less psychological and physical symptoms then those who did not receive adequate social support. Victims of elder abuse who receive a high level of social support experience less depression and report less generalized anxiety and poor health. Providing education to the public, law enforcement, and health care providers could increase reporting of abuse (including emotional abuse). Victims have greater success when abuse is exposed, addressed, and they are provided with the necessary social supports.[9]

Misconceptions and Myths About Mental Health

Kids are Resilient

"Resiliency" is a term often used to describe individuals who have experienced a traumatic or negative, potentially life-altering event and are, or appear to be, functioning well with little to no negative outcomes.[10] Children who are engaged in play after a traumatic event can be perceived as resilient because they appear to be adjusting well post-trauma, since they are engaging in a developmentally appropriate activity. Although children may appear to be managing their stress or trauma because they are found to be engaged in play, this activity does not actually mean that they do not need assistance with processing a traumatic experience. Some children who are thought to be well adjusted post-trauma because of play benefit from violence and risk assessments as well as therapeutic interventions. Children use play to process and manage their emotions and world. Play is also used as a barometer for assessing a child's developmental milestones when used therapeutically as an assessment tool and subsequently as an intervention.[11,12] Frequently, therapists who work with children incorporate play into various treatment modalities that have been effective in treating children exposed to trauma.[13] According to the Substance Abuse and Mental Health Services Administration (SAMHSA), assessing resiliency in children should include the following: (1) cognitive development and problem-solving skills, (2) self-regulation, and (3) relationships with caring adults who are consistent and safe.[14] A child's external appearance or healthy behaviors should not determine resiliency or prevent further inquiry into the impact violence exposure has had on them.

People with Mental Health Problems are Violent and Unpredictable

Mental illness alone is not the only risk factor or the primary determinant of violent behavior. Rather, having a history of childhood abuse, living in an under-resourced community, or lacking resources to meet basic needs are better predictors of violent behavior.[15] Essentially, the experiences in a person's life, along with their privileges or lack thereof and available resources are more predictive than their mental health challenges in determining their propensity for violence. People with mental illness do not commit a statistically significant portion of violent crimes, mass violence, or community violence. A nationally representative community sample of 34 653 people found that 2.9% of people with serious mental illness (eg, major depressive disorder, bipolar disorder, schizophrenia, and schizoaffective disorder) had committed acts of violence 2 and 4 years following the baseline of the study, as compared to 0.8% of people who did not have a diagnosed mental health condition or substance misuse challenges.[16] This is a statistically insignificant finding, meaning there is not a marked or significant causational relationship to mental illness leading to increased perpetuation of violent acts. In one of the most rigorous and widely cited studies on the topic to date, the MacArthur Violence Risk Assessment Study conducted in 2000 identified 2 specific clinical symptoms as being the most predictive of and associated with violent acts among patients who had been discharged from psychiatric facilities.[16] These 2 clinical symptoms were command hallucinations (ie, psychotic voices telling a person to harm others) and psychopathy (characterized by a lack of empathy, poor impulse control, and antisocial deviance). Other factors just as likely to explain violent acts were history of prior violence, a history of childhood physical abuse, having a father who abused substances or committed crimes, displaying antisocial behavior, and scoring high on anger measures. The study also revealed that when a community is unsafe due to high crime, poverty, and a lack of resources, mental illness has no significant bearing on whether or not a person in that community will commit a crime. Markedly, people with severe mental illnesses are over 10 times more likely to be victims of violent crime than the general population.

Mental Health Challenges are a Sign of Weakness, a Choice, or a Result of Low Intelligence

Mental illnesses are comparable to a medical disease in that they must be assessed, managed, and monitored for proper health. Unfortunately, there is a pervasive belief that individuals with mental illness are flawed in character or unintelligent.

Unlike most medical illnesses, where there are usually standardized tests (eg, MRIs, blood tests, biopsies) that offer a visual to confirm and treat an identified "illness," mental illnesses are complex and are often confirmed after prolonged distress by way of presenting symptoms and not always through specific tests.[17] Mental illnesses are the result of converging biological, social, and environmental factors that impact how illness or dysfunction is expressed, the severity of the illness, and the types of treatment required. The formation of stigmas surrounding individuals experiencing mental health distress is primarily due to lack of knowledge.[18] The stigma associated with mental health impacts the care, resources, and empathy those who have a mental illness receive, both from the general public and health care providers.[19] Many individuals with mental illness indicate they have been provided subpar care and are treated with disrespect when seeking out mental health care services.[20] Mental health challenges can affect anyone, with 1 in 5 Americans experiencing mental illness in their lifetime.[21] Access to trauma and violence education for health care providers surrounding the assessment and treatment of mental health challenges can decrease stigma and increase effective and supportive treatments.

Male-Identified or Masculine-Presenting People are Not Typically Victims of IPV

As elaborated on by Mancha & Stewart (see **Chapter 7: The Effects of Violence, Trauma, and Protective Factors on Individuals and Communities**), bidirectional violence occurs in 58% of relationships where IPV is present, with men and women being equally likely to be the primary aggressor and men representing approximately 1/3 of identified victims of IPV. However, there are many barriers present for male-identified and masculine-presenting people in reporting IPV. One of these barriers is the stigma against being a victim of IPV, rooted in sociocultural and individual beliefs about gender and masculinity.[22] These beliefs are formed, in part, by media depictions, media campaigns, and educational materials that do not highlight the full spectrum of identities that experience victimization, narrowing the profile of victims to female-identified people and children. The societally normalized assumption that men and male-identified individuals do not seek out help after being victimized, in and of itself serves to inhibit help-seeking behaviors. Male-identified individuals may believe there are no resources for them, they will not be believed, or that being a male victim is rare, increasing internalized shame. Male-identified individuals often are discredited or invalidated when sharing their experiences with violence due to misconceptions related to not fitting the dominant narrative of who perpetuates or experiences violence.[22] Implicit and conscious biases, prejudice, and narrow views of victimization all contribute to prevailing myths and messaging about who should or does seek help, who is deserving of advocacy and services, and who is impacted by violence.

Asking a Person About Suicide Will Only Increase Their Risk for Suicide

Suicide is the 12th leading cause of death for adults and the third leading cause of death for adolescents in the United States.[23] Though there is a popular belief that asking a person about their risk for suicide will increase the chances they will attempt or complete suicide, decades of evidence does not support this belief. A meta-analysis conducted of 18 studies where participants were directly assessed for suicidality found that there was no increased risk for suicide after assessment.[24] The analysis further identified that, rather than increasing risk, there was a small, noted benefit to exploring suicidal thoughts and behaviors. In 2022, SAMHSA guidelines for helping someone who is thought to be at risk for suicide included directly asking the person about suicide.[25] The guidelines also include the nationally launched #988 Suicide & Crisis Lifeline number that is available 24 hours per day to assist both someone in crisis or someone who is concerned about another person who may be in crisis. One recent study confirmed that screening does reduce suicide attempts and completions.[26] Educating the public and health care providers on the importance of screening individuals for suicide can create an open environment for individuals to share any distress they may be in and provide the opportunity to offer needed resources to increase protective factors.

People Will Not be Honest About IPV, Trauma, or Mental Health, or it Will Make Things Worse if you Ask About Them

Some individuals may not be forthcoming about their experiences with violence and trauma due to fear, stigma, cultural norms around disclosing personal information, or past experiences with medical trauma. People who have experienced violence may feel triggered, anxious, or afraid when health care providers ask about IPV, trauma, or mental health, but assessing for risk and exposure to violence is not what is harmful or problematic. The manner in which a person is being asked impacts their ability to disclose personal information.[27] First impressions made by health care providers who are screening for violence or mental health influence all future decisions involving whether a person is inclined to disclose safety issues or seek out care.[28] Although health care providers are encouraged and often mandated to screen their patients for safety (specifically related to IPV, exposure to trauma, and mental health), many times they are not provided with training on how to implement or operate from a trauma-informed approach when screening patients for safety.[29] With 1 in 5 adults in the United States experiencing mental illness each year,[30] and 70% of adults in the United States having experienced some type of traumatic event at least once in their lives,[31] it is essential that all individuals are screened for trauma and provided with resources as appropriate.

People Cannot Experience Remission of PTSD Symptoms or Recover from Other Mental Health Challenges

There are many definitions for what it means to recover, ranging from a complete cessation or resolution of symptoms to the successful management of symptoms allowing for an individual to live, work, learn, and participate fully in their communities. People have more options than ever before to address the challenges they experience because of mental illness. Rigorously studied therapeutic techniques and interventions, access to medication and innovative advances in medicine, and holistic and nonallopathic treatments such as meditation and community support all contribute to one's ability to engage in meaningful introspection, understanding, and healing. Having restorative, healthful, positive, and resilience-building experiences, in combination with available supports and interventions, facilitates the integration of trauma and supports an individual in understanding how to navigate adversity, stress, and seeking out help. When people are given better educational and employment opportunities, access to healthy and safe environments, have lower health care costs, increased access to trauma- and violence-informed care, and are given adequate resources, they are less likely to experience mental health challenges. Additionally, the duration, recurrence, and intensity of mental health challenges are reduced. For example, a therapeutic technique known as eye movement desensitization and reprocessing (EMDR) has been studied extensively as an effective treatment for PTSD, with robust data revealing significant improvements and reductions in trauma-related symptoms after 3 to 6 months.[32]

Provider Strategies for Prevention, Assessment, and Intervention

An economic assessment from 2018 found that childhood IPV exposure results in an average lifetime cost estimated to be around \$50 000 per person victimized. This amount takes into account increased health care costs (\$11 000), increased criminal costs (\$14 000), and productivity losses (\$26 000).[33] Economic impact, paired with an abundance of research regarding the prevalence of violence to which individuals in the United States are exposed, highlights the tangible and measurable ways violence and victimization influence individual mental health outcomes. Consideration for the allocation, acquisition, or lack of resources that contribute to revictimization, polyvictimization, and the ability to heal from trauma are important in informing the brainstorming of strategies to reduce or prevent these occurrences. The cumulative data on this topic supports the need for increased awareness through public health campaigns and education, enhanced screenings in health care and educational settings, solutions aimed at treating dyads or family systems rather than exclusively individual victims, and strategic preventive measures. The immense cost of treatment, both for medical and mental health, is far higher than the investment required to prevent violence from happening in the first place.

Prevention

The prevention of violence becomes much more complex as violence is encountered. The most significant impact in prevention is addressing risk factors throughout the lifespan to either prevent or mitigate the impact through early intervention. There are some common elements that address prevention of IPV. Some common threads throughout the lifespan that are related to prevention are the development of supportive communities, availability of education on identifying early signs of abuse to provide early interventions and lessen the negative impact of the abuse, and availability of resources for all age groups that can be easily accessed to support the wellbeing of all individuals.

In addition to overall general preventative strategies, the CDC recommends the following strategies for preventing child abuse[34]:

— *Strengthen economic supports to families.* Assessing for food and housing insecurity and economic challenges, providers can help facilitate referrals and access to resources that support a family in meeting their needs to sustain stable employment and housing and nourishing foods consistently.

— *Change social norms to support parents and positive parenting.* Campaigns, policy changes, educational materials, and shifting cultural perspectives on the utilization of corporal punishment can support parents/caregivers in learning and utilizing nonviolent and positive parenting strategies to increase resilience and skill building within children and families.

— *Provide quality care and education early in life.* Many Americans live in communities that lack adequate childcare facilities or preschool options. There are not enough resources for working parents/caregivers to secure a safe environment while they are out of the home, which limits household economic mobility.

— *Enhance parenting skills to promote healthy child development.* When home visitation services are available to people who have children living in the home, there is an increase in skill acquisition amongst family members, as well as an increase in access to preventative or responsive early childhood development specific services.

— *Intervene to lessen harm and prevent future risk.* By offering more robust access to parent/caregiver training programs and health care provider services, it is possible to reduce trauma, abuse, and neglect exposure due to increased education and screening opportunities.

As with children, strategies recommended for providers when working with older adults include:

— Preventative psychoeducation aimed at helping family members recognize signs of abuse in their aging relatives and burnout in themselves

— Assessing caregivers' and aging adults' access to resources and potential or current barriers to needed care and resources

— Connecting older adults to community-based programming such as money management programs to avoid exploitation

Assessment and Intervention

Children who experience polyvictimization reported sexual victimization and assaults differently than peers who had experienced singular victimizations, with the biggest difference being a trend towards identifying caregivers, siblings, and peers as the individual perpetuating violence against them. This trend in reporting can help inform which types of interventions can be most effective for providers to utilize, including discerning whether a child who has been victimized needs support in preventing or recovering from victimization.[2] Implementation of interventions at the community, organizational, and policy level are far more effective in cultivating substantial societal change than interventions focused on the individual. Numerous studies demonstrate the ways in which structural racism, socioeconomic mobility, and other environmental factors contribute to violence exposure and subsequent health outcomes.

Addressing the impact of IPV throughout the lifespan is supported by many insurance plans, including Medicaid and Medicare, which currently cover 1 annual universal IPV screening per provider, per patient across the lifespan. This positively reinforces the importance and necessity of screening as a crucial element in addressing and preventing declining health in patients and clients. One study showed the benefit of routine screenings within the context of analyzing perinatal mood and anxiety disorders. The study found that screening by itself resulted in 22% of women who screened positive for perinatal depression seeking out and accessing mental health care treatment.[35]

Responsive interventions might include offering resources for caregivers to receive respite in their caretaking duties, multidisciplinary team responses to care (behavioral, physical, and mental health services), and helping older adults connect to advocates for legal and fiduciary services.

Future Considerations

The NIH supported the creation of the Adolescent Brain Cognitive Development (ABCD) study, a decade-long longitudinal study which completed enrollment of participants in 2018.[36] This study has the potential to be used for exploring the etiology of violence and the consequences of violence exposure across the lifespan by assessing the trajectory of brain development in children as influenced by environmental factors in addition to social, behavioral, and physical factors.[36] The examination of each developmental stage, through comprehensive analysis of longitudinal research, can help bridge gaps in our understanding as providers, policy makers, and advocates about what types of violence are associated with certain age ranges. When we understand how various environmental, individual, and genetic factors play a role in development, we can concurrently examine the roles trauma and violence exposure have on influencing health outcomes; determine how exposure to substances affects developmental outcomes; and decipher the impact changing state and local policies and laws have on youth drug use and related health and development.[36]

To build community-centered, organization-based interventions, there must be consideration for impact evaluation, performance monitoring, process evaluation, and cost evaluation to determine which programs are effective and worth adopting to drive policies around systemic change. As of the writing of this chapter, many violence prevention strategies target specific types of violence and mostly tend to be short-term educational programs that are designed to change individual attitudes, beliefs, and behaviors.[2] The benefits of these programs are often short-term and necessitate a substantial amount of effort and resources to implement. One article published in 2022 by Translational Behavioral Medicine states,

> "With increasing recognition of the critical role of broader sociocultural forces and the relevant experiences of structural racism and discrimination on violence, particular emphasis has been placed on interventions that work across multiple levels of the socioecological model (e.g., individual, relationship/family, community, societal). Indeed, the CDC's new strategic vision prioritizes community- or societal-level preventive efforts along with identifying root causes that cut across different types of violence and address racial, gender, and economic disparities. Such efforts are critical to achieving health equity."[2]

The implementation of structural prevention strategies requires simultaneously having an awareness of community-level challenges, resources, and needs, while also identifying the systemic challenges that create health disparity outcomes. Attempting to enact change or modifying only the characteristics of a community setting (such as schools, workplaces, and neighborhoods) fails to integrate a collaborative approach or address the multi-level influences that impact health outcomes. When creating and implementing structural-based interventions, integrated across multiple systems (justice, health care, community, and housing), the focus is shifted away from strictly targeting violence reduction methods for individuals or exclusively focusing on psychoeducational community programming. Shifting the focus to interventions that target higher-level structural factors is a more effective approach to sustainable change.

Case Study

Case Study 14-1

A 15-year-old Alaskan Native male who identifies as gay was seen in the emergency department after a suicide attempt. The client reported that after the death of his dearest friend to suicide a month prior to his attempt, he thought that suicide would be the solution for ending his pain. The patient reported that his attempt coincided with the anniversary of the death of his older brother by suicide. He further disclosed that before he shared with his family that he was gay, he was sexually abused from the ages of 9 to 12 years on a routine basis by an uncle. The patient stated that although his parents were supportive when he shared with them his sexual orientation, the rest of the family shunned him. The patient also stated that he was frequently bullied in school and that he frequently skipped classes with his now deceased friend. The patient did also share that he started drinking at the age of 10 and was drinking the day he attempted suicide.

Discussion

During the patient's inpatient psychiatric hospitalization, Child Protective Services were notified related to the reported sexual abuse by the uncle. After the report was made, several of the patient's cousins also reported being sexually abused by the uncle. The uncle was arrested and convicted of child sexual abuse. During family therapy, the parents revealed that the patient's older brother, prior to his suicide, said that he was gay and that they (the parents) did not "handle it well." The parents also stated that they thought supporting the patient would be enough and were ashamed that they did not do more for him. The patient's parents were not aware of the uncle's abuse, but now wonder if he had also abused the patient's older brother.

Summary

The pervasive issue of violence significantly affects all people in the United States, with dire consequences for both physical and mental health. However, some populations are more vulnerable than others. Each year, 1 in 15 children are exposed to IPV, and 90% of these children witness the events directly.[1] This exposure can lead to severe long-term effects including drug addiction, PTSD, and chronic health problems. Similarly, violence ranks among the top causes of death and nonfatal injuries, particularly affecting young people and marginalized communities. Youth experiencing multiple types of victimization face compounded risks. Notably, older adults also suffer increasing rates of abuse, especially post-COVID-19, that impact families and social systems significantly.

Trauma experienced at any life stage, but particularly during childhood, disrupts normal development and increases the risk of long-term health issues. The broader societal impacts of violence are underscored by structural racism, which limits opportunities for adequate housing, education, and economic advancement, disproportionately affecting Black, Latinx, and Indigenous communities.

Effective interventions and prevention strategies must address these multifaceted issues, focusing on structural changes and community-based support. Enhanced screening, public health campaigns, and comprehensive care models that include mental, physical, and social health services are crucial. Understanding and addressing the socioecological factors contributing to violence can lead to more effective, sustainable solutions, ultimately reducing the profound impact of violence across the lifespan.

References

1. Statistics. National Coalition Against Domestic Violence. 2021. https://ncadv.org/statistics
2. Burgdorf CE, Maholmes V, O'Connor S, Blachman-Demner DR. Emerging research areas and contributions of NIH in violence research across the lifespan and throughout different settings. *Transl Behav Med.* 2022;12(9):956-964. doi:10.1093/tbm/ibac052
3. Ford JD, Delker BC. Ployvictimization in childhood and its adverse impacts across the lifespan: introduction to the special issue. *J Trauma Dissociation.* 2018;19(3):275-288. doi:10.1080/15299732.2018.1440479
4. Abuse of older people. World Health Organization. June 13, 2022. https://www.who.int/news-room/fact-sheets/detail/abuse-of-older-people
5. Faugno DK, Mitchell SA, Sievers V, Pederson SL, Volz JM, Speck PM. *Introduction to Forensic Nursing: Principles and Practice.* STM Learning, Inc; 2022.
6. Sanderson M, Cook M, Brown LL, Mallet V, Coker AL. Lifetime interpersonal violence or abuse and diabetes rates by sex and race. *Am J Prev Med.* 2023; 65(5):P783-P791. doi:10.1016/j.amepre.2023.06.007
7. Signs & symptoms of abuse/neglect. Stanford Medicine. 2018. https://childabuse.stanford.edu/screening/signs.html
8. What is complex trauma: a resource guide for youth and those who care about them. The National Child Traumatic Stress Network. March 5, 2018. https://www.nctsn.org/resources/what-complex-trauma-resource-guide-youth-and-those-who-care-about-them
9. Insights on adverse effects of elder abuse. National Institute of Justice. July 13, 2020. https://nij.ojp.gov/topics/articles/insights-adverse-effects-elder-abuse
10. Kaplan HB. Understanding the concept of resilience. In: Goldstein S, Brooks RB, eds. *Handbook of Resilience in Children.* Springer; 2005.
11. Malik F, Marwaha R. *Developmental Stages of Social Emotional Development in Children.* StatPearls; 2022. https://www.ncbi.nlm.nih.gov/books/NBK534819

12. Yogman M, Garner A, Hutchinson J, Hirsh-Pasek K, Golinkoff RM. The power of play: a pediatric role in enhancing development in young children. *Pediatrics.* 2018;142(3):e20182058. doi:10.1542/peds.2018-2058

13. Vanderzee KL, Sigel BA, Pemberton JR, John SG. Treatments for early childhood trauma: decision considerations for clinicians. *J Child Adolesc Trauma.* 2018;12(4):515-528. doi:10.1007/s40653-018-0244-6

14. Childhood resilience. Substance Abuse and Mental Health Services Administration. https://www.samhsa.gov/homelessness-programs-resources/hpr-resources/childhood-resilience

15. DeAngelis T. Mental illness and violence: debunking myths, addressing realities. American Psychological Association. Updated July 11, 2022. https://www.apa.org/monitor/2021/04/ce-mental-illness

16. Torrey EF, Stanley J, Monahan J, Steadman HJ. The MacArthur Violence Risk Assessment Study revisited: two views ten years after its initial publication. *Psychiatr Serv.* 2008;59(2):147-152. doi:10.1176/ps.2008.59.2.147

17. *Diagnostic and Statistical Manual of Mental Disorders.* 5th ed. American Psychiatric Association; 2013.

18. Malla A, Joober R, Garcia A. "Mental illness is like any other medical illness": a critical examination of the statement and its impact on patient care and society. *J Psychiatry Neurosci.* 2015;40(3):147-150. doi:10.1503/jpn.150099

19. Shin WG, Woo CW, Jung WH, et al. The neurobehavioral mechanisms underlying attitudes toward people with mental or physical illness. *Front Behav Neurosci.* 2020;14. doi:10.3389/fnbeh.2020.571225

20. Knaak S, Mantler E, Szeto A. Mental illness-related stigma in healthcare. *Healthc Manag Forum.* 2017;30(2):111-116. doi:10.1177/0840470416679413

21. Powell S. Dispelling myths on mental illness. NAMI: National Alliance on Mental Illness. July 17, 2015. https://www.nami.org/Blogs/NAMI-Blog/July-2015/Dispelling-Myths-on-Mental-Illness

22. Taylor JC, Bates EA, Colosi A, Creer AJ. Barriers to men's help seeking for intimate partner violence. *J Interpers Violence.* 2022;37(19-20):NP18417-NP18444. doi:10.1177/08862605211035870

23. Suicide and self-harm injury. National Center for Health Statistics, Centers for Disease Control and Prevention. Updated April 18, 2024. https://www.cdc.gov/nchs/fastats/suicide.htm

24. Blade CA, Stritzke WG, Page AC, Bown JD. The benefits and risks of asking research participants about suicide: a meta-analysis of the impact of exposure to suicide-related content. *Clin Psychol Rev.* 2018;64:1-12. doi:10.1016/j.cpr.2018.07.001

25. Help prevent suicide. Substance Abuse and Mental Health Services Administration. Updated April 24, 2023. https://www.samhsa.gov/suicide

26. Angelone KM. Suicide risk screenings can save lives. Pew. January 25, 2022. https://www.pewtrusts.org/en/research-and-analysis/articles/2022/01/25/suicide-risk-screenings-can-save-lives

27. Calow N, Bachmeier B, O'Connor AL. Trauma, violence & resilience informed care. Academy of Forensic Nursing. November 12, 2021. https://www.goafn.org/_files/ugd/3ebece_3b33acf7d0e64f5b92366ee3660467b2.pdf

28. *SAMHSA's Concept of Trauma and Guidance for a Trauma-Informed Approach.* Substance Abuse and Mental Health Services Administration; 2014. HHS Publication No. (SMA) 14-4884.

29. Kalra N, Hooker L, Reisenhofer S, DiTanna GL, García-Moreno C. Training healthcare providers to respond to intimate partner violence against women. *Cochrane Database System Rev.* 2021;5. doi:10.1002/14651858.CD012423.pub2

30. Menschner C, Maul A. Key ingredients for successful trauma-informed care implementation. Substance Abuse and Mental Health Services Administration. April 2016. https://www.samhsa.gov/sites/default/files/programs_campaigns/childrens_mental_health/atc-whitepaper-040616.pdf

31. Mental health by the numbers. National Alliance on Mental Illness. June 2022. https://www.nami.org/mhstats

32. Wilson G, Farrell D, Barron I, Hutchins J, Whybrow D, Kiernan MD. The use of eye-movement desensitization reprocessing (EMDR) therapy in treating post-traumatic stress disorder—a systematic narrative review. *Front Psychol.* 2018;9(923). doi:10.3389/fpsyg.2018.00923

33. Clements PT, Fay-Hillier T. The effects of intimate partner violence on children: navigating therapeutic assessment and intervention. *Issues Ment Health Nurs.* 2019;40(6):486-492. doi:10.1080/01612840.2018.1553000

34. Prevention strategies. Centers for Disease Control and Prevention. 2019. https://www.cdc.gov/violenceprevention/childabuseandneglect/prevention.html

35. Turtle A, Bezruchka S. Population health and paid parental leave: what the United States can learn from two decades of research. *Healthcare (Basel).* 2016;4(2):30. doi:10.3390/healthcare4020030

36. Adolescent Brain Cognitive Development℠ Study (ABCD Study®). National Institute on Drug Abuse. May 24, 2021. https://nida.nih.gov/drug-topics/adolescent-brain/longitudinal-study-adolescent-brain-cognitive-development-abcd-study

www.ingramcontent.com/pod-product-compliance
Lightning Source LLC
LaVergne TN
LVHW060032210926
848481LV00013B/3841

9781953119230